GUIDELINES FOR THE IDENTIFICATION AND MANAGEMENT OF LEAD EXPOSURE IN PREGNANT AND LACTATING WOMEN

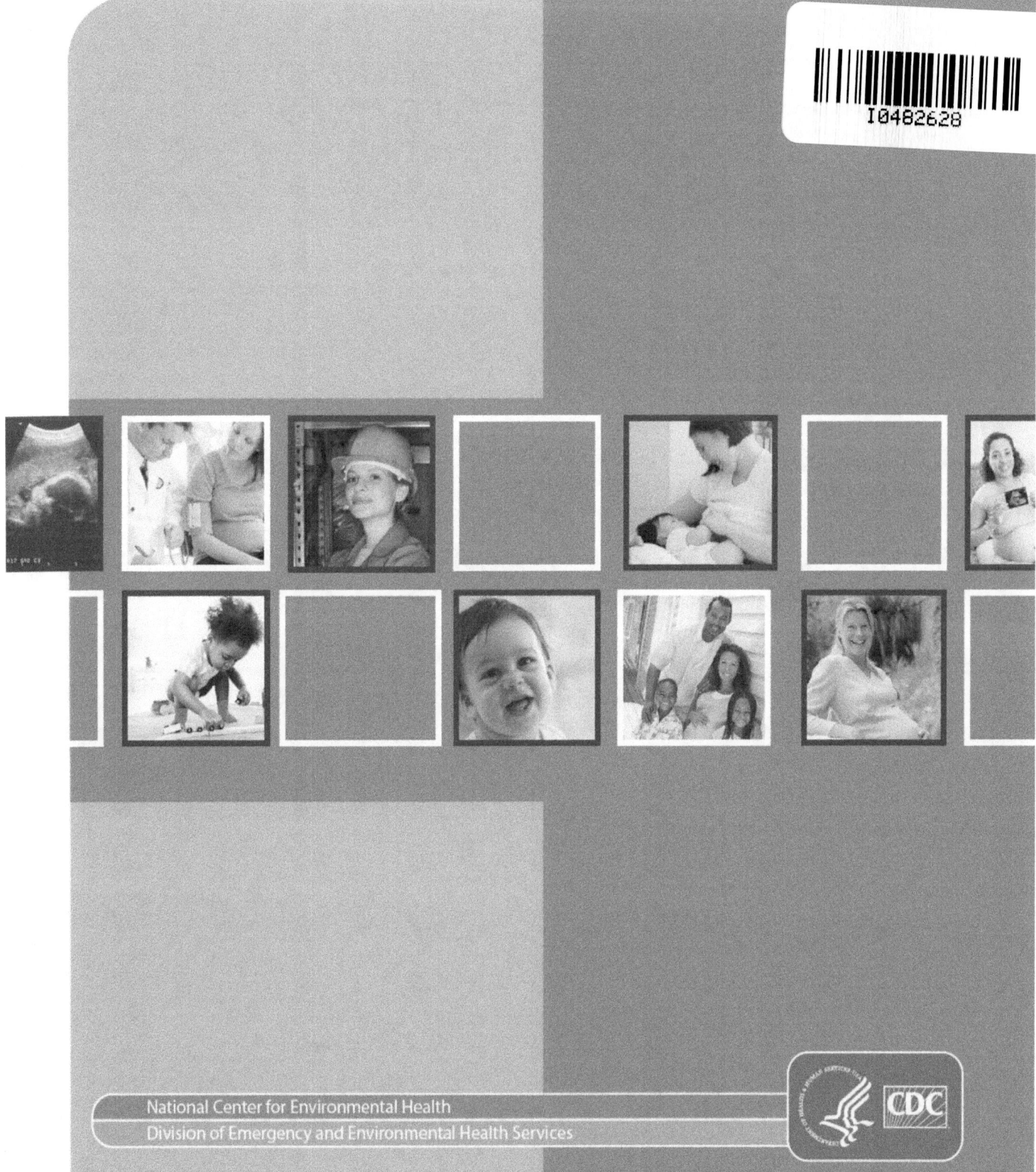

I0482628

National Center for Environmental Health
Division of Emergency and Environmental Health Services

CDC

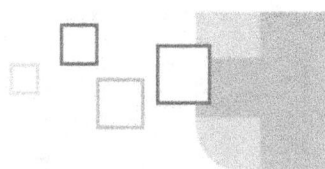

GUIDELINES FOR THE IDENTIFICATION AND MANAGEMENT OF LEAD EXPOSURE IN PREGNANT AND LACTATING WOMEN

Edited by
Adrienne S. Ettinger, ScD, MPH
Anne Guthrie Wengrovitz, MPH

Centers for Disease Control and Prevention

National Center for Environmental Health/Agency for Toxic Substances and Disease Registry
Christopher Portier, PhD
Director

Healthy Homes and Lead Poisoning Prevention Branch
Mary Jean Brown, ScD, RN
Chief

November 2010
U.S. Department of Health and Human Services
Atlanta, GA

This document is dedicated to the memories of Michael W. Shannon, MD, MPH (1953-2009) and Kathryn R. Mahaffey, PhD (1943-2009).

Dr. Shannon was a gifted scientist, a respected leader in medicine and public health, and a tireless advocate for prevention of childhood lead poisoning. His contributions to the scientific literature documenting unrecognized sources of exposure and describing innovative management protocols did much to improve the lives of countless children both in the United States and around the world.

Dr. Mahaffey's early work to ensure that blood samples collected during the National Health and Nutrition Examination Surveys increased understanding of lead poisoning and contributed to the identification of lead in gasoline and paint as primary routes of lead exposure in children. She was actively involved in preventing lead exposure in children for over 35 years and provided invaluable assistance with this document.

The thoughtful contributions of Drs. Shannon and Mahaffey to the CDC Advisory Committee on Childhood Lead Poisoning Prevention will be deeply missed.

TABLE OF CONTENTS

LIST OF FIGURES

LIST OF TABLES

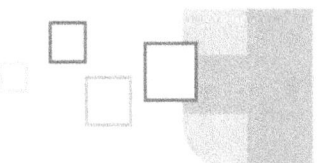

PREFACE

Lead exposure during pregnancy and breastfeeding can result in lasting adverse health effects independent of lead exposure during other life stages. However, to date there has been limited guidance available for clinicians and the public health community regarding the screening and management of pregnant and lactating women exposed to high levels of lead. Recognizing the need for national recommendations, the Centers for Disease Control and Prevention and the Advisory Committee on Childhood Lead Poisoning Prevention convened a workgroup of recognized experts to review the existing evidence for adverse effects of past and current maternal lead exposure on maternal health and fertility and on the developing fetus, infant, and child in prenatal and postnatal states and to propose evidence-based strategies for intervention.

These *Guidelines for the Identification and Management of Lead Exposure in Pregnant and Lactating Women* are based on scientific data and practical considerations regarding preventing lead exposure during pregnancy, assessment and blood lead testing during pregnancy, medical and environmental management to reduce fetal exposure, breastfeeding, and follow up of infants and children exposed to lead *in utero*.

The guidelines also outline a research agenda that will provide crucial information for future efforts to prevent and treat lead exposure during pregnancy and lactation. Further research is needed for a better understanding of lead's effect on pregnancy outcomes and infant development; lead kinetics across the placenta and in breast milk and their relationship to long-term health effects; genetic susceptibility to damage from lead; as well as the pharmacokinetics, effectiveness, and safety of chelating agents in the pregnant woman. Research is also needed to address important clinical and public health needs including validation of risk questionnaires for pregnant women, optimal timing of blood lead testing, and effective strategies for identification and treatment of pica in pregnant women.

I wish to thank the members of the Advisory Committee on Childhood Lead Poisoning Prevention, members of the Lead in Pregnancy Workgroup, and consultants who developed this document and acknowledge their contribution to the health of the nation's children. This document was voted on and approved with one abstention at the October 21-22, 2009, meeting of the Advisory Committee on Childhood Lead Poisoning Prevention. I believe this document represents a major advance in our efforts to prevent lead exposure in those most vulnerable.

Christopher Portier, PhD
Director
National Center for Environmental Health/Agency
   for Toxic Substances and Disease Registry
Centers for Disease Control and Prevention

EXECUTIVE SUMMARY

Despite improvements in environmental policies and significant reductions in U.S. average blood lead levels, lead exposure remains a concern for pregnant and lactating women, particularly among certain population subgroups at increased risk for exposure.

Recent National Health and Nutrition Examination Survey (NHANES) estimates suggest that almost 1% of women of childbearing age (15-44 years) have blood lead levels greater than or equal to 5 μg/dL (Centers for Disease Control and Prevention 2008, unpublished data). As documented in these guidelines, there is good evidence that maternal lead exposure during pregnancy can cause fetal lead exposure and can adversely affect both maternal and child health across a wide range of maternal exposure levels.

However, guidance for clinicians regarding screening and managing pregnant and lactating women exposed to lead has not kept pace with the scientific evidence. There are currently no national recommendations by any medical or nursing professional association that covers lead risk assessment and management during pregnancy and lactation. Currently, New York State, New York City, and Minnesota are the only jurisdictions that have issued lead screening guidelines and follow-up requirements for pregnant women by physicians or other providers of medical care. The lack of national recommendations about testing pregnant women and managing those identified with lead exposure above background levels has created confusion in the clinical and public health sectors. In response to this need, the Centers for Disease Control and Prevention (CDC) Advisory Committee on Childhood Lead Poisoning Prevention (ACCLPP) convened the Lead and Pregnancy Work Group to review the existing evidence for adverse effects of past and current maternal lead exposure on maternal health and fertility and on the developing fetus, infant, and child in prenatal and postnatal states. This document presents ACCLPP's summary of the evidence to date from human studies, conclusions, and CDC recommendations regarding

- prevention of lead exposure for pregnant and lactating women,

- risk assessment and blood lead testing of pregnant women,

- medical and environmental management,

- breastfeeding, and

- follow up of infants and children of mothers with blood lead levels exceeding national norms.

In instances where there is an absence of clear and convincing evidence, recommendations are based on the combined clinical, practical, and research experience of ACCLPP and work group members. This document also identifies research, policy, and health education needs to inform policy and improve care of pregnant and lactating women with lead exposure above background levels. The guidelines do not address all women of childbearing age, nor does it address male reproductive health issues associated with lead exposure.

The evidence that prenatal lead exposure impairs children's neurodevelopment, placing them at increased risk for developmental delay, reduced IQ, and behavioral problems, is convincing. The research also suggests, but is inconclusive, that fetal lead exposure at levels found in the United States results in low birth weight or adverse health conditions in adults who were exposed to lead *in utero*, among others. Further research is needed for a better understanding of several biomedical issues, including pregnancy outcomes and infant development associated with maternal lead exposure during pregnancy, lead kinetics across the placenta and in breast milk and their relationship to long-term health effects, genetic susceptibility to damage from lead, pharmacokinetics and effectiveness of chelating agents in the pregnant woman, among others. Research is also needed to address important clinical and public health needs, like validation of risk questionnaires for pregnant women, optimal timing of blood lead testing during pregnancy, and effective strategies for identification and treatment of pica in pregnant women.

This document provides guidance based on current knowledge regarding blood lead testing and follow-up care for pregnant and lactating women with lead exposure above background levels. Because there is no apparent threshold below which adverse effects of lead do not occur, CDC has not identified an allowable exposure level, level of concern, or any other bright line intended to connote a safe or unsafe level of exposure for either mother or fetus. Instead, CDC is applying public health principles of prevention in recommending follow-up blood lead testing and interventions when prudent. These guidelines recommend follow-up activities and interventions beginning at blood lead levels (BLLs) ≥5 µg/dL in pregnant women. Unlike the BLL level of concern of 10 µg/dL for children, which is a communitywide action level, a BLL of 5 µg/dL in pregnant women serves a different purpose: it flags the occurrence of prior or ongoing lead exposure above background levels, which may not otherwise be recognized. The vulnerability of a developing fetus to adverse effects and the possibility of preventing additional exposures postnatally justify intervention for pregnant women showing evidence of lead exposure above background levels.

CDC does not recommend blood lead testing of all pregnant women in the United States. State or local public health departments should identify populations at increased risk for lead exposure and provide community-specific risk factors to guide clinicians in determining the need for population-based blood lead testing. Routine blood lead testing of pregnant women is recommended in clinical settings that serve populations with specific risk factors for lead exposure. Health care providers serving lower risk communities should consider the possibility of lead exposure in individual pregnant women by evaluating risk factors for exposure as part of a comprehensive occupational, environmental, and lifestyle health risk assessment of the pregnant woman, and perform blood lead testing if a single risk factor is identified. Assessment for lead exposure, based on risk factor questionnaires or blood lead testing, should take place at the earliest contact with the pregnant patient.

For all patients, but especially those with known lead exposures, health care providers should provide guidance regarding sources of lead and help identify potential sources of lead in the patient's environment. Risk factors for lead exposure above background levels in pregnant women differ from those described in young children. Important risk factors for lead exposure in pregnant women include recent immigration, pica practices, occupational exposure, nutritional status, culturally specific practices such as the use of traditional remedies or imported cosmetics, and the use of traditional lead-glazed pottery for cooking and storing food. Lead-based paint is less likely to be an important exposure source for pregnant women than it is for children, except during renovation or remodeling in older homes. Pregnant women with blood lead concentrations of 10 µg/dL or higher should be removed from occupational lead exposure.

Follow-up testing; increased patient education; and environmental, nutritional, and behavioral interventions are indicated for all pregnant women with blood lead levels greater than or equal to 5 µg/dL in order to prevent undue exposure to the fetus and newborns. Since lead exposure at these levels affects only approximately 1% of U.S. women of childbearing age, the recommendations in this guidance document should not significantly impact many individuals or clinical practices.

The essential activity in management of pregnant women with blood lead levels ≥5 µg/dL is removal of the lead source, disruption of the route of exposure, or avoidance of the lead-containing substance or activity. Source identification beyond obtaining a thorough environmental and occupational history should be conducted for BLLs ≥15 µg/dL in collaboration with the local health department, which will conduct an environmental investigation of the home environment in most jurisdictions and an investigation of the work environment (in some jurisdictions). Women who engage in pica behavior, regardless of the substance consumed, may benefit from nutritional counseling. Pregnant and lactating women with a current or past BLL ≥5 µg/dL should be assessed for the adequacy of their diet and provided with prenatal vitamins and nutritional advice emphasizing adequate calcium and iron intake. Chelation therapy during pregnancy or early infancy may be warranted in certain circumstances where the maternal or neonatal blood lead exceeds ≥45 µg/dL and in consultation with an expert in lead poisoning. Insufficient data exist regarding the advisability of chelation for pregnant women with BLL <45 µg/dL. CDC recognizes the important benefits of breastfeeding for both the mother and child and considered the adverse health and developmental effects associated with lead exposure compared to those associated with not breastfeeding. The adverse developmental effects of ≥5 µg/dL in infant blood lead level was of greater concern than the risks of not breastfeeding. Thus, CDC encourages mothers with blood lead levels <40 µg/dL to breastfeed, however, mothers with higher blood lead levels are encouraged to pump and discard their breast milk until their blood lead levels drop below 40 µg/dL. These recommendations are made for the U.S. population and are not appropriate in countries where infant mortality from infectious diseases is high. Specific recommendations regarding appropriate follow-up blood lead testing of the mother and infant are provided.

Summary of Public Health Actions Based on Maternal and Infant Blood Lead Levels

All Women of Child-Bearing Age

Provide anticipatory guidance, provide health education materials, test workers according to established guidelines, and manage elevated BLLs according to adult lead guidelines (OSHA Medical Guidelines)

Pregnant Women

- Provide anticipatory guidance
- Confirm and referrals
- Notify health department
- Environmental assessment & abatement of lead paint hazards
- Consider chelation therapy; Consult with an expert in lead poisoning
- Medical emergency
- Chelation therapy
- Medical removal from occupational exposure

Lactating Women

- Breastfeeding should be encouraged
- Breastfeeding may be initiated if infant's BLLs monitored
- Lactation should be continued, but breast milk should be pumped and discarded until BLLs <40

Neonates (<1 Month of Age)

- Follow-up test within 1 month
- Follow-up test within 2 weeks
- Follow-up test within 24 hours
- Consider chelation therapy; Consult with an expert in lead poisoning

Infants (1 - 6 Months)

- Follow local pediatric lead screening guidelines
- Follow-up test within 3 months
- Follow-up test within 1-3 months
- Follow-up test within 1 month
- Follow-up test within 24 hours
- Consider chelation therapy; Consult with an expert in lead poisoning

Micrograms/Deciliter: 0 5 10 15 20 25 30 35 40 45 50 55 60 65 70

cs211920

MEMBERS OF THE WORK GROUP ON LEAD AND PREGNANCY

Chairperson

Jessica Leighton, PhD, MPH
Deputy Commissioner, New York City Department of Health & Mental Hygiene

Members

David Bellinger, PhD, MSc
Professor of Neurology
Children's Hospital of Boston, Harvard Medical School

Carla Campbell, MD, MS
Philadelphia Department of Public Health and Children's Hospital of Philadelphia

Crystal Cash, MD
Associate Chair for Graduate Education, Department of Family Medicine
Associate Professor of Clinical Medicine
Stritch School of Medicine, Loyola University Chicago
Liaison to the American Academy of Family Medicine

Valerie Charlton, MD, MPH
Chief, Childhood Lead Poisoning Prevention Branch
California Department of Public Health

Joel Forman, MD
Associate Professor of Pediatrics and Community and Preventive Medicine
Vice Chair for Education and Residency Program Director, Department of Pediatrics
Mount Sinai School of Medicine

Nathan Graber, MD
New York City Department of Health and Mental Hygiene

Barbara Hackley, MS, CNM
Yale University of School of Nursing
Liaison to the American College of Nurse Midwives

Howard Hu, MD, MPH, ScD
Chair and Professor of Environmental Health Sciences
University of Michigan School of Public Health

Ezatollah Keyvan-Larijani, MD, DrPH
Maryland Department of Environment
Liaison to the Council of State and Territorial Epidemiologists

Kathryn Mahaffey, PhD (deceased)
U.S. Environmental Protection Agency

Morri Markowitz, MD
Montefiore Medical Center

Ellen O'Flaherty, PhD
University of Cincinnati Medical School (Emeritus Professor)

Michael Shannon, MD, MPH (deceased)
Children's Hospital of Boston
Liaison to the American Academy of Pediatrics

Kevin U. Stephens, Sr., MD, JD
Director, New Orleans Department of Health

Juan Vargas, MD
San Francisco General Hospital
Liaison to the American College of Obstetricians and Gynecologists

Richard P. Wedeen, MD
University of Medicine and Dentistry of New Jersey
Department of Veterans Affairs Health Care System, New Jersey
Liaison to the Association of Occupational and Environmental Clinics

CDC Staff Members

Mary Jean Brown, ScD, RN
Chief, Healthy Homes and Lead Poisoning and Prevention Branch (HHLPPB)
National Center for Environmental Health

Adrienne S. Ettinger, ScD, MPH
Oak Ridge Institute for Science and Education Fellow, HHLPPB
Research Scientist, Harvard School of Public Health

John Osterloh, MD, MS
Division of Laboratory Sciences
National Center for Environmental Health

Elizabeth A. Whelan, PhD
Chief, Industrywide Studies Branch
National Institute for Occupational Safety and Health

ACKNOWLEDGMENTS

Adrienne S. Ettinger, ScD, MPH was supported by the Centers for Disease Control and Prevention (CDC) Research Participation Program with the Oak Ridge Institute for Science and Education (ORISE) through an interagency agreement with the U.S. Department of Energy (DOE). ORISE is managed by Oak Ridge Associated Universities under DOE contract number DE-AC05-00OR22750.

Anne M. Wengrovitz, MPH provided editorial and writing services under contract to CDC.

Kendrin Sonneville, MS, RD provided input on public health nutrition.

MEMBERS OF THE ADVISORY COMMITTEE ON CHILDHOOD LEAD POISONING PREVENTION

Chair

George G. Rhoads, MD, MPH
Associate Dean, School of Public Health
University of Medicine and Dentistry of New Jersey
Piscataway, NJ
Term: 07/19/04-05/31/12

Carla Campbell, MD, MS
The Children's Hospital of Philadelphia
Philadelphia, Pennsylvania
Term: 5/31/02–5/31/07

Designated Federal Official

Mary Jean Brown, ScD, RN
Chief, Healthy Homes and Lead Poisoning Prevention Branch
National Center for Environmental Health
Centers for Disease Control and Prevention
Atlanta, GA

Members

Magaly C. Angeloni, MBA
Program Manager, Childhood Lead Poisoning Prevention Program
Rhode Island Department of Health
Providence, Rhode Island
Term: 06/01/05-05/31/09

William Banner, Jr. MD, PhD
The Children's Hospital at St. Francis
Tulsa, Oklahoma
Term: 10/1/02 – 5/31/05

Helen J. Binns, MD
Children's Memorial Hospital
Chicago, Illinois
Term: 9/30/02-5/31/05

Valerie Charlton, MD, MPH
Chief, Childhood Lead Poisoning Prevention Branch
California Department of Public Health
Richmond, California
Term: 06/01/05-05/31/09

Deborah A. Cory-Slechta, PhD
Professor of Environmental Medicine
University of Rochester School of Medicine & Dentistry
Rochester, New York
Term: 06/01/06-05/31/10

Sher Lynn Gardner, MD, FAAP
Assistant Professor of Pediatrics, Emory University
Atlanta, Georgia
Term: 06/01/06-05/31/10

Walter S. Handy, Jr., PhD
Cincinnati Health Department
Cincinnati, Ohio
Term: 9/30/03–5/31/07

Kimberly Hansen, MD
Pediatric Medical Director
Peoples Community Health Clinic
Waterloo, Iowa
Term: 07/02/08–05/31/12

Ing Kang Ho, PhD
University of Mississippi Medical Center
Jackson, Mississippi
Term: 9/28/03–5/31/07

Richard E. Hoffman, MD
State Epidemiologist
Denver, Colorado 80231
Term: 5/19/97–5/31/2004

Valarie Johnson
Founder, Urban Parent to Parent
Rochester, New York
Term: 06/01/04-05/31/08

Linda Kite
Coordinator, Healthy Homes Collaborative
Los Angeles, California
Term: 03/16/05-05/31/10

Michael J. Kosnett, MD, MPH
Associate Clinical Professor, University of Colorado Health Sciences Center
Denver, CO
Term: 12/12/06-5/31/11

Jessica Leighton, PhD, MPH
Deputy Commissioner, New York City Department of Health and Mental Hygiene
New York, New York
Term: 10/1/03–12/15/09

Tracey Lynn, DVM, MPH
Alaska Department of Health and Social Services
Anchorage, Alaska
Term: 5/31/02–5/31/2006

Sally Odle
President and Owner, SafeHomes, Inc.
Waterbury, Connecticut
Term: 06/24/04-05/31/08

Sergio Piomelli, MD
Director
Pediatric Hematology
Columbia University
New York, NY 10032
Term: 5/31/00–5/31/04

Brenda Reyes, MD, MPH
Bureau Chief, Community & Children's Environmental Health
Environmental Health Division
Houston Department of Health and Human Services
Term: 06/01/08-05/31/12

Megan T. Sandel, MD, MPH
Assistant Professor, Boston Medical Center
Boston, MA
Term: 09/05/08-5/31/10

Catherine M. Slota-Varma, MD (deceased)
Pediatrician
Milwaukee, Wisconsin
Term: 4/18/03–5/31/06

Wayne R. Snodgrass, PhD, MD
Professor, Pediatrics and Pharmacology-Toxicology,
University of Texas Medical Branch
Galveston, Texas
Term: 06/21/04-05/31/08

Kevin U. Stephens, Sr., MD, JD
Director, Department of Health
New Orleans, Louisiana
Term: 09/22/03-5/31/07

Kimberly M. Thompson, ScD
Harvard School of Public Health
Boston, Massachusetts
Term: 5/31/00–5/31/05

Gail Wasserman, PhD
Professor of Clinical Psychology, Columbia University
New York, New York
Term: 6/1/06-5/31/10

Dana Williams, Sr.
Parent
Decatur, Georgia
Term: 07/03/2008-5/31/12

GLOSSARY

abatement: any set of measures designed to permanently eliminate lead-based paint or lead-based paint hazards.

ABLES: Adult Blood Lead Epidemiology and Surveillance program, a CDC-funded state-based program to track laboratory-reported BLLs in adults.

ACCLPP: CDC Advisory Committee on Childhood Lead Poisoning Prevention.

ACOG: American College of Obstetrics and Gynecology.

acute: having or experiencing a rapid onset and short duration.

AI (adequate intake): a recommended average daily nutrient intake level, based on estimations of average nutrient intakes by groups healthy people.

alternative medicines: for these guidelines, alternative medicines are defined as nonstandard therapies not sanctioned in modern Western medicine; typically from other countries; and usually unregulated in the United States, including folk, traditional, botanic, herbal, alternative, and complementary therapies, medicines, agents, and remedies (also "traditional medicines").

anemia: a condition in which there is a reduction of the number or volume of red blood cells or of the total amount of hemoglobin in the bloodstream

antenatal: occurring or existing before birth (also "prenatal").

antepartum: pertaining to the period before delivery or birth.

anticipatory guidance: practical information given to individuals to promote health before a certain milestone, such as pregnancy, is reached.

antioxidant: any substance that reduces damage due to oxygen in the body.

AOEC: Association of Occupational and Environmental Clinics.

apoptosis: a form of cell death in which a programmed sequence of events leads to the elimination of cells without releasing harmful substances into the surrounding area.

asymptomatic: without observable signs or reportable symptoms of illness.

at-risk populations: populations with characteristics, behaviors, or lifestyles (including home, work, and hobbies) that put them at increased risk for lead exposure.

ayurveda: one of India's traditional systems of medicine, involving a holistic system of healing and natural (herbal) medicines, that has been practiced for over 5,000 years.

bioavailable: readily absorbed and used by the body.

biokinetics: the study of movements of or within organisms.

biomarker (biological marker): a measure of exposure to lead, or other substance, that is measured in human tissue and corresponds to absorbed dose.

BLL (blood lead level): the concentration of lead in a sample of blood expressed in micrograms per deciliter (µg/dL) or micromoles per liter (µmol/L) (1 µg/dL = 0.048 µmol/L).

breast milk lead: levels of lead in breast milk; the concentration of lead in a sample of maternal breast milk is usually expressed in micrograms per liter (μg/L).

bone lead: long-lived stores of lead from past exposure that is accumulated in the body's skeletal system; measured in micrograms (μg) of lead/gram bone mineral.

bone mobilization or bone turnover: the process by which the body dissolves part of the bone in the skeleton in order to maintain or raise the levels of circulating calcium in the blood or for pathological reasons, such as immobilization, age-related osteoporosis, or hyperthyroidism.

bone resorption: the break down and wearing away of bone tissue that results in the release of bone minerals into circulation.

care coordination: the formal coordination of the care of a mother or infant with a BLL that exceeds a specific value and making available existing services as needed to the mother-infant pair.

case management: the follow-up care of a pregnant/lactating woman with a blood lead level ≥5 μg/dL, and her newborn infant, if necessary. Case management includes a) client identification and outreach, b) individual assessment and diagnosis, c) service planning and resource identification, d) linkage of clients to needed services, e) service implementation and coordination, f) monitoring of service delivery, g) advocacy, and h) evaluation.

casein: the main protein found in milk and other dairy products.

CDC (Centers for Disease Control and Prevention): part of the U.S. Department of Health and Human Services.

chelation therapy: the use of a chelating agent (chemical compounds that bind to metals) to remove toxic metals, such as lead, from the body.

chronic: being long-lasting and recurrent.

CI (confidence interval): an interval estimate that defines and upper and lower limit with an associated probability.

clearance standards: maximum allowable lead dust levels (established by the U.S. Department of Housing and Urban Development and the U.S. Environmental Protection Agency) on floors and interior window sills after a residence has undergone lead hazard control work.

CLPPP (Childhood Lead Poisoning Prevention Program): CDC-funded state or local program to prevent childhood lead poisoning.

conception: union of the sperm and the egg which marks the onset of pregnancy (also "fertilization").

confirmatory test: a venous blood lead test performed after a previous capillary, filter paper, or venous blood lead test to verify the results before interventions occur.

congenital anomaly: a structural or functional abnormality of the human body that develops before birth but is usually identified in the period just after birth or in early life.

contraindication: a condition that makes a particular treatment or medical procedure inadvisable.

creatinine: a chemical waste product generated from muscle processes that create and use energy in the human body; measured to determine if kidneys are functioning properly.

cumulative: increasing by successive additions over a period of time.

dyad: two individuals or units regarded as a pair, such as the mother-infant pair.

DRI (dietary reference intake): a set of dietary reference values introduced in the 1990s with the primary goal of preventing nutrient deficiencies, but also reducing the risk for chronic diseases such as osteoporosis, cancer, and cardiovascular disease.

EAR (estimated average requirement): nutrient intake levels expected to satisfy the needs of 50% of the people in a particular age group.

encephalopathy: any diffuse disease of the brain that alters brain function or structure. Lead exposure is one of many possible causes of encephalopathy. Lead encephalopathy is a life-threatening emergency associated with high blood lead levels and often characterized by coma, seizures, ataxia, apathy, bizarre behavior, and poor physical condition.

endogenous: developing or originating from within the body.

endothelium: a thin layer of cells that line the body's hollow organs including blood vessels.

environmental investigation: an investigation of the residence (or other place where person spends significant amounts of time) by trained personnel to identify lead hazards.

exchange transfusion: simultaneous withdrawal of the recipient's blood and transfusion with the donor's blood.

exogenous: developing or originating from outside the body.

EPA (U.S. Environmental Protection Agency; U.S. EPA): federal agency charged with protecting human health and the environment by writing and enforcing regulations based on laws passed by Congress.

FDA (U.S. Food and Drug Administration; U.S. FDA): federal agency responsible for assuring the safety, efficacy, and security of human and veterinary drugs, biological products, medical devices, the U.S. food supply, cosmetics, and products that emit radiation.

fecundity: the potential reproductive capacity of an organism or population, as measured by the number of reproductive cells capable of reproducing (e.g., eggs and sperm).

ferritin: the body's major iron-carrying protein, which is measured to monitor iron status.

fertility: the ability to conceive and have children through normal sexual activity.

Fetal Origins of Adult Disease (or Barker) hypothesis: the suggestion that prenatal adverse nutritional or environmental conditions affect fetal development and have lifelong health and developmental consequences.

fetus: the unborn human offspring from the end of the 8th week after conception (when the major structures have formed) until birth.

first trimester (of pregnancy): time period extending from the first day of the last menstrual period through 12 weeks of gestation. The first trimester is a critical window of fetal development that is important for the formation and development of organs and organ systems.

follow-up test: a blood lead test used to monitor the status of a person with a previously blood test indicating excessive exposure to lead.

gestation: period of time from conception to birth.

gestational age: the age of a fetus or newborn, counting from the time of fertilization, usually measured in weeks, and calculated from the first day of the last menstrual period.

gestational hypertension: a type of high blood pressure that first occurs during pregnancy.

hemoglobin: a protein in red blood cells that transports oxygen.

hematopoiesis: the formation or production of all types of blood cells.

HUD (U.S. Department of Housing and Urban Development): federal agency that develops and executes policies on housing and cities.

hyperuricemia: a buildup of excess uric acid (a waste product) in the blood.

immigration: the one-way inward movement of individuals into a population or population area, usually to a country or region, to which one is not originally born.

infant: a child in the earliest period of life (for the purposes of this document, from 0 to 6 months of age).

IOM (Institute of Medicine): a nonprofit agency established in 1970 under the charter of the National Academy of Sciences that provides independent, objective, evidence-based advice to policymakers, health professionals, the private sector, and the public.

interim controls: a set of measures designed to temporarily reduce human exposure to lead-based paint hazards.

in utero: "within the uterus" (womb) where the unborn baby develops.

iron deficiency: a disorder that occurs when there is not enough iron in the body, causing problems with red blood cell production, muscle function, and numerous other effects, including growth and developmental impairment.

K-x-ray fluorescence: a noninvasive (outside the body) technique for the measurement of lead in bone.

lactation: the period after childbirth when milk is produced and secreted from the mother's breasts to provide nourishment to the baby.

lead-based paint: paint or other surface coating that contains lead equal to or exceeding 1.0 milligram per square centimeter or 0.5 percent by weight (5,000 parts per million), as defined by 302(c) of the Lead-Poisoning Prevention Act (42 U.S.C. 4822(c)) and TSCA section 401(9) (15 U.S.C. 2681(9)).

lead-based paint hazard: any condition that causes exposure to lead from lead-contaminated dust, lead-contaminated soil, or lead-contaminated paint that is deteriorated or present in accessible surfaces, friction surfaces, or impact surfaces that would result in adverse human health effects as established by the appropriate federal agency.

lead-glazed ceramic pottery: ceramic ware or pottery manufactured mainly by artisans and small family businesses using a centuries-old tradition of low-temperature-fired lead glazes to vitrify the surface and color the objects, and often imported from Mexico and other countries.

lead-safe: housing or building units with no lead-based paint hazards as determined by a lead risk assessment or by dust sampling at the conclusion of lead hazard control activities.

lead-safe work practices: low-technology/best practices techniques, methods, and processes that minimize the amount of dust and debris created during the remodeling, renovation, rehabilitation, or repair of pre-1978 housing that are used to control, contain, and clean up lead dust and deteriorated lead-based paint hazards in a manner that protects both the workers and the occupants of the unit.

low birth weight: a baby that weighs less than 2,500 grams at birth.

LPWG (Lead and Pregnancy Work Group): subgroup of the CDC Advisory Committee on Childhood Lead Poisoning Prevention.

medical management: for this guidelines, medical management is the care provided by a health care provider to a pregnant/lactating woman or infant whose blood lead levels indicate exposure to lead above background levels. Medical management includes clinical evaluation for complications of lead exposure, family lead education and referrals, chelation therapy if appropriate, follow-up testing at appropriate intervals, and communication with local health department as necessary.

μg/dL (micrograms per deciliter): a unit of measure for blood lead concentration.

milk-to-plasma ratio: used to express the relative efficiency of passive transfer of a chemical from the blood into milk.

neonate: a newborn infant, less than 1 month of age.

neurodevelopment: normal growth and progression of the nervous system during the life of an organism, measurement of which usually incorporates aspects of intellectual and behavioral attainment.

normotensive: blood pressure in the normal range for a healthy individual given their age.

nutrient: substances that are vital to health and give us energy, growth, help repair body tissues, and regulate body functions. The two major nutrient groups are macronutrients (protein, carbohydrates, fat) and micronutrients (vitamins, minerals).

nutrition: the way the human body takes in and uses foods. Substances or ingredients in food that are sources of nutrition are called nutrients.

NHANES (National Health and Nutrition Examination Survey): a periodic assessment of the health and nutritional status of a representative sample of adults and children in the United States conducted by the CDC National Center for Health Statistics.

NIOSH (National Institute for Occupational Safety and Health): the part of CDC responsible for conducting research and making recommendations for the prevention of work-related illnesses and injuries.

OSHA (Occupational Safety and Health Administration): the main federal agency charged with promulgation and enforcement of safety and health regulations.

observational study: a type of study in which free-living individuals are observed and certain outcomes are measured with no attempt made to affect the outcome (for example, no treatment is given).

organogenesis: the formation of organs within a developing fetus that occurs within the first trimester of pregnancy (prior to 16 weeks gestation).

PCP (primary care provider): the health professional who oversees a patient's care, usually a physician, nurse practitioner, or physician's assistant.

pica: a pattern of deliberate ingestion of nonfood items.

placenta: a temporary organ joining the mother and fetus; it is attached to the wall of the uterus (womb) to transfer oxygen and nutrients to the baby during pregnancy.

plasma: the protein-containing fluid portion of the blood.

plasma lead: lead in the protein-containing fluid portion of the blood and available to cross cell membranes.

postnatal: the time period that occurs after birth, usually referring to the baby.

postpartum: the time period that occurs after birth, usually referring to the mother.

ppb (parts per billion): Represents the concentration of something in water or soil. One ppb represents one microgram of something per liter of water (μg/L), or one microgram of something per kilogram of soil (μg/kg).

ppm (parts per million): Represent the concentration of something in water or soil. One ppm represents one milligram of something per liter of water (mg/L) or 1 milligram of something per kilogram soil (mg/kg).

preeclampsia: a condition in pregnancy characterized by a sharp rise in blood pressure, protein in the mother's urine, and swelling of the hands and feet; this condition has negative consequences for both the mother and baby if not identified and treated promptly.

pregnancy: the period from conception to birth when a woman carries a developing fetus (baby) in her uterus (womb), usually lasting about 9 months (40 weeks).

pre- (or post-) menopause: before (or after) the end of a woman's reproductive years; regular menstrual periods stop in menopause.

preterm delivery: the birth of a baby before 37 weeks gestation.

prevalence: the proportion of individuals in a population having a specific health condition.

primary prevention: preventing a problem before it occurs. Primary prevention of lead poisoning eliminates lead sources before exposure, thus preventing exposure.

primigravid: a woman who is pregnant for the first time.

primiparous: relating to a woman who has given birth only once.

proteinuria: excess protein in the urine.

puberty: onset of the biological capacity for reproduction

RCT (randomized [placebo-controlled] clinical trial): a study in which participants are assigned by chance to different treatment groups and the outcomes between the groups are compared.

RD (registered dietician): a certified professional with the combined education and experience to conduct dietary assessments and advise clients on issues related to diet and nutrition.

RDA (recommended dietary allowance): used from 1941 until 1989 to evaluate food choices that would meet the nutrient requirements of groups or populations with the primary goal of preventing diseases caused by nutrient deficiencies.

renal: having to do with the kidneys.

renovation: construction and/or home or building improvement measures (e.g., window replacement, weatherization, remodeling, repairing).

risk factor questionnaire: a set of questions designed to elicit responses from an individual that can identify their characteristics that can increase that person's chances of, in these guidelines, being exposed to lead from various sources.

screening (blood lead screening): for lead poisoning, a laboratory test for lead that is performed on the blood of an asymptomatic person to determine if that person has evidence of lead exposure above background levels.

secondary prevention: responding to a problem after it has been detected. Secondary prevention of lead poisoning involves identifying persons with confirmed lead exposure and eliminating or reducing additional lead exposure.

spontaneous abortion (or miscarriage): the loss of a fetus before the 20th week of pregnancy.

Tanner scale or Tanner stage: used to define physical measurements of a child's development based on external primary and secondary sex characteristics, such as the size of the breasts or genitalia and development of pubic hair.

targeted screening: blood lead testing of some, but not all, individuals in a population or group designated as being at increased risk for lead exposure.

threshold: an established dose or level below which an effect does not occur.

TTDI (maximum total tolerable daily intake): a term used by the FDA to caution against excessive intake of nutrients that can be harmful in large amounts.

toxicokinetics: the fate and transport of chemicals in the human body.

traditional medicines: see alternative medicines.

umbilical cord: the tubal structure (consisting of two arteries and one vein) that connects the fetus (baby) to the placenta, supplying blood, oxygen and nutrients to the baby during pregnancy.

universal screening: the blood lead testing of all persons in a population or group, such as pregnant women or city residents.

U.S. PHSTF (U.S. Preventive Health Services Task Force): An independent panel of experts in primary care and prevention that systematically reviews the evidence of effectiveness and develops recommendations for clinical preventive services.

WIC: Special Supplemental Nutrition Program for Women, Infants, and Children.

KEY POINTS

- Lead exposure remains a public health problem for certain groups of women of childbearing age and for the developing fetus and nursing infant. Prenatal lead exposure has known influences on maternal health and infant birth and neurodevelopmental outcomes.

- Bone lead stores are mobilized in pregnancy and lactation for women with prior lead exposure, which is a concern since lead released into maternal blood and breast milk can adversely affect the fetus or newborn.

- Certain population subgroups of women at increased risk for exposure have been identified and may be highly exposed, particularly the following: workers in certain occupations; foreign-born recent immigrants; and those practicing certain behaviors associated with lead exposure, such as pica or renovation of older homes.

- Identifying pregnant women with a history of lead poisoning or who are currently exposed to lead above background levels and preventing additional lead exposure can help prevent adverse health outcomes in these children.

Despite improvements in environmental policies and significant reductions in U.S. average population blood lead levels, lead exposure remains a concern for pregnant and lactating women among certain population subgroups at increased risk for exposure. There is increasing awareness that unintended exposures to environmental contaminants, such as lead, adversely affect maternal and infant health, including the ability to become pregnant, maintain a healthy pregnancy, and have a healthy baby. In the United States, women of childbearing age represent approximately 42% of the total population (American Community Survey 2004) and at any given time almost 9% are pregnant (Crocetti et al. 1990). In the 2003-2006 National Health and Nutrition Examination Survey (NHANES) survey, the 95th percentile for blood lead levels among women aged 15-49 was 2.4 micrograms per deciliter (μg/dL). As Figure 1-1 indicates, blood lead levels among women aged 15-49 have dropped substantially since the 1976-1980 NHANES. Recent NHANES estimates suggest that almost 1% of women of childbearing age (15-49 years) have blood lead levels greater than or equal to 5 μg/dL (Centers for Disease Control and Prevention 2008, unpublished data).

Lead exposure remains a public health problem for subpopulations of women of childbearing age and for the developing fetus and nursing infant for several important reasons. First, prenatal lead exposure has known influences on maternal health and infant birth and neurodevelopmental outcomes (Bellinger 2005). Research findings suggest that prenatal lead exposure can adversely affect maternal and child health across a wide range of maternal exposure levels. In addition, adverse effects of lead are being identified at lower levels of exposure than previously recognized in both child and adult populations (Canfield et al. 2003; Jusko et al. 2008; Lanphear et al. 2005; Menke et al. 2006; Navas-Acien et al. 2007; Tellez-Rojo et al. 2006).

Second, bone lead stores are mobilized during periods of increased bone turnover such as pregnancy and lactation. Over 90% of lead in the adult human body is stored in bone (Barry 1975; Barry and Mossman 1970), and may result in redistribution of cumulative lead stores from bone into blood during periods of heightened bone turnover, such as pregnancy and lactation (Gulson et al. 2003; Roberts and Silbergeld 1995). Since bone lead stores persist for decades, women and their infants may be at risk for continued exposure long after exposure to external environmental sources has been terminated.

Finally, there is evidence that a significant number of pregnant women, and presumably their infants, are being exposed to lead in the United States today. It is clear that exposed subgroups do exist and some may be highly exposed, particularly recent immigrants (Graber et al. 2006; Klitzman et al. 2002); workers in specific high-risk occupations (Calvert and Roscoe 2007); and those practicing certain behaviors, such as pica (Hackley and Katz-Jacobson 2003; Shannon 2003), use of culturally-specific remedies and products (Centers for Disease Control and Prevention 2004; Saper et al. 2004, 2008), and renovating older homes (Marino et al. 1990; Jacobs et al. 2002). Women living near hazardous wastes site or active smelters (Garcia-Vargas et al. 2001) and residents in countries still using leaded gasoline (Albalak et al. 2003) may also be highly exposed.

Although lead exposure remains an important potential risk to the fetus, until now, little emphasis has been placed on developing guidelines for prenatal health care providers and women of childbearing age. There are currently no national recommendations or guidelines by any obstetric, family practice, pediatric, or nursing groups that cover lead risk assessment and management during pregnancy and lactation. Currently, New York State, New York City, and Minnesota are the only jurisdictions known to have issued lead screening regulations and follow-up recommendations for pregnant women by physicians or other health care providers (Minnesota Department of Health 2004; New York City Department of Health and Mental Hygiene 2006) [see Appendix I]. Other states have considered implementation of similar regulations or guidelines, and federal legislation has also been proposed. However, scientific discussion in this area has been limited.

Because no national recommendations exist, the Centers for Disease Control and Prevention (CDC) and local and state lead poisoning prevention programs have not been able to consistently respond to concerns from medical providers about when to test pregnant or lactating women for lead exposure and how to manage pregnant or lactating women who have been identified with lead exposure above background levels that have resulted from widespread ambient lead contamination and naturally occurring lead in the earth's crust. In response to this need, the Lead and Pregnancy Work Group was convened in April 2004 by the CDC Advisory Committee on Childhood Lead Poisoning Prevention (ACCLPP) to review the existing evidence for adverse effects of past and current maternal lead exposure on maternal health and fertility and on the developing fetus, infant, and child, and to develop recommendations on blood lead testing and management for pregnant and lactating women with lead exposure above background levels.

For the purposes of the review of existing scientific literature, the work group was divided into three subgroups: Prevalence, Risk, and Screening; Maternal, Pregnancy, and Child Outcomes; and Management, Treatment, and Other Interventions. The subgroups were asked to review the literature, summarize findings, and address the issues outlined in Appendix II. These guidelines do not include findings from animal studies, except when there are limited human data and consistent findings confirmed from multiple animal studies.

This document presents ACCLPP's summary of the evidence, provides guidance for preventing and treating lead exposure in pregnant and lactating women, and identifies research, policy, and education needs to improve health outcomes and care provided to pregnant women and their infants. These guidelines do not address all women of childbearing age, nor do they address male reproductive health issues associated with lead exposure.

Figure 1-1. Distribution of Blood Lead Levels in U.S. Women of Childbearing Age (15-49 Years)

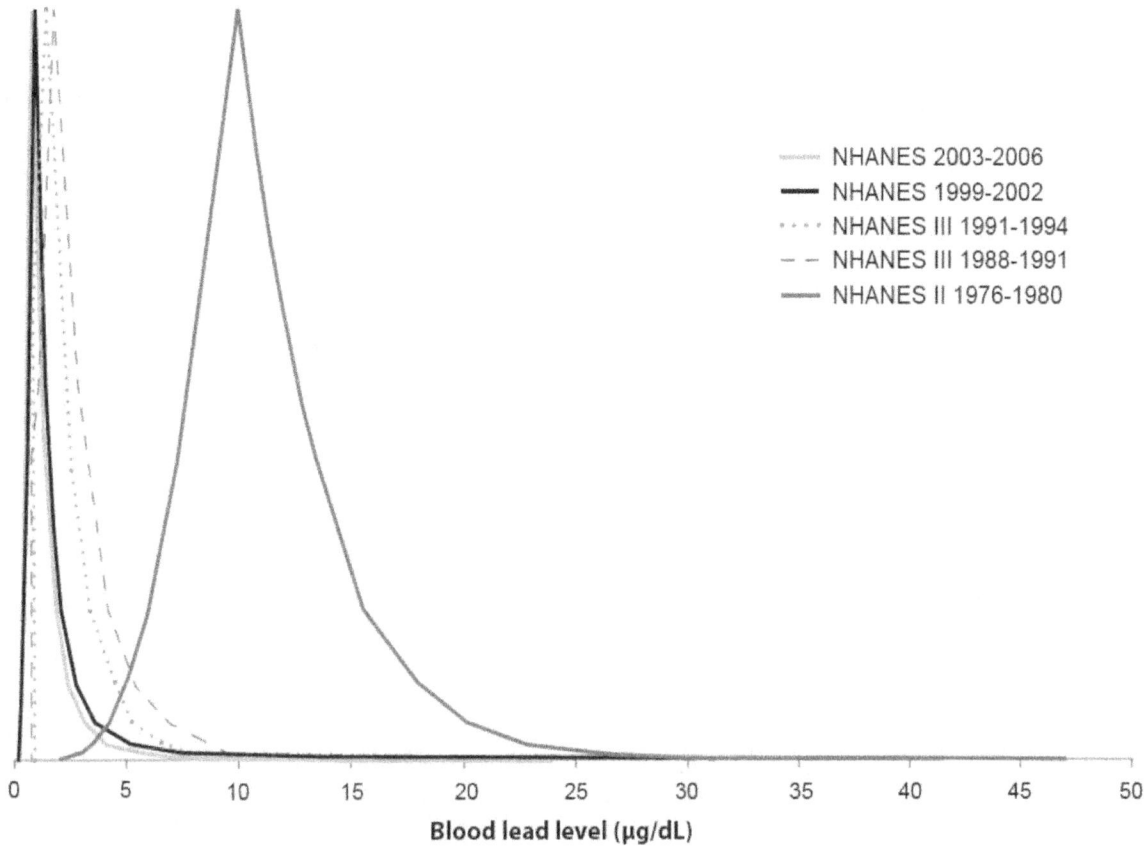

KEY POINTS

- For centuries, exposure to high concentrations of lead has been known to pose health hazards. Recent evidence suggests that chronic low-level lead exposure also has adverse health effects in both adults and children and no blood lead threshold level for these effects has been identified.

- CDC has not identified an allowable exposure level, level of concern, or any other bright line intended to connote a safe or unsafe level of exposure for either mother or fetus. Instead, CDC is applying public health principles of prevention to intervene when prudent.

- Epidemiologic and experimental evidence suggest that lead is a potent developmental toxicant, but many details regarding lead's mechanism of action have not been determined.

- Recent epidemiologic cohort studies suggest that prenatal lead exposure, even with maternal blood lead levels below 10 μg/dL, is inversely related to fetal growth and neurodevelopment independent of the effects of postnatal exposure, though the exact mechanism(s) by which low-level lead exposure, whether incurred prenatally or postnatally, might adversely affect child development remains uncertain.

- Lead may adversely impact sexual maturation in the developing female and may reduce fertility, but the scientific evidence is limited.

- Lead exposure has been associated with increased risk for gestational hypertension, but the magnitude of the effect, the exposure level at which risk begins to increase, and whether risk is more associated with acute or cumulative exposure, remain uncertain.

- Evidence is limited to support an association between blood lead levels from 10-30 μg/dL and spontaneous abortion. There are also few and inconsistent studies on the association between blood lead levels and preterm delivery.

- The available data are inadequate to establish the presence or absence of an association between maternal lead exposure and major congenital anomalies in the fetus.

INTRODUCTION

For centuries, exposure to high concentrations of lead has been known to pose health hazards. High levels of exposure can result in delirium, seizures, stupor, coma, or even death. Other overt signs and symptoms may include hypertension, peripheral neuropathy, ataxia, tremor, headache, loss of appetite, weight loss, fatigue, muscle and joint aches, changes in behavior and concentration, gout, nephropathy, lead colic, and anemia. In general, symptoms tend to increase with increasing blood lead levels. A substantial body of recent epidemiologic and toxicologic research demonstrates that multiple health effects can occur at low to moderate blood lead levels previously without recognized harm. Health effects of chronic low-level exposure in adults include cognitive decline, hypertension and other cardiovascular effects, decrements in renal function, and adverse reproductive outcome (Agency for Toxic Substances and Disease Registry 2007).

This chapter focuses on the effects of maternal lead exposure on reproductive health, maternal health, pregnancy outcome, infant growth, and child neurodevelopment. Although the studies described in this chapter focus on maternal exposures, paternal influences may also influence reproductive outcomes. Issues related to male-mediated reproductive toxicity for lead have been reviewed elsewhere (Apostoli et al. 1998; Jensen et al. 2006). In these guidelines, the discussion of scientific literature focuses on findings in humans. However, there also exists an extensive body of literature on the health effects of lead in experimental animals, which, while not cited, generally supports the human data. The reader is referred to other sources (Agency for Toxic Substances and Disease Registry 2007; U.S. Environmental Protection Agency 2006) for recent reviews of the experimental animal data.

An area of active study is the relationship between toxic exposures (such as lead) and fetal programming of growth and chronic disease. According to the Barker hypothesis (Barker 1990), now known more broadly as "fetal origins of adult disease," poor development *in utero*—for example, low birth weight—increases the risk for obesity, hypertension, and cardiovascular disease during adulthood (Barker 1995; Khan et al. 2003). These epidemiologic findings highlight the importance of the intrauterine environment and are consistent with experimental evidence of long-term "programming" in early life. For example, because exposure to developmental toxicants, including lead, is associated with low birth weight, lead exposure to the fetus may increase the risk for later cardiovascular disease. Evidence supporting the fetal origins hypothesis is mounting rapidly (Ingelfinger and Schnaper 2005). However, evidence of effects from *in utero* lead exposure on adult disease are currently too limited to provide conclusive information.

IMPACT OF LEAD EXPOSURE ON SEXUAL MATURATION AND FERTILITY

Few studies have examined possible lead-related effects on sexual maturation and fertility. Delay in puberty is an important yet understudied health outcome that may be associated with relatively low blood lead levels. Two studies have examined this outcome using cross-sectional data from the third NHANES (NHANES III). Selevan et al. (2003) analyzed blood lead and pubertal development by race in girls ages 8-18 years of age. Blood lead levels as low as 3 µg/dL were associated with 2 to 6 month delays in Tanner stage measurements (breast and pubic-hair development) and menarche in African-American and Mexican-American girls, while Non-Hispanic white girls experienced non-statistically significant delays in all pubertal measures. Wu et al. (2003) found that higher blood lead levels were significantly associated with delayed attainment of menarche and pubic hair development, but not breast development, even after adjustment for race/ethnicity, age, family size, residence, income, and body mass index. The cross-sectional design of NHANES III limits the ability to assess the temporal relation between blood lead and markers of puberty.

The studies on time-to-pregnancy associated with lead exposure have not been conclusive. One study of time-to-pregnancy did not suggest adverse effects of lead on fecundity at maternal blood lead concentrations less than 29 µg/dL. However, above this level, an association with longer time-to-pregnancy was found, but this was based on eight subjects (Sallmen et al. 1995). In a study of environmental lead exposure and reproductive health in Mexico City, no association was observed between maternal blood lead levels (mean = 9 µg/dL) and time-to-pregnancy in the first year (Guerra-Tamayo et al. 2003). However, in the subset of women with blood lead levels above 10 µg/dL, the likelihood of not achieving pregnancy after one year was five times higher (95% confidence interval [CI] 1.9-19.1) compared to women with blood lead levels below 10 µg/dL.

Summary of Evidence: Sexual Maturation and Fertility

Although studies are limited, there is some suggestion that blood lead at relatively low levels may lead to alterations in onset of sexual maturation and reduced fertility. These findings underscore the importance of considering sensitive markers of human fecundity in relation to lead exposure and should be confirmed in studies that can address the methodologic limitations of previous research.

IMPACT OF LEAD EXPOSURE ON MATERNAL HYPERTENSION DURING PREGNANCY

There is some evidence that maternal physiologic parameters in pregnancy can be modulated by low levels of lead exposure (Tabacova et al. 1994; Takser et al. 2005; Tellez-Rojo et al. 2004). However, the definitive relationship between lead exposure and maternal health outcomes in pregnancy is unclear. Lead is an established risk factor for hypertension in adults (Hertz-Picciotto and Croft 1993; Kosnett et al. 2007). Hypertension is one of the most common complications of pregnancy. There is substantial evidence that lead damages the vascular endothelium (Vaziri and Sica 2004) and that endothelial dysfunction is an important mediator of hypertension and preeclampsia in pregnancy (Karumanchi et al. 2005).

The most widely used classification of high blood pressure in pregnancy is that of the National High Blood Pressure Education Program Working Group (2000). This classification distinguishes between new hypertension arising during the pregnancy after 20 weeks (gestational hypertension) and preexisting hypertension (chronic hypertension).

It is important to differentiate between non-proteinuric hypertension and hypertension plus proteinuria (preeclampsia), as adverse clinical outcomes are more closely related to the latter. Severe hypertension usually defined as a systolic blood pressure of ≥180 mm Hg or diastolic blood pressure of ≥110 mm Hg, even in the absence of proteinuria, has been associated with adverse maternal and perinatal outcomes.

Gestational Hypertension

Hypertension in pregnancy is defined as a systolic blood pressure of 140 mm Hg or higher or diastolic pressure of 90 mm Hg or higher that occurs after 20 weeks gestation in a woman with previously normal blood pressure. Increasing levels of lead in blood have been associated with gestational hypertension. Among 3,851 women delivering at a Boston hospital from 1979-1981, incidence of pregnancy hypertension and elevated blood pressure at delivery increased significantly as blood lead increased (mean blood lead 6.9 ± 3.3 µg/dL). During delivery, lead levels correlated with both systolic (Pearson r = 0.081, p = 0.0001) and diastolic (r = 0.051, p = 0.002) blood pressure. Using a reference level of 0.7 µg/dL, the relative risk doubled when blood lead level approached 15. There was no association, however, between blood lead level and risk for preeclampsia in this study (Rabinowitz et al. 1987).

Rothenberg et al. (1999a) found that blood lead was a statistically significant predictor of maternal blood pressure among 1,627 women immigrants (mean blood lead 2.3 µg/dL) but not among nonimmigrants (mean blood lead 1.9 µg/dL).

In a cross-sectional analysis of third trimester primigravid women in Malta (N = 143), investigators compared normotensive women to those with gestational hypertension (Magri et al. 2003). Those with hypertension (mean blood lead 9.6 ± 6 µg/dL, N = 30) had significantly higher blood lead levels compared to normotensive controls (mean blood lead 5.8 ± 3 µg/dL, N = 93). A study of women with gestational age ranging from 30-41 weeks in Tehran, Iran, was conducted to assess the relationship between blood lead levels and gestational hypertension (Vigeh et al. 2004). Postpartum blood lead levels were significantly higher among 55 cases with hypertension (mean 5.7 ± 2.0 µg/dL) in comparison to 55 age-matched normotensive controls (mean 4.8 ±1.9 µg/dL).

The prevalence of gestational hypertension has been shown to be increased even at blood lead levels less than 5 µg/dL. Sowers et al. (2002) studied a cohort of 705 women aged 12-34 years who presented for prenatal care at one of three clinics in New Jersey with with mean (standard error) blood lead level equal to 1.2 ± 0.03 µg/dL and found maternal blood lead significantly associated with gestational hypertension.

Associations have also been found between gestational hypertension and bone lead. Rothenberg et al. (2002) reported on a prospective cohort study of 1,006 women aged 16-44 years enrolled during their third trimester in south central Los Angeles. This study included postpartum measures of tibia and calcaneus bone lead in addition to maternal blood lead levels. They found that each 10 µg/g increase in calcaneus bone lead (range -30.6 to 49.9 µg/g) was associated with an almost two-fold increased risk for third-trimester hypertension, a

0.70-mm Hg increase in third-trimester systolic blood pressure, and a 0.54-mm Hg increase in third-trimester diastolic blood pressure.

Preeclampsia

Preeclampsia, a pregnancy-specific disorder associated with increased maternal and perinatal morbidity and mortality, is defined as a) systolic blood pressure ≥140 mm Hg and/or diastolic blood pressure ≥90 mm Hg beginning after the 20th week of gestation and b) proteinuria ≥300 mg per 24 hours. Preeclampsia is usually associated with edema, hyperuricemia, and a fall in glomerular filtration rate. Blood lead levels have been associated with the risk for preeclampsia, although the evidence is less clear than for gestational hypertension. Dawson et al. (2000) observed significant differences between normotensive (N = 20) and hypertensive or preeclamptic (N = 19) pregnancies with respect to red blood cell lead content. They found maternal blood pressure to be directly proportional to RBC lead content; however, the selection criteria and study population in this small group at increased risk are not well-defined, so selection bias and confounding cannot be ruled out.

In the 2004 study by Vigeh et al. noted above, there were no significant differences in blood lead concentrations among hypertensive subjects with proteinuria (N = 30) and those without proteinuria (N = 25). In another study by Vigeh et al. (2006), among 396 postpartum women in Tehran, 31 with preeclampsia had significantly higher blood lead levels (mean 5.09 ± 2.01 µg/dL) compared to 365 normotensive controls (mean 4.82 ± 2.22 µg/dL) and significantly higher umbilical cord blood lead levels (mean 4.30 ± 2.49 µg/dL compared to 3.5 ± 2.09 µg/dL) (Vigeh et al. 2006). A 13-fold increased risk for preeclampsia compared to normotensive controls (mean blood lead 3.52 ± 2.09 µg/dL) was observed for every log-unit increase (~3 µg/dL) in blood lead. The 1987 study by Rabinowitz et al. of 3,851 women delivering in Boston found no association between blood lead level and risk for preeclampia (Rabinowitz et al. 1987).

Summary of the Evidence: Effects on Maternal Hypertension

Gestational hypertension and preeclampsia have been associated with adverse maternal and perinatal outcomes. Lead exposure has been associated with increased risk for gestational hypertension but the magnitude of the effect, the exposure level at which risk begins to increase, and whether risk is most associated with acute or cumulative exposure, remain uncertain. It is unclear whether lead-induced increases in blood pressure during pregnancy lead to severe hypertension or preeclampsia. However, even mild gestational hypertension can be expected to lead to increased maternal and fetal monitoring, medical interventions, and additional health care costs. Also, causality is unclear since preexisting hypertension reduces renal function, which in turn could result in the retention of lead.

IMPACT OF LEAD EXPOSURE ON PREGNANCY OUTCOMES

Spontaneous Abortion

There is consistent evidence that the risk for spontaneous abortion is increased by maternal exposure to high levels of lead. In her review of studies on the association between elevated blood lead levels and spontaneous abortion, Hertz-Picciotto (2000) includes a detailed summary of studies involving high blood lead levels, which come primarily from the literature on industrial exposures in Europe during the 19th century. Yet few studies have addressed the risk for spontaneous abortion at lower levels of exposure. Of those studies that have addressed this issue, most reports provide limited evidence to support an association between maternal blood lead levels of 0 to 30 µg/dL and increased risk for spontaneous abortion (Laudanski et al. 1991; Lindbohm et al. 1992; McMichael et al. 1986; Murphy et al. 1990; Tabacova and Balabaeva 1993). However, the lack of evidence for an association at these low-to-moderate blood lead levels may be due to methodologic deficiencies in these studies, such as small sample sizes, lack of control for confounding, problems in case ascertainment, and/or limitations in exposure assessment (Hertz-Picciotto 2000).

The strongest evidence to date is a prospective study of pregnant women in Mexico City, which addressed most of the deficiencies of the prior studies and demonstrated a statistically significant dose-response relationship between maternal blood lead levels (average 11.0 μg/dL) and risk for spontaneous abortion (Borja-Aburto et al. 1999). Odds ratios for spontaneous abortion for the blood lead groups 5-9, 10-14, and >15 μg/dL were 2.3, 5.4, and 12.2, respectively, in comparison to the reference group (<5 μg/dL) (p for trend = 0.03) with an estimated increased odds for spontaneous abortion of 1.8 (95% CI = 1.1–3.1) for every 5 μg/dL increase in blood lead. In another study of pregnant women (N = 207) from Mexico City (mean BLL 6.2 μg/dL), a 0.1% increment in the maternal plasma-to-blood lead ratio was associated with a 12% greater incidence of reported history of spontaneous abortion (p = 0.02) (Lamadrid-Figueroa et al. 2007). On average, women with no spontaneous abortions had higher blood lead levels than women with one or more reported spontaneous abortions (6.5 vs. 5.8 μg/dL); however, with each additional abortion experienced, women had an 18% greater plasma-to-blood lead ratio on average (p < 0.01). Women with a larger plasma-to-whole blood lead ratio may be at higher risk for miscarriage due to a greater availability of lead in plasma, which more readily crosses the placental barrier.

Preterm Delivery, Low Birth Weight, Length, and Head Circumference

Andrews et al. (1994) reviewed the epidemiologic literature through the early 1990s on prenatal lead exposure in relation to gestational age and birth weight. These studies are somewhat contradictory, most likely due to methodologic differences in study design, sample size, and/or degree of control for confounding. The more recent and well-designed studies suggest that maternal lead exposure during pregnancy is inversely related to fetal growth, as reflected by duration of pregnancy and infant size. Irgens et al. (1998), using a registry-based approach, found that women occupationally exposed to lead were more likely to deliver a low birth weight infant than women not exposed to lead (odds ratio [OR] = 1.1, 95% CI = 0.98–1.29). A case-control study in Mexico City found cord blood lead to be higher in preterm infants (mean 9.8 μg/dL) compared to term infants (mean 8.4 μg/dL) (Torres-Sanchez et al. 1999). A birth cohort study, also conducted in Mexico City, found maternal bone lead burden to be inversely related to birth weight (Gonzalez-Cossio et al. 1997) and birth length and head circumference at birth (Hernandez-Avila et al. 2002). A study by Rothenberg et al. (1999) among Mexican-Americans found that over the 1–35 μg/dL range of maternal blood lead at 36 weeks of pregnancy, the estimated reduction in 6-month infant head circumference was 1.9 cm (95% CI = 0.9–3.0 cm).

Congenital Anomalies

Very few studies have examined maternal lead exposure and risk for congenital malformations and, with one exception, none included biologic measures of lead exposure. Needleman et al. (1984) conducted a record review and reported an association between cord blood lead and minor congenital anomalies, but major anomalies did not show a similar association. In a case-control study, Bound et al. (1997) found an increased risk between living in an area with water lead levels greater than 10 μg/L (ppb) and delivering a child with a neural tube defect. Irgens et al. (1998) found, in a registry-based study, women occupationally exposed to lead were more likely to deliver an infant with a neural tube defect than women not exposed to lead (OR = 2.87, 95% CI = 1.1–6.4). In a case-control study conducted within the Baltimore-Washington Infant Study (Jackson et al. 2004), an association was observed between maternal occupational lead exposure and total anomalous pulmonary venous return although this relationship was not statistically significant (OR = 1.57, 95% CI = 0.64–3.47).

Summary of the Evidence: Pregnancy Outcomes

Overall, increased risk for spontaneous abortion appears to be associated with blood lead levels ≥30 μg/dL. Limited evidence suggests that maternal blood lead levels less than 30 μg/dL could also increase the risk for spontaneous abortion, although these findings remain to be confirmed in further research. Maternal lead exposure may increase the risk for preterm delivery and low birth weight, although data are limited and a blood lead level at which the risks begin to increase has not been determined. The available data are inadequate to establish the presence or absence of an association between maternal lead exposure and major congenital anomalies in the fetus.

IMPACT OF LEAD EXPOSURE ON INFANT GROWTH AND NEURODEVELOPMENT

Infant Growth

Few studies have investigated the effects of prenatal lead exposure on infant growth. Two studies suggest an association between maternal lead exposure and decreased growth. In one study, maternal bone lead levels were negatively associated with infant weight at one month of age and with postnatal weight gain between birth and 1 month (Sanin et al. 2001). In another study, postnatal linear growth rate was negatively related to prenatal blood lead level, although only when infants' postnatal lead exposure was elevated (Shukla et al. 1989). Infants born to a mother with prenatal blood lead concentration greater than 7.7 µg/dL (the median level in the cohort) and whose blood lead increased 10 µg/dL between 3 and 15 months of age were about 2 cm shorter at 15 months of age ($p = 0.01$). Greene and Ernhart (1991) also reported negative associations between prenatal lead level and birth weight, birth length, and head circumference, although none were statistically significant. Data on the association between prenatal lead exposure and infant growth is limted and thus inconclusive.

Lead and Neurodevelopment

Neurotoxic effects of lead are observed during episodes of acute lead poisoning in both children and adults. It remains unclear, however, whether prenatal or postnatal lead exposure is more detrimental to neurodevelopment. A number of chemicals, including lead, have been shown, in experimental animal models as well as in humans, to cause morphological changes in the developing nervous system (Costa et al. 2004). Given the incomplete blood-brain barrier in the developing nervous system, children might be more susceptible to insults during the prenatal and early postnatal periods (Bearer 1995; Rodier 1995; Weiss and Landrigan 2000).

Animal research indicates that the central nervous system is the organ system most vulnerable to developmental chemical injury (Rodier 2004), with vulnerabilities that pertain to processes critical to neurodevelopment, such as the establishment of neuron numbers; migration of neurons; establishment of synaptic connections, neurotransmitter activity, receptor numbers; and deposition of myelin. Neurons begin forming even before the neural tube closes. Most cerebral neurons form during the second trimester of gestation and migrate to their adult location well before birth (Goldstein 1990). Neuronal connections, however, are sparse at birth compared to adulthood. During the first 24 months of life, synaptic density and cerebral metabolic rate increase dramatically and by age 3 years are two-fold greater than those in the adult. The proliferation of synapses (synaptogenesis) is critical for the formation of basic circuitry of the nervous system (Rodier 1995). Synaptic "pruning" during early childhood establishes the final number of neurons.

Lead is known to interfere with synaptogenesis and, perhaps, with pruning (Goldstein 1992). It interferes with stimulated neurotransmitter release at synapses in the cholinergic, dopaminergic, noradrenergic, and GABergic systems (Cory-Slechta 1997; Guilarte et al. 1994). It substitutes for calcium and zinc as a second messenger in ion-dependent events. These disturbances in neurotransmitter release would thus be expected to disrupt the normal organization of synaptic connections (Bressler and Goldstein 1991).

The brain is protected from large molecular compounds in the blood by the blood-brain barrier, created by tight junctions between endothelial cells in cerebral blood vessels (Goldstein 1990). The development of this barrier function begins *in utero* and continues through the first year of life (Goldstein 1990). The brain is one of the target organs for lead and lead exposure *in utero* and the first year of life may dirupt the development of the blood-brain barrier.

These lead-induced biochemical disturbances in the brain are accompanied by impaired performance on a wide variety of tests of learning and memory in a variety of animal models and no threshold for these impairments has been identified (White et al. 2007).

Epidemiologic Evidence for Neurodevelopmental Effects of Lead

A large number of studies provide convincing evidence that prenatal lead exposure impairs children's neurodevelopment (Table 2-1). In most of the early prospective studies, many children had prenatal exposures exceeding 10 µg/dL. Several studies reported significant inverse associations with neurobehavior (Bellinger et al. 1987; Dietrich et al. 1987a,b; Ernhart et al. 1987; Shen et al. 1998; Wasserman et al. 2000). One study found that the early developmental delays were largely overcome if postnatal lead exposures were low in the preschool years, but appeared to be more persistent among children whose postnatal blood lead levels were also greater than 10 µg/dL (Bellinger et al. 1990). Other studies found that the effects of prenatal exposure were independent of changes in postnatal blood lead levels (e.g., Wasserman et al. 2000). These inverse associations persisted into adolescence and beyond, as maternal blood lead levels during pregnancy predicted teenage attention and visuoconstruction abilities (Ris et al. 2004), teenage self-reported delinquent behaviors (Dietrich et al. 2001), and increased arrest rates between the ages of 19 and 24 (Wright et al. 2008). A relationship between prenatal blood lead levels and the onset of schizophrenia between the late teens and early 20s is also seen (Opler et al. 2004, 2008). Some studies, however, did not find evidence of prenatal lead effects (e.g., Baghurst et al. 1992; Bellinger et al. 1992; Cooney et al. 1989a, 1989b; Dietrich et al. 1990, 1993; Ernhart et al. 1989; McMichael et al. 1988).

More-recent prospective studies have included children with lower prenatal exposures, and continue to detect inverse associations with neurodevelopment. Wasserman et al. (2000) found independent adverse effects of both prenatal and postnatal blood lead on IQ among Yugoslavian children age 3-7 years. Prenatal lead exposure was associated with a deficit of 1.8 IQ points for every doubling of prenatal maternal blood lead after controlling for postnatal exposure and other covariates. In a study conducted in Mexico City, Gomaa et al. (2002) found that umbilical cord blood lead and maternal bone lead levels were independently associated with covariate-adjusted scores at 2 years of age on the Mental Development Index score of the Bayley Scales of Infant Development with no evidence of a threshold. Maternal blood lead level early in the second trimester and in the third trimester was a significant predictor for some measures of mental and psychomotor development at age 2 years (Wigg et al. 1988). In another study in Mexico City, maternal plasma lead level in the first trimester was a particularly strong predictor of neurodevelopment at age 2 years (Hu et al. 2006). When this cohort was assessed at 24 months, inclusion of umbilical cord blood lead level in the model indicated that it was a significant predictor of psychomotor development even when analyses were restricted to children whose lead levels never exceeded 10 µg/dL (Tellez-Rojo et al. 2006). Schnaas et al. (2006) found that prenatal lead exposure around 28-36 weeks gestation (third trimester) was a stronger predictor of reduced intellectual development at ages 6–10 years than second trimester (12-20 weeks) exposure, but that study did not measure prenatal exposure in the first trimester of pregnancy. Jedrychowski et al. (2008) found a higher risk of scoring in the high-risk group on the Fagan Test of Infant Intelligence at age 6 months when umbilical cord blood was higher. Low-level umbilical cord blood lead levels can also negatively impact responses to acute stress (Gump et al. 2008).

In another study conducted in Mexico City, third trimester increases in maternal blood lead levels were associated with decreased ability of newborns to self-quiet and be consoled during the first 30 days of life (Rothenberg et al. 1989). In addition, greater prenatal and perinatal lead exposure was associated with altered brainstem auditory evoked responses (Rothenberg et al. 1994, 2000).

Threshold Levels and Persistence of Effects

No threshold has been found for the adverse effects of lead on neurodevelopment (Centers for Disease Control and Prevention 2004). Recent evidence, in fact, suggests that the dose-effect relationship might be supralinear, with steeper dose responses at levels below 10 µg/dL than above 10 µg/dL (Bellinger and Needleman 2003; Canfield et al. 2003; Jusko et al. 2008; Kordas et al. 2006; Lanphear et al. 2000; Tellez-Rojo et al. 2006). In the largest study of this issue, Lanphear et al. (2005) pooled data on 1,333 children who participated in seven international population-based longitudinal cohort studies and were followed from birth or infancy until 5-10 years of age. Among children with a maximal blood lead level <7.5 μg/dL, the decline in full-scale IQ for a given increase in blood lead was significantly greater than the decline observed among children with a maximal level ≥7.5 μg/dL. Nonlinear relationships were also detected in the Yugoslavia (Wasserman et al. 2000) and Mexico City (Schnaas et al. 2006) studies which suggest that the effects of prenatal exposure may also be more pronounced at blood lead levels less than 10 μg/dL.

Evidence from several of the prospective studies suggests that the adverse effects of early childhood lead exposure on neurodevelopment persist into the second decade of life (Bellinger et al. 1992; Fergusson et al. 1997; Ris et al. 2004; Tong et al. 1996; Wasserman et al. 2000) and are unrelated to changes in later blood lead level (Burns et al. 1999; Tong et al. 1998;). Administration of the chelating agent succimer to children with blood lead levels of 20-44 μg/dL did not prevent or reverse neurodevelopmental toxicity (Dietrich et al. 2004; Rogan et al. 2001).

Summary of the Evidence: Infant Growth and Neurodevelopment

Data on the association between prenatal lead exposure and infant growth are limted and thus inconclusive. The findings of recent cohort studies offer suggest that prenatal lead exposure at maternal blood lead levels below 10 μg/dL is inversely related to neurobehavioral development independent from the effects of postnatal exposure. While the lead-associated differences in test score are small when viewed as a potential change in an individual child's score, they acquire substantially greater importance when viewed as a shift in the mean score within a population (Bellinger 2004). The mechanism(s) by which low-level lead exposure, whether incurred prenatally or postnatally, might adversely affect neurobehavioral development remains uncertain, although experimental data support the involvement of many pathways.

Because there is no apparent threshold below which adverse effects of lead do not occur, CDC has not identified an allowable exposure level, level of concern, or any other bright line intended to connote a safe or unsafe level of exposure for either mother or fetus. Instead, CDC is applying public health principles of prevention to intervene when prudent. Specific recommendations are presented throughout the rest of these guidelines.

Table 2-1. Summary of Studies Estimating Association of Prenatal Lead Exposure with Neurodevelopmental Effects

Year	Study	Study Site	Study Type	N	Estimate of Prenatal Exposure Measured	Lead Levels (in μg/dL)	Outcome Measure(s)	Age at Outcome	Results
2008	Low-level prenatal and postnatal blood lead exposure and adrenocortical responses to acute stress in children (Gump et al. 2008)	Oswego, NY	Cohort study	154	Umbilical cord blood lead level (BLL)	Range: <1.0–6.3	Cortisol response to acute stress (the glucocorticoid product of hypothalamic–pituitary–adrenal (HPA) activation)	9.5 years	Relatively low prenatal blood lead levels, e.g., BLL <10 μg/dL, can alter adrenocortical response to acute stress.
2008	Prenatal low-level lead exposure and developmental delay of infants at age 6 months (Krakow inner city study) (Jedrychowski et al. 2008)	Krakow, Poland	Cohort study	452	Umbilical cord BLL	Mean cord BLL 1.42, 95% CI = 1.35–1.48	Fagan Test of Infant Intelligence (FTII)	6 months	Estimated risk for scoring in high-risk group of developmental delay (FTII classification 3) due to higher lead blood levels was two-fold greater (odds ratio [OR] = 2.33, 95% confidence interval [CI] = 1.32–4.1) than for lower lead blood levels after adjusting for potential confounders (gestational age, gender of the child, and maternal education).
2008	Prenatal exposure to lead, delta-aminolevulinic acid, and schizophrenia: further evidence (Opler et al. 2008)	Oakland, CA, Providence, RI, and Boston, MA	Pooled case control	200 (119 from Oakland, 81 from New England)	Maternal delta-ALA from second trimester frozen blood samples	Dichotomized to estimated (from delta-aminolevulinic acid [ALA]) maternal BLLs in 2nd trimester of ≥15 or <15	Schizophrenia (includes schizophrenia, schizoaffective disorder schizotypal personality disorder, delusional disorder, and nonaffective psychoses not otherwise specified)	15–22 years (not included in this report, but from Opler et al. [2004])	OR for schizophrenia associated with exposure, corresponding to 15 μg/dL of blood lead was 1.92 (95% CI = 1.05–3.87, p = 0.03).

Year	Study	Study Site	Study Type	N	Estimate of Prenatal Exposure Measured	Lead Levels (in µg/dL)	Outcome Measure(s)	Age at Outcome	Results
2008	Association of prenatal and childhood blood lead concentrations with criminal arrests in early adulthood (Wright et al. 2008)	Cincinnati, OH	Cohort study	250	Maternal prenatal BLL at 1st or early 2nd trimester	Mean (standard deviation (SD)) BLL = 8.3 (3.8); Median 7.8 (5th to 95th percentile 2.9–16).	Number of criminal arrests since turning 18 years of age	19-24 years	Increased arrest rates associated with prenatal BLL, relative risk (RR) = 1.40 (95% CI = 1.07 – 1.85).
2006	Fetal lead exposure at each stage of pregnancy as a predictor of infant mental development (Hu et al. 2006)	Mexico City, Mexico	Cohort study	146	Maternal prenatal plasma lead	Plasma lead mean (SD): 1st trimester 0.016 (0.014), N = 119; 2nd trimester 0.014 (0.011), N = 136; 3rd trimester 0.016 (0.024), N = 132	Bayley Mental Development Index (MDI)	24 months	Single-trimester models of MDI scores suggested a negative relationship between prenatal lead and MDI at 24 months adjusting for covariates. Maternal plasma lead in 1st trimester most strongly associated with MDI (β = −4.13, p = 0.03)
2006	Fetal lead exposure at each stage of pregnancy as a predictor of infant mental development (Hu et al. 2006)	Mexico City, Mexico	Cohort study	146	Maternal prenatal BLL	BLL mean (SD): 1st trimester 7.1 (5.1), N = 119; 2nd trimester 6.1 (3.2), N = 136; 3rd trimester 6.9 (4.2), N = 132; delivery 7.3 (4.3), N = 111	Bayley MDI	24 months	Single-trimester models of MDI scores suggested a negative relationship between prenatal lead and MDI at 24 months adjusting for covariates. Maternal blood lead in 1st trimester most strongly associated with MDI (β = −3.77, p = 0.03).
2006	Fetal lead exposure at each stage of pregnancy as a predictor of infant mental development (Hu et al. 2006)	Mexico City, Mexico	Cohort study	146	Umbilical cord BLL	Umbilical cord lead (mean 6.2 SD 3.9) (for N = 83 only)	Bayley MDI	24 months	Umbilical cord blood lead was not statistically significantly associated with MDI (β = −0.35, p = 0.88), but this exposure measure was only available on a subset of subjects.

Year	Study	Study Site	Study Type	N	Estimate of Prenatal Exposure Measured	Lead Levels (in µg/dL)	Outcome Measure(s)	Age at Outcome	Results
2006	Reduced intellectual development in children with prenatal lead exposure (Schnaas et al. 2006)	Mexico City, Mexico	Cohort study	150	Maternal BLL (12-20 weeks)	Geometric mean 8.2; 3.0–20.7, 5th–95th percentile	Full-scale IQ (FSIQ) as assessed using the Wechsler Intelligence Scale for Children–Revised (WISC-R; Spanish version) under standardized conditions	6-10 years	Multivariate regression analysis showed IQ reduction associated with BLL increase (β = -1.45, 95% CI = -4.75 to 2.00), but was not statistically significant (p = 0.42).
2006	Reduced intellectual development in children with prenatal lead exposure (Schnaas et al. 2006)	Mexico City, Mexico	Cohort study	150	Maternal BLL (28-36 weeks)	Geometric mean 7.8; 2.5–24.6, 5th–95th percentile	FSIQ as assessed using WISC-R; Spanish version under standardized conditions	6-10 years	Multivariate regression analysis showed IQ reduction associated with BLL increase (β = -4.00, 95% CI = -6.37 to -1.65) and was statistically significant (p = 0.001).
2006	Reduced intellectual development in children with prenatal lead exposure (Schnaas et al. 2006)	Mexico City, Mexico	Cohort study	112	Maternal BLL (at delivery)	Not reported	FSIQ as assessed using WISC-R; Spanish version under standardized conditions	6-10 years	Multivariate regression analysis showed IQ reduction associated with BLL increase (β = -1.29, 95% CI = -4.41 to 1.83) but was not statistically significant (p = 0.41).
2006	Reduced intellectual development in children with prenatal lead exposure (Schnaas et al. 2006)	Mexico City, Mexico	Cohort study	109	Umbilical cord BLL	Not reported	FSIQ as assessed using WISC-R; Spanish version under standardized conditions	6-10 years	Multivariate regression analysis showed IQ reduction associated with BLL increase (β = -0.95, 95% CI = -3.65 to 1.75) but was not statistically significant (p = 0.49).

Year	Study	Study Site	Study Type	N	Estimate of Prenatal Exposure Measured	Lead Levels (in µg/dL)	Outcome Measure(s)	Age at Outcome	Results
2004	Prenatal lead exposure, delta-aminolevulinic acid, and schizophrenia (Opler et al. 2004)	Oakland, CA	Nested case control	119	Maternal delta-ALA from 2nd trimester frozen blood samples	Dichotomized to estimated (from delta-ALA) maternal BLLs in 2nd trimester of ≥15 and <15	Schizophrenia (includes schizophrenia, schizoaffective disorder schizophrenia, schizotypal personality disorder, delusional disorder, and nonaffective psychoses not otherwise specified)	15-22 years	OR for schizophrenia associated with exposure, corresponding to 15 µg/dL of blood lead was 2.43 (95% CI = 0.99-5.96; p = 0.051).
2004	Early exposure to lead and neuropsychological outcome in adolescence (Ris et al. 2004)	Cincinnati, OH	Prospective cohort study	195	Prenatal maternal BLL	Mean BLL 4-35	Neuropsychological measures: memory, learning/ IQ, attention, visuoconstruction, and fine-motor	15-17 years	Prenatal BLL associated with decreased neuropsychological measures in the attention and visuoconstructional domains at mid-adolescence.
2002	Maternal bone lead as an independent risk factor of fetal neurotoxicity: a prospective study (Gomaa et al. 2002)	Mexico City, Mexico	Prospective cohort study	197	Maternal tibia bone lead 1 month after delivery (cortical bone)	Mean 11.5, SD 11.0, range <1-85.9	MDI and Psychomotor Development Index (PDI) scores as assessed using the Bayley Scales of Infant Development II (BSID-II; Spanish version)	24 months	Higher tibia lead levels were associated with lower MDI scores, but this association was not statistically significant.
2002	Maternal bone lead as an independent risk factor of fetal neurotoxicity: a prospective study (Gomaa et al. 2002)	Mexico City, Mexico	Prospective cohort study	197	Maternal patella bone lead 1 month after delivery (trabecular bone)	Mean 17.9, SD 5.2, range <1-76.6	MDI and PDI scores as assessed using BSID-II; Spanish version	24 months	In relation to the lowest quartile of trabecular bone lead, the 2nd, 3rd, and 4th quartiles were associated with 5.4 (p = 0.05), 7.2 (p = 0.01) and 6.5 (p = 0.02) point decrements in adjusted MDI scores, respectively.

Year	Study	Study Site	Study Type	N	Estimate of Prenatal Exposure Measured	Lead Levels (in µg/dL)	Outcome Measure(s)	Age at Outcome	Results
2002	Maternal bone lead as an independent risk factor of fetal neurotoxicity: a prospective study (Gomaa et al. 2002)	Mexico City, Mexico	Prospective cohort study	197	Umbilical cord BLL	Mean 6.7, SD 3.4, range 1.2 to 21.6	MDI and PDI scores as assessed using BSID-II; Spanish version	24 months	A 2-fold increase in cord blood lead level was associated with a 3.1-point decrement in MDI score
2001	Early exposure to lead and juvenile delinquency (Dietrich et al. 2001)	Cincinnati, OH	Prospective cohort study	157	Prenatal BLL (end of 1st trimester)	Mean 8.9, SD 3.9; range was not reported	Delinquency	15-17 years	Prenatal exposure to lead was significantly associated with a covariate-adjusted increase in the frequency of parent-reported delinquent and antisocial behaviors (β = 0.194, SE = 0.089, Partial r2 = 0.045; p = 0.032), and with a covariate-adjusted increase in frequency of self-reported delinquent and antisocial behaviors. Partial r2 = (β = 0.192, SE = 0.076, 0.049, p = 0.002).
2000	Brainstem auditory evoked response at five years and prenatal and postnatal blood lead (Rothenberg et al. 2000)	Mexico City, Mexico	Prospective cohort study	100	Maternal BLL (20 weeks)	Abstract: geometric mean 7.7; range 1–30 5. Table, with BAER Geometric mean 8.1 SD +8.1/–4.0	Brainstem auditory evoked response (BAER) interval	BAER: 5 years	Using multiple linear regression, both conduction intervals I-V and III-V had significant or marginally significant relationships with 20-week maternal blood lead level. The nonlinear model showed I-V and III-V interpeak intervals decreased as 20-week blood lead rose from 1 to 8 µg/dL, and then increased as blood lead rose from 8 to 30.5 µg/dL.

Year	Study	Study Site	Study Type	N	Estimate of Prenatal Exposure Measured	Lead Levels (in µg/dL)	Outcome Measure(s)	Age at Outcome	Results
2000	The Yugoslavia prospective lead study: contributions of prenatal and postnatal lead exposure to early intelligence (Wasserman et al. 2000)	Mitrovica and Pristina, Yugoslavia	Prospective cohort study	390	Maternal BLL (mid-pregnancy)	Means: exposed 18 2; controls 5.25	Early intelligence as assessed by McCarthy GCI (ages 3 and 4); Wechsler Preschool and Primary Scale of Intelligence–Revised (WPPSI–R IQ) (age 5); Wechsler Intelligence Scale for Children-version III (WISC-III IQ) (age 7)	3-5, 7 years	With adjustment for covariates, a significant decrement was detected: 6.05 points in IQ for each log unit increase in prenatal BLL (SE 1.35, p < 0.001). A 50% rise in prenatal BLL was associated with a 1.07 point decrement in IQ (95% CI = 0.60, 1 53). The association between prenatal BLL and IQ is not linear; the strongest postnatal effects are noted at the lower levels of prenatal exposure.
2000	The Yugoslavia prospective lead study: contributions of prenatal and postnatal lead exposure to early intelligence (Wasserman et al. 2000)	Mitrovica and Pristina, Yugoslavia	Prospective cohort study	390	Prenatal (average of mother's log10 BLL at mid-pregnancy and at delivery)	Means: exposed 19 5; controls 5.13	Early intelligence as assessed by McCarthy GCI (ages 3 and 4); WPPSI-R IQ (age 5); WISC-III IQ (age 7)	3-5, 7 years	With adjustment for covariates, a significant decrement was detected: 6.05 points in IQ for each log unit increase in prenatal BLL (SE 1.35, p < 0.001). A 50% rise in prenatal BLL was associated with a 1.07 point decrement in IQ (95% CI: 0.60, 1 53). The association between prenatal BLL and IQ is not linear; the strongest postnatal effects are noted at the lower levels of prenatal exposure.
2000	The Yugoslavia prospective lead study: contributions of prenatal and postnatal lead exposure to early intelligence (Wasserman et al. 2000)	Mitrovica and Pristina, Yugoslavia	Prospective cohort study	390	Umbilical cord BLL	Means: exposed 20.4; controls 5.01	Early intelligence as assessed by McCarthy GCI (ages 3 and 4); WPPSI-R IQ (age 5); WISC-III IQ (age 7)	3-5, 7 years	With adjustment for covariates, a significant decrement was detected: 6.05 points in IQ for each log unit increase in prenatal BLL (SE 1.35, p < 0.001). A 50% rise in prenatal BLL was associated with a 1.07 point decrement in IQ (95% CI: 0.60, 1 53). The association between prenatal BLL and IQ is not linear; the strongest postnatal effects are noted at the lower levels of prenatal exposure.

Year	Study	Study Site	Study Type	N	Estimate of Prenatal Exposure Measured	Lead Levels (in µg/dL)	Outcome Measure(s)	Age at Outcome	Results
1998	Low-level prenatal lead exposure and neurobehavioral development of children in the first year of life: a prospective study in Shanghai (Shen et al. 1998)	Shanghai, China	Prospective cohort study	133	Umbilical cord BLL	Geometric mean: 9.2, range 1.6 to 17.5, 95% CI = 8.86 to 9.54. High lead group mean 13.4, SD 2.0; Low lead group mean 5.3, SD 1.4	Child development as assessed by the MDI and PDI of the Bayley Scales of Infant Development	3, 6, and 12 months	At all three ages, after controlling for confounders, the MDI scores were inversely related to the infants' cord blood lead levels (at 3, 6, 12 months, p = 0.0187, 0.0315, and 0.0279, respectively); however, no significant association between cord blood lead levels and the PDI scores was detected.
1994	Prenatal and perinatal low level lead exposure alters brainstem auditory evoked responses in infants (Rothenberg et al. 1994)	Mexico City, Mexico	Prospective cohort study	25-29	Maternal BLL (12, 20, 28, 36 weeks)	Not reported	Infant BAER	Median: 9 days (range 2-39 days); 3 months	For neonates, the I-V interpeak interval is increased with increasing maternal BLL at 12 weeks. Latencies of peaks I and III are decreased with increasing maternal BLL at 20 weeks, and the III-V interpeak interval is increased with increasing maternal BLL at 20 weeks. The III-V interpeak interval is increased with increasing maternal BLL at 28 and 36 weeks. At 3 months, maternal BLL at 20 and 36 weeks were associated with increased III-IV interpeak intervals. These findings are statistically significant (p < 0.1). Infant spatial localization of sound may be compromised by mid-pregnancy lead exposure.

Year	Study	Study Site	Study Type	N	Estimate of Prenatal Exposure Measured	Lead Levels (in µg/dL)	Outcome Measure(s)	Age at Outcome	Results
1994	Prenatal and perinatal low level lead exposure alters brainstem auditory evoked responses in infants (Rothenberg et al. 1994)	Mexico City, Mexico	Prospective cohort study	25	Maternal BLL (at delivery)	Not reported	Infant BAER	Median: 9 days (range 2-39 days)	The III-V interpeak interval is increased with increasing maternal BLL at delivery. This finding is statistically significant ($p < 0.1$). Infant spatial localization of sound may be compromised by prenatal mid-pregnancy lead exposure.
1994	Prenatal and perinatal low level lead exposure alters brainstem auditory evoked responses in infants (Rothenberg et al. 1994)	Mexico City, Mexico	Prospective cohort study	27	Umbilical cord BLL	Not reported	Infant BAER	Median: 9 days (range 2-39 days); 3 months	For neonates, the III-V interpeak interval is increased with increasing cord BLL. At 3 months, cord BLL was associated with increased III-IV interpeak intervals. These findings are statistically significant ($p < 0.1$). Infant spatial localization of sound may be compromised by prenatal midpregnancy lead exposure.
1993	The developmental consequences of low to moderate prenatal and postnatal lead exposure: Intellectual attainment in the Cincinnati lead study cohort following school entry (Dietrich et al. 1993)	Cincinnati, OH	Prospective cohort study	217	Maternal BLL (end of 1st trimester)	Mean 8.3, SD 3.7	Full Scale IQ (FSIQ), Performance IQ (PIQ), and Verbal IQ (VIQ) as assessed by WISC-R	6.5 years	Covariate-adjusted regression coefficients for BPb indices and the Wechsler scales demonstrated that PreBPb was unrelated to intellectual attainment at 6.5 years (FSIQ: $\beta = 0.15$, SE 0.21; PIQ $\beta = 0.06$, SE 0.23; VIQ: $\beta = 0.16$, SE 0.21; all $p > 0.1$).
1992	Environmental exposure to lead and children's intelligence at the age of seven years: the Port Pirie study (Baghurst et al. 1992)	Port Pirie, Australia	Prospective cohort study	494	Maternal BLL (average antenatal)	Geometric mean concentrations by quartile: I 6.2 (low); II 8.7; III 10.6; IV 14.3 (high)	IQ as measured by WISC-R	7 years (median age: 186 days after 7th birthday)	Inverse relationship between full-scale IQ at age 7 years and antenatal BLLs (unadjusted), but not statistically significant after adjustment for multiple covariates ($\beta = -1.4$, SE 2.0, $p = 0.48$).

Year	Study	Study Site	Study Type	N	Estimate of Prenatal Exposure Measured	Lead Levels (in µg/dL)	Outcome Measure(s)	Age at Outcome	Results
1992	Environmental exposure to lead and children's intelligence at the age of seven years: the Port Pirie study (Baghurst et al. 1992)	Port Pirie, Australia	Prospective cohort study	494	Umbilical cord BLL	Geometric mean concentrations by quartile: I 4.3 (low); II 7.4; III 9.9; IV 15.0 (high); overall mean 8.9	IQ as measured by WISC-R	7 years (median age: 186 days after 7th birthday)	Inverse relationship between full-scale IQ at age 7 years and cord BLLs (unadjusted), but not statistically significant after adjustment for multiple covariates (β = 0.6, SE 1.4, p = 0.68).
1992	Low level lead exposure, intelligence and academic achievement: a long-term follow-up study (Bellinger et al. 1992)	Boston, MA	Prospective cohort study	148	Umbilical cord BLL	Categorized into: low <3; medium 6-7; high ≥10; no mean, SD, range given	WISC-R and the Kaufman Test of Educational Achievement (K-TEA)	10 years	Cord BLL was inversely associated with crude full-scale IQ (low: β = -1.29, SD 3.03; medium β = -1.52, SD 3.01 [high: β = 1.0]; p = 0.86), and with adjusted full-scale IQ (low: β = -0.48, SD 2.65; medium -2.55 β = 2.56, SD [high: β = 1.0]; p = 0.57). but the association failed to meet statistical significance.
1990	Antecedents and correlates of improved cognitive performance in children exposed in utero to low levels of lead (Bellinger et al. 1990)	Boston, MA	Prospective cohort study	170	Umbilical cord BLL	Categorized into: low <3; medium 6-7; high ≥10; no mean, SD, range given	Cognitive function as assessed by MDI scores from the Bayley Scales of Infant Development at age 2 and by GCI score from the McCarthy Scales of Children's Abilities at 57 months	24 months; 57.8 months (median age)	Elevated prenatal lead is associated with lower MDI scores at 2 years old. Recovery from 2 to 5 years of age is modified by sociodemographic factors and BLL at 2 years.
1990	Lead exposure and neurobehavioral development in later infancy (Dietrich et al. 1990)	Cincinnati, OH	Prospective cohort study	237	Maternal BLL (50% first trimester, 49% 2nd trimester, 1% 3rd trimester)	Mean 8.0, SD 3.7, Range 1-27	Behavioral development as assessed by Bayley MDI	24 months	No statistically significant relationships between prenatal blood lead variables and Bayley MDI were found.

Year	Study	Study Site	Study Type	N	Estimate of Prenatal Exposure Measured	Lead Levels (in µg/dL)	Outcome Measure(s)	Age at Outcome	Results
1989	Low level exposure to lead: the Sydney lead study (Cooney et al. 1989a)	Sydney, Australia	Prospective cohort study	207	Maternal BLL (at delivery)	Geometric mean 9.1, SD 1.3	GCI score from the McCarthy Scales of Children's Abilities and motor subscale	48 months	Prenatal BLL was not significantly associated with developmental indices at 48 months of age with limited control for potential confounding variables.
1989	Low level exposure to lead: the Sydney lead study (Cooney et al. 1989a)	Sydney, Australia	Prospective cohort study	207	Umbilical cord BLL	Geometric mean 8.1, SD 1.4	GCI score from the McCarthy Scales of Children's Abilities and motor subscale	48 months	Umbilical cord BLL was not significantly associated with developmental indices at 48 months of age with limited control for potential confounding variables.
1989	Neurobehavioral consequences of prenatal low level exposure to lead (Cooney et al. 1989b)	Sydney, Australia	Prospective cohort study	215-274	Maternal BLL (at delivery)	Geometric mean, 9.1; range 0-29 (70% ≤10)	Development assessed by the MDI and PDI scores of the Bayley Scales of Infant Development at 6, 12, and 24 months, and GCI score from the McCarthy Scales of Children's Abilities and motor subscale at 36 months	6, 12, 24, and 36 months	Analyses do not support a relationship between maternal BLL in this range and developmental deficits to the age of 3 years.
1989	Neurobehavioral consequences of prenatal low level exposure to lead (Cooney et al. 1989b)	Sydney, Australia	Prospective cohort study	215-274	Umbilical cord BLL	Geometric mean, 8.1; range 0-29 (80% ≤10)	Development assessed by the MDI and PDI scores of the Bayley Scales of Infant Development at 6, 12, and 24 months, and GCI score from the McCarthy Scales of Children's Abilities and motor subscale at 36 months	6, 12, 24, and 36 months	Analyses do not support a relationship between cord BLL in this range and developmental deficits to the age of 3 years.

Year	Study	Study Site	Study Type	N	Estimate of Prenatal Exposure Measured	Lead Levels (in µg/dL)	Outcome Measure(s)	Age at Outcome	Results
1989	Low level lead exposure in the prenatal and early preschool periods: intelligence prior to school entry (Ernhart et al. 1989)	Cleveland, OH	Prospective cohort study	135	Maternal BLL (at delivery)	Mean 6.5, SD 1.8, range 2.7-11.8	Cognitive development as assessed by the Wechsler Preschool and Primary Scale of Intelligence (WPPSI)	4 years 10 months	Maternal BLL was significantly correlated with the WPPSI full scale and subscale IQ scores when unadjusted (r values -0.23 to -0.25, p<0.01), but not statistically significant when adjusted for covariates.
1989	Low level lead exposure in the prenatal and early preschool periods: intelligence prior to school entry (Ernhart et al. 1989)	Cleveland, OH	Prospective cohort study	118	Umbilical cord BLL	Mean 5.89, SD 2.10, range 2.8-14.7	Cognitive development as assessed by WPPSI	4 years 10 months	Cord BLL is significantly correlated with the WPPSI full scale and subscale IQ scores when unadjusted (r values -0.20 to -0.22, p<0.05), but not statistically significant when adjusted for covariates.
1989	Neurobehavioral deficits after low level lead exposure in neonates: the Mexico City pilot study (Rothenberg et al. 1989)	Mexico City, Mexico	Prospective cohort study	42	Maternal BLL (36 weeks)	Mean (SD) range (µg/dL): 15.0 (6.4) 5.5-42	Brazelton Neonatal Behavioral Assessment Scale (NBAS)	48 hours; 15 and 30 days	Change in maternal BLL between 36 weeks and birth predicted NBAS regulation of state as identified by the neonatal behavioral assessment scale at 15 days (partial r2 = 0.068, p = 0.049), regulation of state at 30 days (partial r2 = 0.061, p = 0.055), and autonomic regulation at 30 days (partial r2 = 0.048, p = 0.073).
1989	Neurobehavioral deficits after low level lead exposure in neonates: the Mexico City pilot study (Rothenberg et al. 1989)	Mexico City, Mexico	Prospective cohort study	42	Maternal BLL and umbilical cord lead (at delivery)	Mean (SD) range (µg/dL): maternal BLL 15.5 (5.7) 6.0-33.5; umbilical cord 13.1 (6.0) 3.0-33.5	Brazelton NBAS	48 hours; 15 and 30 days	Difference in maternal and umbilical cord lead at delivery predicted NBAS regulation of state as identified by the neonatal behavioral assessment scale at 30 days (partial r2 = 0.071, p = 0.042).

Year	Study	Study Site	Study Type	N	Estimate of Prenatal Exposure Measured	Lead Levels (in µg/dL)	Outcome Measure(s)	Age at Outcome	Results
1988	Port Pirie cohort study: childhood blood lead and neuropsychological development at age two years (Wigg et al. 1988)	Port Pirie, Australia	Prospective cohort study	509-586	Maternal BLL (14-20 weeks; 3rd trimester)	Not reported	Development as assessed by the MDI and PDI scores of the Bayley Scales of Infant Development	24 months	Maternal BLL was negatively correlated with mental and psychomotor development, with some measures achieving statistical significance: 14-20 weeks gestation: MDI -0.06, PDI -0.05; after 20 weeks gestation: MDI -0.08 (p <0.05), PDI 0.02; average prepartum MDI -0.11 (p <0.05), PDI -0.06 (Pearson correlation coefficients, unadjusted for covariates).
1988	Port Pirie cohort study: childhood blood lead and neuropsychological development at age two years (Wigg et al. 1988)	Port Pirie, Australia	Prospective cohort study	524	Maternal BLL (at delivery)	Not reported	Development as assessed by the MDI and PDI scores of the Bayley Scales of Infant Development	24 months	Maternal BLL at delivery was negatively correlated with mental and psychomotor development, but was not statistically significant: MDI -0.03, PDI -0.02 (Pearson correlation coefficients, unadjusted for covariates).
1988	Port Pirie cohort study: childhood blood lead and neuropsychological development at age two years (Wigg et al. 1988)	Port Pirie, Australia	Prospective cohort study	520	Umbilical cord BLL	Geometric mean 8.3, 95% CI = 8.0-8.6	Development as assessed by the MDI and PDI scores of the Bayley Scales of Infant Development	24 months	Cord BLL was negatively correlated with mental and psychomotor development; but was not statistically significant: MDI -0.04, PDI -0.04 (Pearson correlation coefficients, unadjusted for covariates).

Year	Study	Study Site	Study Type	N	Estimate of Prenatal Exposure Measured	Lead Levels (in µg/dL)	Outcome Measure(s)	Age at Outcome	Results
1987	Longitudinal analyses of prenatal and postnatal lead exposure and early cognitive development (Bellinger et al. 1987)	Boston, MA	Prospective cohort study	182–201	Umbilical cord BLL	Mean 6.6, SD 3.2, range 0–37. Categorized into: low, <3; medium, 6–7; high, >= 10	Development as assessed by the MDI of the Bayley Scales of Infant Development	6, 12, 18, 24 months	At all ages, infants who had higher cord BLLs had lower crude MDI scores than infants in the other two groups; this relationship was stronger when adjusted for covariates. Estimated difference between low exposure and high exposure group was 4.8 points (95% CI = 2.3, 7.3); between medium exposure and high exposure group was 3.8 (95% CI = 1.3, 6.3).
1987	Low-level fetal lead exposure effect on neurobehavioral development in early infancy (Dietrich et al. 1987)	Cincinnati, OH	Prospective cohort study	266	Maternal BLL (50% first trimester, 49% 2nd trimester, 1% 3rd trimester)	Mean 8.0, SD 3.7, range 1–27	Development as assessed by the MDI and PDI scores of the Bayley Scales of Infant Development	3 and 6 months	In multiple regression analysis, at 3 months, MDI decreased by 0.34 for each increase of 1 µg/dL of prenatal lead (SE = 0.17, p = 0.05); at 6 months, MDI decreased by 0.76 for each increase of 1 µg/dL of prenatal lead (SE = 0.34, p = 0.02). No significant effects of prenatal lead exposure on PDI were found after adjustment for covariates.
1987	Low-level fetal lead exposure effect on neurobehavioral development in early infancy (Dietrich et al. 1987)	Cincinnati, OH	Prospective cohort study	96	Umbilical cord BLL	Mean 6.4, SD 4.5, range 1–28	Development as assessed by the MDI and PDI scores of the Bayley Scales of Infant Development	3 and 6 months	In multiple regression analysis, at 3 months, MDI decreased by 0.6 for each increase of 1 µg/dL of umbilical cord lead (SE = 0.26, p = 0.02); at 6 months, MDI decreased by 0.66 for each increase of 1 µg/dL of umbilical cord lead, but was not statistically significant at the 0.05 level (SE = 0.37, p = 0.08). No significant effects of prenatal lead exposure on PDI were found after adjustment for covariates.

Year	Study	Study Site	Study Type	N	Estimate of Prenatal Exposure Measured	Lead Levels (in µg/dL)	Outcome Measure(s)	Age at Outcome	Results
1987	Low-level lead exposure in the prenatal and early preschool periods: early preschool development (Ernhart et al. 1987)	Cleveland, OH	Prospective cohort study	119-145	Maternal BLL (at delivery)	Mean 6.5, SD 1.8, range 2.7-11.8	Bayley MDI and PDI and modified Kent Infant Development (KID) scale at 6 months; Bayley MDI at 1 year and 2 years; Stanford-Binet Intelligence scale at 3 years	6 months; 1, 2, and 3 years	Maternal BLL was statistically significantly associated with 6 month MDI, PDI, and KID in unadjusted analyses, but these associations were not significant after control for covariates.
1987	Low-level lead exposure in the prenatal and early preschool periods: early preschool development (Ernhart et al. 1987)	Cleveland, OH	Prospective cohort study	109-127	Umbilical cord BLL	Mean 5.99, SD 2.11, range 2.8-14.7	Bayley MDI and PDI and modified KID scale at 6 months; Bayley MDI at 1 year and 2 years; Stanford-Binet Intelligence scale at 3 years	6 months; 1, 2, and 3 years	Umbilical cord BLL was not statistically significantly associated with 6 month or later MDI, PDI, and KID.

Abbreviations: 95% CI: 95% confidence interval; BAER: brainstem auditory evoked response; BLL: blood lead level; BSID-II: Bayley Scales of Infant Development; delta-ALA: delta-aminolevulinic acid; FSIQ: full-scale IQ; FTII: Fagan Test of Infant Intelligence; GCI: general cognitive index; HPA: hypothalamic-pituitary-adrenal; KID: Kent Infant Development; K-TEA: Kaufman Test of Educational Achievement; MDI: mental development index; NBAS: Neonatal Behavioral Assessment Scale; OR: odds ratio; PDI: psychomotor development index; PIQ: performance IQ; RR: relative risk; SD: standard deviation; VIQ: verbal IQ; WISC-III IQ: Wechsler Intelligence Scale for Children-version III; WISC-R: Wechsler Intelligence Scale for Children-Revised; WPPSI: Wechsler Preschool and Primary Scale of Intelligence; WPPSI-R IQ: Wechsler Preschool and Primary Scale of Intelligence-Revised.

Key Points

- No single test is available to establish total body lead burden; biological markers (bio-markers) must be used to estimate maternal lead body burden and to assess lead dose to the fetus or infant during pregnancy or breastfeeding.

- Blood lead is the most well-validated and widely available measure of lead exposure. However, a single blood lead test may not reflect cumulative lead exposure and may not be sufficient to establish the full nature of the developmental risk to the fetus/infant. Repeat testing may be necessary.

- Bone is a potential endogenous source of lead exposure and studies have demonstrated that some of the previously acquired maternal bone lead stores are mobilized during pregnancy and lactation. However, bone lead measurement is almost exclusively a research tool.

- Lead readily crosses the placenta by passive diffusion and has been measured in the fetal brain as early as the end of the first trimester, so primary prevention of exposure is particularly important to reduce risk.

- Lead has been detected in the breast milk of women in population-based studies; however, the availability of high-quality data to assess the risk for toxicity to the breastfeeding infant is limited.

- Given the difficulty of accurately and precisely measuring trace amounts of lead in human breast milk, routine measurement of breast milk lead is not warranted for routine clinical application at this time.

INTRODUCTION

The purpose of this chapter is to discuss biological markers (biomarkers) that have been proposed to assess lead body burden and to summarize our present understanding of the biokinetics of lead during pregnancy and lactation. There is no single test available to establish total body lead burden, since lead may be in all body fluids and tissues including bone. Biomarkers must be used to estimate lead body burden and to assess lead dose to the fetus during pregnancy and to the infant during lactation. Figure 3-1 shows the major lead exposure pathways from mother to infant.

BIOLOGICAL MARKERS OF LEAD EXPOSURE

Certain biomarkers of lead dose to the fetus during pregnancy have been validated as measures of exposure. These include measurement of lead collected from maternal venous blood during pregnancy and umbilical cord blood at delivery, and measurement of lead in maternal bone using the noninvasive technique of K-x-ray fluorescence (Hu and Hernandez-Avila 2002). Each of these biomarkers provides an independent level of information regarding fetal lead exposure; together, they are critical to understanding whether lead toxicity varies based on timing of exposure, cumulative versus acute dose, and partitioning of lead between red cells and plasma (Hu and Hernandez-Avila 2002; Tellez-Rojo et al. 2004).

Variability in individual blood lead levels and limitations in the accuracy of measurement techniques including limits of detection, rounding, analytical methods, and regression to the mean pose challenges to reliable assessment of blood lead levels, particularly when blood lead levels are low. Laboratory instruments introduce measurement error, as do certain blood lead sampling methods (e.g., capillary samples may be prone to contamination due to lead dust on the skin surface). Venous blood lead tests produce the most reliable results. Capillary samples have a high level of sensitivity but lower specificity and may produce a higher number of false positives.

Other biomarkers have been used or proposed, usually because of the relative ease and noninvasiveness of collection procedures. These include hair, nails, teeth, saliva, urine, feces, meconium, placenta, and sperm. However, the utility of these alternatives as biomarkers for internal dose has not been demonstrated. In addition to the absence of consistent, validated analytic methods and standard reference materials for these biomarkers, they would also have to overcome the challenge of external contamination (Barbosa et al. 2005).

Whole Blood Lead

Blood lead has been the most commonly used and readily available biomarker of exposure to date with standard units of measurement in micrograms per deciliter (1 μg/dL = 0.0484 μmol/L). Following removal of the subject from environmental exposure, the decline in blood lead concentration occurs relatively rapidly at first; the initial half-life of lead in blood is about 35 days (Rabinowitz et al. 1976). This initial rapid drop is followed by a slow continuing decline over several months to years. In addition to lead from exogenous sources, blood lead represents the contribution of past environmental exposure being mobilized from endogenous bone stores. It is this reservoir of lead that determines the slow decline in blood lead after the first few weeks following removal from exposure.

Umbilical cord whole blood lead collected at delivery has been widely used as a measure of fetal exposure (Harville et al. 2005; Satin et al. 1991; Scanlon 1971; Rothenberg et al. 1996;). Lead readily crosses the placenta by passive diffusion (Goyer 1990; Silbergeld 1986) and fetal blood lead concentration is highly correlated with maternal blood lead concentration (Goyer 1990).

However, a single blood lead test may not reflect cumulative lead exposure and may not be sufficient to establish the full nature of the developmental risk to the fetus/infant. Physiologic changes, such as decreasing hematocrit, saturation of red cell lead-binding capacity, and increased bone resorption or intestinal absorption of lead, may influence the interpretation of blood lead levels during pregnancy. In addition, it is well known from the experimental literature that the vulnerability of developing organ systems, including the brain, to environmental toxicants can vary widely over the course of pregnancy (Mendola 2002). Thus, it is plausible that lead exposure may be particularly neurotoxic during a specific trimester (Hu et al. 2006; Schnaas et al. 2006).

Plasma Lead

The overwhelming majority of lead in blood is bound to erythrocytes (DeSilva 1981), but plasma is the blood compartment from which lead is available to cross cell membranes (Cavalleri et al. 1978). An understanding of how plasma lead concentration is related to whole blood lead concentration is important. Plasma lead concentrations in the range of 0.1%-5.0% of whole blood lead concentration have been reported (DeSilva 1981; Manton and Cook 1984; Ong et al. 1986). Although whole blood lead levels are highly correlated with plasma lead levels, lead levels in bone and other tissues (particularly trabecular bone) exert an additional independent influence on plasma lead levels (Hernandez-Avila et al. 1998). Recent data suggest that the plasma-to-whole blood lead ratio may vary quite widely among and within individuals (Hu 1998; Lamadrid-Figueroa et al. 2006), raising questions about the use of maternal whole blood lead as a proxy for plasma lead and fetal exposure (Chuang et al. 2001; Goyer 1990; Hu et al. 2006).

However, the measurement of maternal plasma lead is not likely to become a clinically useful tool. The methods required to measure plasma lead accurately are laborious and require specialized equipment and ultraclean techniques (Smith et al. 1998). Moreover, recent data suggest that the gain in using measurements of plasma lead during pregnancy to predict fetal/infant outcomes is only modest (Hu et al. 2006). Consequently, this biomarker may be a useful research tool in efforts to understand and detect the health impacts of environmental lead exposure, but cannot be recommended at this time as a clinical tool.

Bone Lead

Bone is a dynamic reservoir for lead, in constant exchange with blood and soft tissue elements (Rabinowitz 1991; Tsaih et al. 1999). Lead is incorporated into the hydroxyapatite crystalline structure of bone, much like calcium, and may also transfer into bone matrix exclusive of incorporation into hydroxyapatite (Marcus 1985). Because over 90% of lead in the adult human body is stored in bone (Barry 1975; Barry and Mossman 1970), there is the possibility of redistribution of cumulative lead stores from bone into blood during periods of heightened bone turnover, such as pregnancy and lactation (Roberts and Silbergeld 1995). Lead in bone has a half-life of years to decades and therefore reflects cumulative lead exposure (Hu et al. 1998). Measurement of lead in bone using a noninvasive, in vivo X-ray fluorescence (XRF) technique makes epidemiologic evaluation of the impact of retained body burden of lead possible (Hu 1998).

The amount of lead in bone depends on the individual's lead exposure history. Smith et al. (1996) determined that bone contributed 40%-70% of the lead in blood of environmentally exposed subjects who were undergoing total hip or knee joint replacement, indicating that the skeleton can be an important endogenous source of lead exposure. By examining the lead isotopic ratio in a small number of pregnant women who were recent immigrants to Australia (and pregnant Australian controls), Gulson and his colleagues (1997) were able to show that the skeletal contribution to maternal blood lead increased during pregnancy and lactation. Lead in maternal diet and bone lead were the main contributors to circulating maternal blood lead levels (Gulson 1998a). The relative contribution of bone lead to blood lead will vary depending on the exposure history of the individuals.

The measurement of bone lead requires special equipment and trained operators and is used mainly in research settings. Therefore, it is unlikely that this method will have widespread clinical application. However, this biomarker is a useful tool in research efforts to understand and detect the health impacts of cumulative lead exposure.

Breast Milk Lead

Detectable levels of lead in breast milk have been documented in population studies of community-dwelling women with no known source of occupational or elevated environmental lead exposure (Abadin et al. 1997; Anderson and Wolff 2000). Given the correlation of breast milk lead levels with maternal and infant blood lead levels (Ettinger et al. 2004a, 2004b), milk lead can be used as an indicator of both maternal and neonatal exposures (Hallén et al. 1995). In studies of lead in human breast milk, concentrations have been observed ranging over three levels of magnitude, from <1 to greater than 100 µg/L (ppb) (Chatranon et al. 1978; Ettinger et al. 2004a; Gulson et al. 1997; Larsson et al. 1981; Murthy and Rhea 1971; Namihira et al. 1993). These differences are partially attributable to true differences in population exposures across time and geographic location (Solomon and Weiss 2002). However, it is also likely that a variety of methodological factors affect the analytic variability and validity of the reported results. Breast milk lead levels from published studies with extremely high values should be reviewed with caution due to the high potential for environmental contamination during sample collection, storage, and analysis. Documented sources of breast milk contamination include the use of lead acetate ointment (Knowles 1974), lead in nipple shields (Knowles 1974; Newman 1997), foil from alcohol wipes used in sample collection (Hu et al. 1996), and latex laboratory gloves (Friel et al. 1996). Pretreatment of biological materials is also subject to unintentional addition of contaminants from chemical reagents, digestion devices, and atmospheric particles (Coni et al. 1990; Stacchini et al. 1989).

Inaccuracies of the laboratory analytic methods, particularly poor analytic sensitivity at low concentrations, also affect measurement of trace lead in human milk. Measurement of lead in breast milk is complicated by the fat content of human milk, which changes during feeding and over the course of lactation (Sim and McNeil 1992). Any partitioning of lead into the fat layer of milk must be accounted for in the analysis, which leads to the problem of either further contamination or loss during the intensive dry ashing procedure frequently used to prepare milk samples for analysis. Precise and accurate analysis is challenging due to difficulty in identifying a method that will digest samples with 100% efficiency (Ettinger et al. 2004a, 2004b). Gulson et al. (1998b) reviewed and compared the results of a number of studies of the relationship of breast milk lead to maternal blood lead published over the past 15 years, and concluded that the line of best fit through the data "that are considered to represent the realistic relationships between lead in maternal blood and breast milk" defines an array of slope of less than 3%. The implication is that those studies yielding ratios greater than 3% suffered from significant contamination.

Given the difficulty of accurately and precisely measuring trace lead in human breast milk, routine measurement of breast milk lead is not warranted for clinical application. It will only be practical in research settings or in certain extenuating circumstances, assuming that a qualified laboratory can be identified.

BIOKINETICS OF LEAD DURING PREGNANCY

Changes in Maternal Blood Lead Levels During Pregnancy

There are several case reports of elevated blood lead measurements in pregnancy (Mayer-Popken et al. 1986; Rothenberg et al. 1992; Ryu et al. 1978; Shannon 2003). Most cross-sectional studies investigating blood lead levels during pregnancy have shown a tendency for blood lead levels to decrease at least through the first half of pregnancy (Alexander and Delves 1981; Bonithon-Kopp et al. 1986; Gershanik et al. 1974). Baghurst (1987) found no difference in BLLs between different stages of pregnancy (weeks 14-20, weeks 30-36, and delivery). However, Farias et al. (1996) found BLLs were associated with gestational week of measurement, with levels declining after week 12.

Rothenberg et al. (1994), attempting to model kinetics over the course of pregnancy, showed a significant drop in blood lead levels from weeks 12 to 20. However, from 20 weeks to delivery, an analysis for linear trend confirmed a significant increase in blood lead levels in the later part of pregnancy. Schell et al. (2000) also reported changes in hematocrit-corrected blood lead levels over the course of pregnancy. Blood lead levels declined between the first and second trimesters and increased over the remaining course of pregnancy through delivery. Hertz-Picciotto et al. (2000) followed 195 women over the course of pregnancy and also found a U-shaped pattern of maternal blood lead concentration across pregnancy. The late pregnancy increases were steeper among women with low dietary calcium intake in both the younger and older age groups. Most recently, Lamadrid-Figueroa and colleagues (2006) found increased plasma lead levels for a given whole-blood lead value as pregnancy progresses for whole-blood lead levels greater than approximately 11.0 μg/dL, but not for those less than 10.0 μg/dL.

Transfer of Lead to the Fetus

That lead reaches human fetal tissues has been known for many years (Barltrop 1969; Kehoe et al. 1933; Thompsett and Anderson 1935). Barltrop (1969) collected serial fetal blood lead measurements from each trimester throughout pregnancy and found no recognizable pattern but was able to show that maternal blood lead concentration was highly correlated with umbilical cord lead, suggesting transplacental movement of lead to the fetus. In fact, lead readily crosses the placenta by passive diffusion (Goyer 1990; Silbergeld 1986) and lead has been measured in the fetal brain as early as the end of the first trimester (13 weeks) (Goyer 1990).

Bone Lead as an Endogenous Source of Exposure

Two early studies implicated bone lead as an endogenous source of exposure during pregnancy. Thompson et al. (1985) documented a case of increased maternal and infant blood lead in a woman with a history of childhood lead poisoning, but no exposure during pregnancy or for 30 years prior. Manton (1985) reported a rise in his wife's blood lead levels over the course of her pregnancy along with changes in the specific lead-isotopic ratios, indicating that contributions to her blood lead during pregnancy did not correspond to an external source.

Recent studies have documented that bone lead stores are mobilized during pregnancy and lactation (Gulson et al. 1997; Hernandez-Avila et al. 1996; Hu et al. 1996; Rothenberg et al. 2000). By examining the lead isotopic ratio in a small number of pregnant women who were recent immigrants to Australia (and pregnant Australian controls), Gulson and colleagues (1997) were able to show that the skeletal contribution to blood lead increased over pregnancy. Rothenberg et al. (2000) followed over 300 Hispanic-American women with serial blood lead levels over the course of pregnancy and found that whole blood lead concentrations were significantly influenced by bone lead. Markowitz and Shen (2001) reported a case of declining bone lead concentration in conjunction with an increase in blood lead levels over the course of pregnancy and the early postpartum period. Riess and Halm (2007) described a case report suggesting that bone sources at high levels can lead to an increase in BLL.

Animal studies support the human data. Using stable lead isotopes in monkeys, researchers found that a 29%-56% decrease in bone lead mobilization in the first trimester was followed by an increase in the second and third trimesters (Franklin et al. 1997). The increases were up to 44% over baseline levels. Further analysis of maternal bone and fetal bone and tissues revealed that from 7%-39% of lead in the fetal skeleton originated from maternal bone.

BIOKINETICS OF LEAD DURING LACTATION

Maternal bone turnover increases during lactation (Sowers et al. 2002), which has raised the concern that maternal blood lead concentrations might increase significantly during lactation. It has been estimated that up to 5% or more of bone mass is mobilized during lactation (Hayslip et al. 1989; Sowers 1996); therefore, the possibility exists for redistribution of cumulative lead stores from bone into plasma, thus returning lead to the maternal circulation.

Gulson et al. (1998a) found that mobilization of lead from bone continued after pregnancy into the postpartum period for up to 6 months during lactation and occurred at levels higher than during pregnancy. They concluded that the major sources of lead in breast milk were maternal bone and diet. Manton et al. (2003) observed sustained elevations of from 1 to 4 μg/dL in maternal blood lead concentration during the first 6 to 8 months of lactation, after the expected normal postpartum reduction in plasma volume, in 6 nursing mothers with prepregnancy blood lead concentrations of less than 2 μg/dL. These elevations were followed by gradual declines over the next year in the two women who continued to breastfeed to 18 months postpartum. Isotope ratio analysis suggested that the additional lead originated from maternal bone.

Osterloh and Kelly (1999) found no relationship between decreasing vertebral or femoral neck bone densites and the changes in maternal blood lead concentration at intervals over 6 months of lactation in 58 mainly poor Hispanic mothers with low mean blood lead concentrations of 2.35 μg/dL at enrollment in the study (32 to 38 weeks of gestation). However, at higher blood concentrations, Téllez-Rojo et al. (2002) observed an incremental increase of 1.4 μg/dL in blood lead concentration in women who were breastfeeding exclusively relative to women who had stopped lactation. These women had blood lead concentrations up to 23.4 μg/dL at delivery and were followed through 7 months postpartum. Bonithon-Kopp et al. (1986) found that women over 30 had significantly higher levels of breast milk lead than women between 20 and 30 years of age. Since bone accumulates lead with age, it is possible that the higher breast milk lead levels in the older women were associated with higher bone lead levels. Maternal bone lead levels have since been shown to be positively associated with breast milk lead concentrations (Ettinger et al. 2004a, 2006).

PREDICTORS OF UMBILICAL CORD BLOOD LEAD LEVELS

Umbilical cord blood lead has been widely used as a measure of fetal exposure (Rabinowitz et al. 1984; Rothenberg et al. 1996; Scanlon 1971). Numerous studies suggest that maternal blood lead and umbilical cord lead levels, measured concurrently at delivery, are highly correlated (Baghurst et al. 1991; Graziano et al. 1990;

Harville et al. 2005; Rothenberg et al. 1996), suggesting a near-perfect linear relationship. Most data indicate that umbilical cord lead is approximately 0.85 of maternal blood lead at parturition (Carbonne et al. 1998; Goyer 1990; Graziano et al. 1990). Thus, fetal-infant lead level, as measured in umbilical cord blood, is often lower than the maternal blood lead at delivery. However, some studies have shown umbilical cord lead to be higher than maternal blood lead levels at delivery and investigated the determinants for such differences (Harville et al. 2005; Rothenberg et al. 1996).

Rothenberg et al. (1996) studied Mexican women of low-to-middle socioeconomic status from 12 weeks of pregnancy to delivery to determine factors that explain the relationship between cord and maternal blood lead. They found from 245 paired maternal-cord blood lead samples that mothers with occasional alcohol use during pregnancy, high milk intake, and more spontaneous abortions delivered babies with lower cord blood lead and that maternal age, use of lead-glazed pottery, and canned foods was associated with increased cord blood lead. They found cord blood lead levels were higher than maternal blood lead levels at delivery in 33% of the cases, predominantly influenced by older maternal age and lower milk consumption. The authors suggested that the measurable influence of maternal blood lead on delivery cord blood lead is limited to the four to eight weeks prior to delivery. Also, many factors suspected of influencing bone lead also influenced cord blood lead, some of them independently of their effect on maternal delivery blood lead.

Harville et al. (2005) studied factors influencing the difference between maternal and cord blood lead levels to determine why some infants receive higher exposures relative to their mother's body burden than do others. They found that higher maternal blood pressure and alcohol consumption were associated with higher cord lead relative to the lead of the mother. Higher maternal hemoglobin and presence of the sickle cell trait were associated with lower cord blood lead in comparison to mother's blood lead, suggesting that iron status may be an important factor in the maternal-fetal transfer of lead across the placenta.

Chuang et al. (2001) modeled the interrelations of lead levels in bone, venous blood, and umbilical cord blood with exogenous lead exposure through maternal plasma lead in peripartum women. An interquartile range increase in either patella (trabecular) or tibia (cortical) bone lead was associated with an increase in cord blood lead by about 1 $\mu g/dL$. An increase of 0.1 $\mu g/m3$ in air lead was associated with an increase in the mean level of fetal cord blood lead by 0.67 $\mu g/dL$. With 1 additional day of lead-glazed ceramic use per week in the peripartum period, the mean cord blood lead level increased by 0.27 $\mu g/dL$. The models suggested that the contributions from endogenous (bone) and exogenous (environmental) sources were relatively equal, and that maternal plasma lead varies independently from maternal whole blood lead.

Figure 3-1. Major Lead Exposure Pathways from Mother to Infant

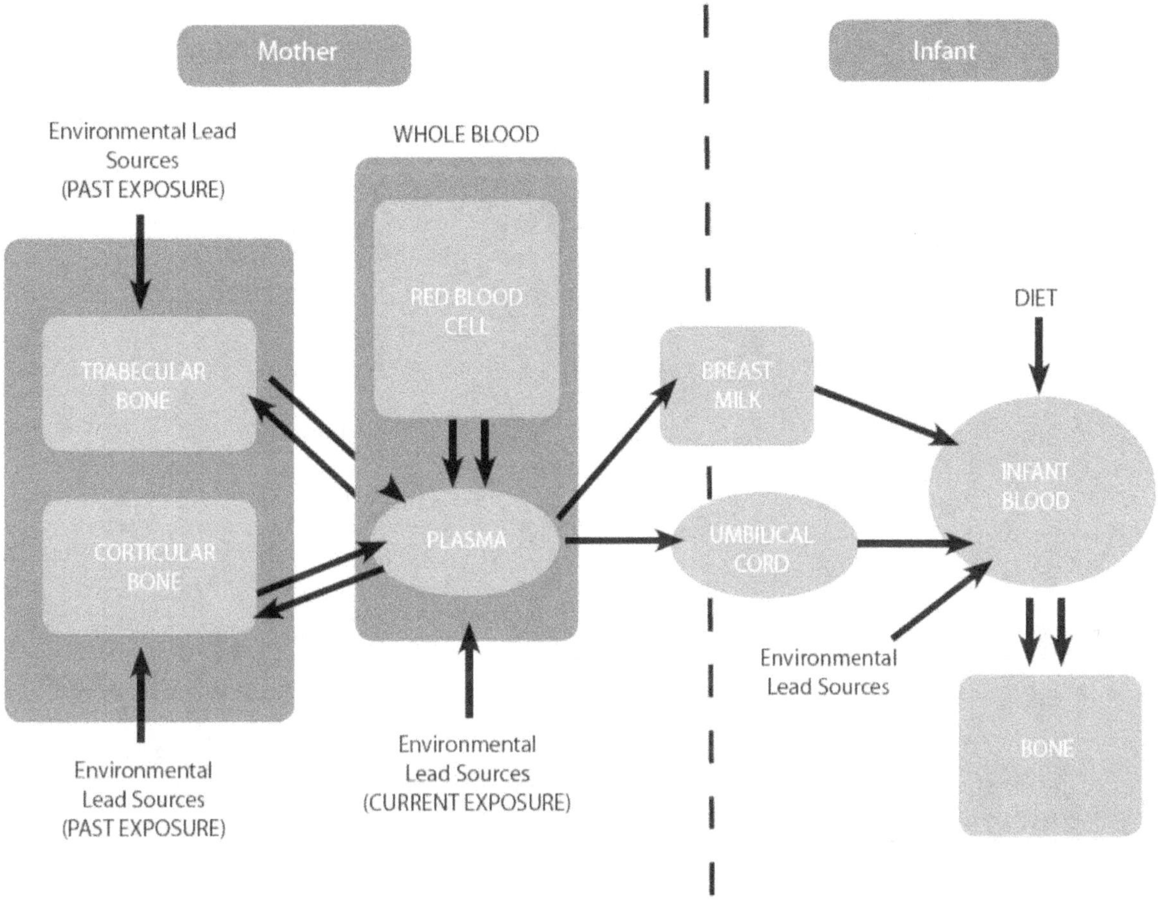

KEY POINTS

- Risk factors for lead exposure in pregnant women differ from those described for young children.

- Common risk factors for pregnant women include recent immigration status, practicing pica, occupational exposure, use of alternative remedies or cosmetics, use of traditional lead glazed pottery, and nutritional status.

- Pica during pregnancy appears to occur more frequently in sections of the South and in immigrant communities where this behavior is a culturally acceptable practice.

- Lead-based paint is less likely to be an important exposure source for pregnant women than it is for children, except during renovation or remodeling of homes built before 1978.

- Sources of lead exposure in the United States vary by population subgroup and geography; therefore, public health agencies should be consulted for community-specific risk data.

- Fetal exposure to lead through maternal bone lead mobilization is possible for women with significant prior lead exposure; however, most women with blood lead levels typical in the United States are unlikely to contribute substantial burdens to their infants.

INTRODUCTION

This chapter discusses the distribution of blood lead levels in women of childbearing age, risk factors relevant to this population, and sources of lead exposure. Information on the distribution of blood lead levels in pregnant women in the United States is derived from cross-sectional surveys, case reports, and epidemiological studies. From the direct, albeit limited, information on the distribution of blood lead levels in pregnant women, along with the available complementary information on blood lead levels in women of childbearing age and in occupational settings, it is evident that the risk factors for lead exposure in pregnant women differ from those described in young children. Health care providers and public health departments need to understand the risk factors specific to pregnant women in order to identify sources of lead in pregnant women, provide patient education and counseling, and intervene to prevent or reduce exposures.

For pregnant women, recent immigration and practicing pica are major risk factors for blood lead levels ≥5 µg/dL. Occupational lead exposure and nutritional status are also important risk factors warranting assessment. Certain culturally specific practices, such as the use of alternative remedies or imported cosmetics and the use of traditional lead glazed pottery for cooking and storing food, are important risk factors for lead exposure in pregnant women (Centers for Disease Control and Prevention 2004; Saper et al. 2004, 2008). Some population groups, such as immigrants, are more likely to be at risk for exposure from these sources. Shannon (2003) identified seven severely lead poisoned women who were exposed to sources of lead including ingestion of soil, pottery, or paint chips; household renovations; and use of herbal remedies. Lead-based paint is less likely to be an important exposure source for pregnant women than it is for children, except during renovation or remodeling in homes built before 1978.

Additionally, recent evidence has shown that bone resorption increases during pregnancy in all women (see Chapter 3). Although not an issue for most women with blood lead levels typical in the United States, fetal exposure to lead through maternal bone lead mobilization may be a concern for women with significant lead exposure earlier in life, either in the United States or in their countries of origin.

EPIDEMIOLOGY OF BLOOD LEAD LEVELS IN U.S. WOMEN

Distribution of Blood Lead Levels Among U.S. Women of Childbearing Age

Lee et al. (2005) studied determinants of blood lead in U.S. women of childbearing age using data from NHANES III (1988-1994). The geometric mean blood lead level among women aged 20-49 years (N = 4,393) was 1.78 µg/dL (range 0.7-31.1). Approximately 30%, 6%, and <1% of the women had blood lead levels ≥2.5 µg/dL, ≥5 µg/dL, and ≥10 µg/dL, respectively. A number of factors were associated with higher blood lead levels including higher maternal age, Black or Hispanic race/ethnicity, living in the Northeast region or in urban areas, lower educational level, poverty, lower hematocrit, alcohol use, cigarette smoking, and higher serum protoporphyrin level. Number of live births, breastfeeding history, year house was built, and type of drinking water were not significantly associated with differences in blood lead. Subjects in the first phase of the survey (1988-1991) had significantly higher weighted mean blood lead levels (2.0 µg/dL) than those in the second phase 1991-1994 (1.6 µg/dL), suggesting a decreasing trend in population average blood lead levels over time (p<0.01).

NHANES data from 1999-2002 showed an even lower geometric mean blood lead level of 1.2 µg/dL among women age 20-59 (Centers for Disease Control and Prevention 2005). Mean blood lead levels were significantly higher in Blacks (1.4 µg/dL) and intermediate in Mexican Americans (1.3 µg/dL). The percentage of women 15-49 years old with blood lead levels ≥10 µg/dL is 0.3% and ≥5 µg/dL is 0.9% (Centers for Disease Control and Prevention 2008, unpublished data).

McKelvey et al. (2007) studied blood lead among New York City adults using data from the 2004 New York City Health and Nutrition Examination Survey (NYC HANES). Further analyses performed by the authors (unpublished) specific to women 20-49 years of age (N = 755) found that the geometric mean blood lead level was 1.30 µg/dL (range 0.33-27.3). Approximately 10.5%, 1.4%, and 0.2% of the women had blood lead levels ≥2.5 µg/dL, ≥5 µg/dL, and ≥10 µg/dL, respectively. Blood lead was positively associated with: age; non-Hispanic Black, White, or Asian race/ethnicity, compared to Hispanic; foreign birth; and former and current smoking. Blood lead was inversely proportional to educational level. After multivariable adjustment, Asian race/ethnicity was the strongest predictor of blood lead level. In a separate study focused solely on immigrant mothers who gave birth in New York City in 2003, Graber et al. (2006) found that mean blood lead levels decreased with age by 0.032 µg/dL per year (see Case Study 4-1).

Reported Occupational Exposures Among U.S. Women of Childbearing Age

CDC's state-based Adult Blood Lead Epidemiology and Surveillance (ABLES) program tracks laboratory-reported BLLs in adults (age 16 years and older) from 37 states who have been tested through workplace monitoring programs or on the basis of clinical suspicion of lead exposure above background levels. The lowest reportable BLL varies by state and some states only report elevated results, not all test results. In the 10 states that reported BLLs of any level in 2004, information was reported on 10,527 women of childbearing age (16-44 years). Among these women, 13% (1,370) had BLLs ≥5 µg/dL; 4.5% (476) had BLLs ≥10 µg/dL, and fewer than 1% (86) had BLLs ≥25 µg/dL. Of the women with BLLs ≥5 µg/dL, 32.3% reported occupational exposures; of those employed, the majority were in the manufacturing sector. Because testing practices vary by employer and clinician, reporting practices vary by state, and all lead exposed women may not be tested, these data should not be used to estimate population-based rates of specific blood lead levels in the general population of women (Centers for Disease Control and Prevention 2007).

RISK FACTORS FOR LEAD EXPOSURE IN U.S. WOMEN OF CHILDBEARING AGE

Recent immigration to the United States and pica behavior are risk factors that have been shown to be associated with lead exposure above background levels in pregnant women, although they are actually behaviors that serve as proxies for other sources of lead. Women with a friend or relative identified with lead exposure above background levels are also more likely to have increased blood lead levels (Handley et al. 2007). In addition, the unique physiology of pregnancy and lactation has been shown to result in increased bone turnover and, thus, higher maternal BLLs. Nutrition may play a role in the extent to which lead is absorbed and the extent of bone turnover. An understanding of these factors is useful in assessing the sources of lead exposures in pregnant women and in developing interventions to prevent and/or interrupt lead exposure. Figure 4-1 presents common risk factors for lead exposure by pregnant women in the United States.

Recent Immigration to the United States

A number of studies have identified immigrant status as a primary risk factor for lead poisoning in women and young children in the United States (Klitzman et al. 2002; Tehranifar et al. 2008). Immigrant status is a risk factor for blood lead levels much higher than concurrent blood lead levels in U.S. women of childbearing age in at least three ways. First, women from countries where relatively high lead exposure is endemic may carry high cumulative body burdens of lead. (Appendices III and V provide information about lead sources and culturally specific products associated with specific countries or regions.) Brown et al. (2000) investigated determinants of bone and blood lead concentrations in women in Mexico City during the early postpartum period and found that maternal age and time spent living in Mexico City, an area with high ambient lead contamination, were strong predictors of bone lead levels. Second, immigrants may transport lead-containing products, cultural practices, and behaviors with them from their countries of origin. Third, some recent immigrants may live in poor conditions that increase their risk for exposure to lead-based paint and other lead hazards from renovation and repair. In addition, since immigrant women may face cultural, linguistic, economic, and legal barriers to early prenatal care, these risk factors may be compounded by delays in identification and management of lead poisoning.

Data on 75 pregnant women identified with blood lead levels ≥15 µg/dL were provided in the Annual Report 2006 for Preventing Lead Poisoning in New York City. Of these 75 women, 99% were foreign born (68% were from Mexico) and 73% reported using imported products during pregnancy, including foods, spices, herbal medicines, pottery, and cosmetics. None of the women were exposed to lead at work.

Klitzman et al. (2002) reported on thirty-three pregnant women in New York City with blood lead levels of 20 µg/dL or higher identified from 1996-1999 by the New York City Department of Health and Mental Hygiene blood lead surveillance program. Ninety percent of individuals were foreign born, the majority being from Mexico (57%), with a median time in the United States of 6 years (range 1 month to 20 years). Two-thirds of the women had levels between 20 and 29 µg/dL and possible sources of exposure were identified in 97% of these cases. Overall, thirteen (39%) reported pica behavior; 7 (21%) reported using imported pottery for cooking; and 8 (24%) reported consuming imported spices, tea, and/or food. Other sources identified included vitamins and supplements, lead-based paint hazards, and previous history of exposure to lead.

Graber et al. (2006) conducted a retrospective record review of pregnant women seeking prenatal care from January 2003 to June 2005 at an inner-city women's health center serving a largely immigrant population in Elmhurst Hospital, Queens, New York City. Of the 4,814 women seeking care, 91% were foreign born and 9% were U.S. born. These data from an inner-city medical clinic suggest that prenatal lead exposure disproportionately occurs during the pregnancies of immigrant women from certain countries and occurs at a prevalence high enough to warrant universal blood lead testing (see Case Study 4-1).

Handley et al. (2007) studied 214 women in 2002-2003 who were enrolled in health department clinics in Monterey, California, for their prenatal care. The study population was 95% Latina and 87% were born in Mexico. Sixty-six of the women were born in Oaxaca, Mexico. The prevalence of blood lead levels ≥10 µg/dL in the study population was 12%, much higher than concurrent blood lead levels in the U.S. population in general. Women with blood lead levels ≥10 µg/dL were more likely to be born in Oaxaca (96%), more likely to eat foods imported from Mexico (84%), and more likely to report having a friend or relative with "lead in their blood" (28%). This study identified home-prepared grasshoppers (chapulines) sent from Oaxaca as a source of lead exposure.

Case Study 4-1. Prenatal Lead Exposure in New York City Immigrant Communities: The Elmhurst Queens Experience

Of the 124,345 babies born in New York City in 2003, 52% were to mothers who were born outside of the United States (New York Vital Statistics). Since many of the sources of lead for pregnant women are related to cultural practices, past exposures, and certain occupations, the prevalence of elevated blood lead levels among pregnant women in New York City is likely to be higher than U.S. averages. A retrospective record review of pregnant women seeking prenatal care at an inner-city women's health center was conducted in order to describe the epidemiology of blood lead levels among pregnant women in an inner-city, primarily immigrant population. Computerized registration and laboratory data for pregnant women seeking prenatal care from January 2003 to June 2005 at the Women's Health Center at Elmhurst Hospital, Queens, New York, were reviewed.

Distribution of Age and Blood Lead Levels (BLLs) for U.S.- and Foreign-Born Pregnant Women in Elmhurst, Queens, NY (January 2003-June 2005)

	U.S. Born	Foreign Born	All Women
N (%)	446 (9.3)	4,368 (90.7)	4,814
Age (years)	23.7	28.3	27.8
Age Range	14-43	13-52	13-52
Mean BLL (µg/dL)	1.2	2.4	2.3
BLL Range	0-17	0–31	0-31
% with BLL ≥10 µg/dL	0.2	1.2	1.1
% with BLL ≥5 µg/dL	1.6	11.5	10.6

Note: All difference between the two groups were statistically significant (p<0.001)

One hundred countries of origin were represented in the sample. Pregnant women who were born outside of the United States were 8.2 times (95% CI = 3.8 to 17.3) more likely to have a BLL ≥5 µg/dL. Those women with the highest mean BLLs and percent with BLLs ≥5 µg/dL were from Bangladesh (4.39 µg/dL, 36.6%), Mexico (3.23 µg/dL, 20.9%) and Pakistan (2.86 µg/dL, 17.6%).

Women from countries where leaded gasoline is still in use had higher mean BLLs (3.42 µg/dL) and percent of women with BLLs ≥5 µg/dL (24.6%) in comparison to women from countries where leaded gasoline is no longer in use (1.42 µg/dL, 1.9%). Mean BLL decreased with age by 0.032 µg/dL per year (p< 0.001). Mean BLL increased by 0.14 µg/dL (p<0.05) from 2003 to 2005 as did the percent of women with BLLs ≥10 µg/dL. BLLs did not vary by time of year.

From Graber N, Gabinskaya T, Forman J, Gertner M. 2006. Prenatal lead exposure in New York City Immigrant communities [poster]. In: Pediatric Academic Societies (PAS) 2006 Annual Meeting, April 29-May 3, 2006, San Francisco.

Pica

Although formal pica definitions vary, the behavior common to all definitions of pica is a pattern of deliberate ingestion of nonfood items. Some definitions focus solely on the eating behavior (e.g., Medline defines pica as "a pattern of eating non-food materials (such as dirt or paper)" (Medline Plus 2009). Western medicine has viewed pica as aberrant and unhealthy behavior, an eating disorder, or a psychiatric diagnosis. For example, the American Psychiatric Association defines pica as the "compulsive eating or appetite for nonnutritive substances, either non-food items (e.g., clay, soil) or some food ingredients (e.g., starch, ice), which persists for more than one month" (American Psychiatric Association 1994). However, respected non-Western community institutions have historically accepted pica as a way to improve health. Pica has been practiced by people worldwide for medicinal, religious, and cultural reasons since antiquity (Abrahams and Parsons 1996; Hunter and de Kleine 1984). The Greeks and Romans used clay to treat various medical conditions. Certain Catholic sects in Central America have sold clay tablets inscribed with Christian scenes for centuries. These clay tablets, known as tierra santa, which are blessed before sale and believed to have health-giving properties, are available throughout Mexico and Central America. Clay tablets are also produced and sold throughout many parts of Africa and are eaten—generally not for religious or health-related purposes, but for their taste and texture.

While pica appears to be relatively rare in the United States, it is a common practice in many parts of the world, particularly in Africa, Asia, and Central America. Prevalence rates have been reported to be as high as 50% to 74% in parts of Africa (Nchito et al. 2004; Sule and Madugu 2001), and 23% to 44% in Latin America (Lopez et al. 2004). In the United States, pica appears to occur more frequently in sections of the South and in immigrant communities where this behavior is a culturally acceptable practice. Prevalence studies of pica in U.S. subpopulations have found 34% in Mexican-born women living in California (Simpson et al. 2000), and 14% (Smulian et al. 1995) to 38% (Corbett et al. 2003) in low-income rural African-American women.

In some studies, women felt that not giving in to pica cravings could harm their fetus and lead to miscarriage, illness, or an unhappy baby (Simpson et al. 2000). Since pica is viewed negatively by the Western medical community (American Psychiatric Association 1994), individuals who engage in pica may be reluctant to disclose that they consume nonfood items if asked directly about the practice. A review of 13 studies published between 1950 and 1987 (Horner et al. 1991) estimated that the risk for pica increases if pica is practiced by other family members and is increased six-fold if the woman had a prepregnancy history of pica. Other factors that may influence whether women are comfortable disclosing pica use include being able to converse in their native language, being able to discuss the practice in private, and being questioned about the practice in an accepting manner by someone from their own community (Simpson et al. 2000).

Materials ingested as pica can be benign or potentially harmful and include ice, paper, dirt, clay, starch, ashes, and small stones as well as substances contaminated with lead or other toxic substances. Pica behavior has been associated with anemia and other nutritional deficiencies in cross-sectional studies, although pica has not been confirmed to be caused by nutritional deficiencies; pica has been associated rarely with more serious side effects, such as gastrointestinal blockages (Edwards et al. 1994; Geissler et al. 1998). Cases of lead poisoning have also been reported if the substances consumed are contaminated with lead. Most commonly these substances have been reported to be lead-contaminated soil and pottery [see Appendix III for a description of commonly ingested substances with pica].

In a case study of one Hispanic pregnant woman in California, Hamilton et al. (2001) found blood lead levels of 119.4 μg/dL in the woman and 113.6 μg/dL in the cord blood at delivery. The woman practiced a form of pica in which she broke a lead-glazed clay pot from Mexico into small pieces and ate several pieces daily. The researchers found that this practice was apparently not uncommon in Mexican women. Shannon (2003) reviewed seven cases of severely lead-poisoned women (BLLs ≥45 μg/dL) over a 3-year period and identified an additional eight cases from the medical literature. He found that severe lead poisoning in these mainly Hispanic women occurred most often because of ingestion of lead-contaminated clay, soil, and pottery. Presenting features were mostly subtle, consisting of only malaise and anemia.

Mobilization of Endogenous Bone Lead in Pregnancy

Although, the majority of U.S. women of childbearing age are unlikely to have bone lead stores large enough to result in large elevations in maternal blood lead concentrations, at least one recent case report suggested that bone sources at high levels can lead to an increase in BLL (Riess and Halm 2007). There also is evidence that with closely spaced multiple pregnancies, maternal blood lead levels in subsequent pregnancies are lower and the increases in maternal blood lead occurring during late pregnancy and lactation are lower relative to those in the first pregnancy (Manton et al. 2003; Rothenberg et al. 1994). This observation is consonant with observations from the lead industry in the nineteenth and early twentieth century (Legge 1901; Legge and Goadby 1912; Paul 1860), which held that if a lead-poisoned woman had a child, her symptoms would be assuaged. This limited evidence suggests that the greatest concern about lead exposure may be during the first pregnancy, although this observation is probably meaningful only at very high lead levels.

Dietary and Lifestyle Factors

Nutritional status may make women more susceptible to lead exposures. Adequate dietary intake of certain key nutrients (calcium; iron; zinc; vitamins C, D, and E) is known to decrease lead absorption (Mahaffey 1990). Iron deficiency anemia is associated with elevated blood lead levels and may increase lead absorption and also has an additional independent negative impact on fetal development. Calcium deficiency may increase bone turnover since maternal bone is a major source of calcium for the developing fetus and nursing infant. Chapter 7 provides a fuller discussion of nutritional issues. Both alcohol use and cigarette smoking have also been associated with higher lead levels and should be avoided during pregnancy and lactation.

SOURCES OF LEAD EXPOSURE

While various sources of lead exposure in pregnant women in the United States have been identified, these sources vary according to population subgroup and geography. Thus, assessment and reduction of sources must be specific to the community. The sources discussed below are those that have been identified in previous research and should be used as a guide for clinical and public health interventions. Figure 4-2 summarizes general advice for pregnant women to avoid lead exposure, although additional advice may be warranted due to specific local risk factors.

Occupational Sources

Lead is used in more than 100 industries [see Appendix IV for a list of major lead-using industries]. Occupations in which workers may be directly exposed to lead at significant levels include construction; smelting; auto repair; work on firing ranges; painting; manufacturing of ceramics, electrical components, batteries, wire and cable, plastics, pottery, and stained glass; battery and scrap metal recycling; mining; and all types of ferrous and nonferrous metals production. In addition, women and children may be exposed to lead through the inadvertent carriage of lead dust from the workplace on workers' clothing, shoes, or bodies, also known as take-home exposure. Lead dust carried from work settles on surfaces in the vehicle and home, where it can be ingested or inhaled by young children with normal mouthing behavior and by household members handling workers' clothing (Hipkins et al. 2004). The National Institute for Occupational Safety and Health documented cases of take-home lead exposure in a 1995 Report to Congress in response to the Workers' Family Protection Act (National Institute for Occupational Safety and Health 1995).

While BLLs in occupationally exposed individuals have fallen dramatically since lead industry standards were revised in 1978 (Anderson and Islam 2006), occupational exposures are still a source of lead exposure in women (Centers for Disease Control and Prevention 2007). According to reports from the ABLES Program, a total of 442 (32.3%) of the 1,370 females with BLLs >5 µg/dL had occupational exposures (Centers for Disease Control and Prevention 2007). ABLES data from the New York State Department of Health indicate that 46% (62 of 135) of women of childbearing age with moderate BLLs (10-25 µg/dL) reported occupational exposure as the primary source of lead exposure (Fletcher et al. 1999). Automobile battery manufacturing and lead battery recovery industries pose the highest risks although workers in the construction trades can also have significant exposures to lead (Centers for Disease Control and Prevention 2007; Fletcher et al. 1999). Laborers and painters have been found to have higher BLLs than other construction trade groups such as plumbers and electricians (Reynold et al. 1999). Construction work that is associated with higher BLLs includes bridge renovation; residential remodeling; and activities such as welding, cutting, and rivet busting (Reynold et al. 1999).

The Occupational Safety and Health Administration (OSHA) has lead standards for general industry (29 CFR 1910.1025) (Occupational Safety and Health Administration 1984) and construction (29 CFR 1926.62) (Occupational Safety and Health Administration 1993). Currently, under the OSHA standards, a worker must be included in a lead medical surveillance program if he/she is exposed to airborne lead levels of 30 µg/m3 or higher (8-hour time-weighted average) for more than 30 days per year. Partly to diminish the risk that a lead worker takes lead home on his clothing or body (take-home exposure), the lead standards contain provisions requiring access to showers, work clothes, and changing rooms at the workplace. Some workers potentially exposed to high levels of lead may not receive adequate medical surveillance because their work does not result in air lead levels that trigger the required surveillance. Additionally, certain occupations are exempt from the workplace protections established by OSHA. Exempted workers include some public employees and the self-employed. Self employed workers might include those in cottage industries such as battery reclamation, automobile/radiator repair, pottery and ceramics, and stained glass. These job categories may not be monitored for lead exposures. In some cases, the home itself may function as a cottage industry workplace, increasing the potential for lead exposure to all family members. Undocumented immigrant workers are a particularly vulnerable group in that their access to lead exposure monitoring and protective measures may be limited.

Occupational exposure to lead also remains a problem in developing countries where industries are less likely to be regulated and little environmental monitoring is done. Studies have documented the impact of cottage industries on lead exposure in international settings, including: backyard battery repair and recycling of batteries (Matte et al. 1989) and radiators (Dykeman et al. 2002) and the production of low-temperature fired lead-glazed ceramics (Fernandez et al. 1997; Hibbert et al. 1999) and tiles (Vahter et al. 1997).

Lead-glazed Ceramic Pottery

Of all the culturally specific practices and products that may put pregnant women at risk for lead exposure, the use of traditional lead-glazed ceramic pottery for cooking and storing food is perhaps the most well-documented in the literature (Hernandez-Avila et al. 1991, 1996; Romieu et al. 1994). Lead-glazed ceramics production is a mostly home-based or cottage industry in Mexico where lead monoxide (greta; 93% lead by weight) is used to make a glaze that is often set in low-temperature (<1,000 degrees), wood-fired kilns. Pottery produced in this manner can leach large amounts of lead into food and beverages being cooked, served, or stored. This traditional pottery is used throughout the country across all levels of socioeconomic status. Acute high-dose exposures from foods and beverage contaminated by traditional Mexican pottery have been reported (Matte et al. 1994) and long-term use of lead-glazed ceramics may result in chronic low-to-moderate lead poisoning and elevated body burden of lead (Hernandez-Avila et al. 1991). Cases of lead poisoning have been reported after the consumption of crushed lead-glazed pottery, mainly among Hispanic women (Shannon 2003).

Herbal and Alternative Remedies

Lead has been found in some alternative medicines and therapeutic herbs traditionally used by East Indian, Indian, Middle Eastern, West Asian, and Hispanic cultures (Garvey et al. 2001; Saper et al. 2004, 2008). These alternative medicines can contain herbs, minerals, metals, or animal products. Lead and other heavy metals are put into certain folk medicines intentionally because these metals are thought to be useful in treating some ailments. They have also been reported to be added to increase the weight of the product for substances sold by weight. Sometimes lead unintentionally gets into the folk medicine during grinding, coloring, or other methods of preparation. Lead has been found in powders and tablets given for arthritis, infertility, upset stomach, menstrual cramps, colic, and other illnesses. Case Study 4-2 describes lead poisoning associated with ayurvedic medicines.

Most of the published literature relating herbal therapies and alternative medicines to elevated BLLs has been in case reports of children or adults (Ernst 2002; Lynch and Braithwaite 2005), not specifically in women of childbearing age or pregnant or lactating women. Many of the alternative therapies used were self-administered, rather than recommended by a traditional healer or health care provider. In a case study of one 45-year old Korean man who drank Chinese herbal tea for medicinal purposes, Markowitz et al. (1994) found a blood lead level of 76 µg/dL. The lead exposure was found to be hai ge fen (clamshell powder), one of 36 ingredients in the tea, which had become contaminated with lead. In another report, Cheng et al. (1998) described that six of eight children found to be taking herbal medicines had BLLs >10 µg/dL. Use of greta was described in a 2-year-old boy identified with a blood lead level of 83 µg/dL in a CDC report (1993). A review of 1991-1992 California data yielded 40 cases with BLLs >20 µg/dL where children had received ethnic remedies. Over 80% of these children had Hispanic surnames (Centers for Disease Control and Prevention 1993). Tait et al. (2002) reported on a 24 year-old woman from India who immigrated to Australia and delivered a child there with a neonatal BLL that was the highest recorded for a surviving infant in the country (cord BLL was 158.3 µg/dL). An exposure assessment revealed the mother's long-term ingestion of lead-contaminated herbal tablets as the source.

Use of herbal and alternative remedies is not confined to immigrant communities and reported use is substantial among the general population, as documented in several studies. Eisenberg found in a 1990 national U.S. survey that 34% of English-speaking adults >18 years of age reported use of at least one unconventional therapy (Eisenberg et al. 1993). Only 10% reported receiving these alternative therapies from a traditional healer or health care provider and 72% did not tell their medical doctor that they used unconventional therapy. Highest use was in non-Black individuals between the ages of 25 to 49 with relatively higher education and income. A follow-up survey conducted in 1997 found that use had increased to 42% (Eisenberg et al. 1998). More than 60% did not tell their medical doctors that they used alternative therapies. A 2001 New York City study found that 47% of women used medicinal therapies (Factor-Litvak et al. 2001). In a questionnaire survey of herbal medicine use among 734 women who had recently or were about to give birth in Massachusetts, Hepner et al. (2002) found that 7.1% reported the use of herbal remedies mostly on the advice of their health care provider. Although the rates of reported use of herbal and alternative remedies vary, symptomatic cases of lead poisoning have been reported from these sources.

Case Study 4-2. Lead Poisoning Associated with Ayurvedic Medications, California (2003)

Lead poisoning can occur from use of alternative or folk remedies. Ayurveda is a traditional form of medicine practiced in India and other South Asian countries. Ayurvedic medications can contain herbs, minerals, metals, or animal products and are made in standardized and nonstandardized formulations.

A woman aged 31 years visited an emergency department with nausea, vomiting, and lower abdominal pain 2 weeks after a spontaneous abortion. One week later, she was hospitalized for severe, persistent microcytic anemia with prominent basophilic stippling that was not improving with iron supplementation. A heavy metals screen revealed a BLL of 112 µg/dL; a repeat BLL 10 days later was 71 µg/dL, before initiation of oral chelation therapy. A zinc protoporphyrin measurement performed at that time was >400 µg/dL. Her husband's BLL was 6 µg/dL. No residential or occupational lead sources were identified, but the woman reported taking nine different ayurvedic medications prescribed by a practitioner in India for fertility during a 2-month period, including one pill four times daily. She discontinued the medications after an abnormal fetal ultrasound 1 month before her initial BLL. Analysis of her medications revealed 73,900 ppm lead in the pill taken four times daily and 21, 65, and 285 ppm lead in three other remedies. Her BLL was 22 µg/dL when she was tested 9.5 months after the initial BLL testing.

From Centers for Disease Control and Prevention. 2004. Lead poisoning associated with ayurvedic medications—five states, 2000-2003. MMWR Morb Mortal Wkly Rep 53;582-4.

Imported Cosmetics

Kohl, also known as 'al kohl' or 'surma', is a gray or black eye cosmetic applied to the conjunctival margins of the eyes that can contain up to 83% lead. It is used in the Middle East, India, Pakistan, and some parts of Africa for medicinal and cosmetic reasons (Parry and Eaton 1991). It is believed to strengthen and protect the eyes against disease. These cosmetics have been associated with elevated lead levels in children (Mojdehi and Gurtner 1996; Sprinkle 1995) and may also be used by women of childbearing age (Moghraby et al. 1989), especially those who are recent immigrants to the United States. [See Appendix V For a detailed list of alternative medicines, herbs, and cosmetics that may contain lead.]

Foods and Other Consumer Products

Lead can enter the food chain from contaminated soil or water, deposition from the air, or contact with food containers and processing. In the United States, dietary intakes of lead have been reduced due to: the removal of lead from gasoline; the elimination of lead-soldered cans and lead-based printing ink on candy wrappers and bread bags; and changes to agricultural practices, such as banning of lead-arsenate pesticides (Bolger et al. 1991, 1996). The U.S. Food and Drug Administration (FDA) maximum total tolerable daily intake (TTDI) of lead is 6 µg/day for children under 6 years of age, 25 µg/day for pregnant women, and 75 µg/day for other adults (Bolger et al. 1996; Carrington et al. 1996; U.S. Food and Drug Administration 1993). These values were established when dietary intake levels were higher than current estimates. Several scientists have suggested that this standard be revised and made more rigorous, which would lower the TTDI for children to 1 µg/day (Carrington et al. 1996; Ross, et al. 2000). Nonetheless, results from the Total Diet Study (sometimes called the market basket study)—an ongoing assessment by FDA that determines levels of various contaminants and nutrients in foods—indicate that current levels of lead in the U.S. food supply are quite low (available at http://www.cfsan.fda.gov/~comm/tds-toc.html). The estimated daily dietary intake in the United States is currently estimated to be in the range of 2 to 10 µg.

On occasion, imported foods and food products brought to the United States have been identified with elevated levels of lead. For instance, Lozeena is an orange powder used to color rice and meat that contains 7.8%-8.9% lead (U.S. Centers for Disease Control and Prevention 1998). FDA has issued warnings about tamarind candy lollipops (labeled Dulmex brand "Bolirindo") imported from Mexico due to high levels of lead that may be associated with the product, especially in the wrapper (U.S. Food and Drug Administration 1993, 2001). Analysis of these wrappers, which children may chew on or lick, showed between 21,000 to 22,000 parts per million (ppm) of lead while the lollipop sticks contained more than 400 ppm of lead, and the candy itself contained approximately 0.2 ppm of lead. Recently, the FDA revised the recommended maximum lead level for lead in candy to 0.1 ppm (U.S. Food and Drug Administration 2006). Traditional food products that are contaminated with lead may be brought into the U.S. through unregulated routes (Handley et al. 2007). Chapulines (grasshoppers) from Mexico, for example, have been found to contain high levels of lead and have been the subject of a health alert by the California Department of Health Services (California Department of Health Services 2003). "Natural" calcium supplements derived from animal bone may contain lead (Ross et al. 2000; Scelfo and Flegal 2000). Waterfowl may ingest lead shot, become contaminated, and possibly be consumed by unsuspecting hunters and their families (Levesque et al. 2003). In addition, regular ingestion of game meat harvested with lead ammunition may be be a source of lead exposure (Kosnett 2009).

Lead in Drinking Water

Control measures taken during the last two decades, including actions taken under the requirements of the 1986 and 1996 amendments to the Safe Drinking Water Act and the Environmental Protection Agency's (EPA) Lead and Copper Rule (U.S. Environmental Protection Agency 1991, 1997a), have greatly reduced exposures to lead in tap water. Even so, lead still can be found in some metal water taps, interior water pipes, or pipes connecting a house to the main water pipe in the street (Centers for Disease Control and Prevention 2004b). Lead found in tap water usually comes from the corrosion of older fixtures or from the solder that connects pipes. When water sits in leaded pipes for several hours, lead can leach into the water supply. Most studies show that consumption of lead-contaminated water alone would not be likely to elevate blood lead levels in most adults to a level that is toxicologically significant, even exposure to water with a lead content close to the EPA action level for lead of 15 parts per billion (ppb) (U.S. Environmental Protection Agency 1991). Risk will vary, however, depending upon the individual, the circumstances, and the amount of water consumed. For example, infants who drink formula prepared with lead-contaminated water may be at higher risk because of the large volume of water they consume relative to their body size and the higher percentage of lead they absorb (Baum and Shannon 1997). [See related discussion on lead in reconstituted infant formula, Chapter 9.] Officials in communities that are considering changes in water additives or that have implemented such changes in water disinfection should assess whether these changes might result in increased lead in residential tap water (Centers for Disease Control and Prevention 2004b; Miranda 2007). EPA has asked all state health and environmental officials to monitor lead in drinking water at schools and day care centers.

Lead Paint: Home Repair, Renovation, and Remodeling Activities

Lead-based paint was commonly used in homes built before 1950, and was not banned from sale for residential use in the United States until 1978. Recent studies estimate that more than 38 million U.S. homes still contain some lead-based paint, with two-thirds of the houses built before 1960 containing lead-based paint hazards (Jacobs et al. 2002). Lead-based paint hazards were concentrated in homes with incomes less than $30,000 (35% vs. 19% in homes with incomes >$30,000) and in the Northeast and Midwest where the prevalence was twice as high as in the South and West.

Lead in paint and house dust are the most common sources of exposure in U.S. children (Lanphear et al. 1998). Among adults, however, exposure to lead-based paint and construction-related lead hazards occurs mainly during home repair, renovation, and remodeling activities conducted by the residents themselves or due to improper work practices of tradesmen and contractors (Centers for Disease Control and Prevention 2009;

Feldman 1978; Fischbein et al. 1981; Jacobs 1998; Jacobs et al. 2003; Marino et al. 1990; Reisman et al. 2002; U.S. Department of Housing and Urban Development 1995).

Two basic circumstances increase the risk for an adult's exposure to lead-based paint: if paint has deteriorated, and when paint has been disturbed during remodeling or renovation. Paint deterioration can be caused by moisture problems, poor maintenance, or other problems. The paint on moveable building components (friction and impact surfaces such as windows and doors) pose higher risks because routine opening/closing can damage the paint on their surfaces over time and lead-based paint was used on these components historically. Property owners should take precautions when repainting surfaces with deteriorated paint or performing any remodeling or renovation work that disturbs painted surfaces (such as scraping off paint or tearing out walls) (U.S. Environmental Protection Agency 1997b).

The U.S. government defines lead-based paint hazards as not only encompassing lead-based paint, but also dangerous levels of lead in settled dust and bare soil. Testing for lead-based paint hazards can be done either by obtaining dust wipe samples from the floor and window sills or by using a portable x-ray fluorescence analyzer (XRF) to document the presence of lead in paint. EPA's 2001 hazard standard (40 CFR 745) set the benchmark for floor dust lead level at 40 µg/ft2 and 250 µg/ft2 for interior window sills.

Lead-contaminated Soil

Soil may contain lead from deteriorating, exterior lead-based paint or other sources such as deposition from years of leaded gasoline use or industrial emissions. Lead-contaminated soil can be tracked into the home and mixed with household dust, which may also contain lead from interior paint sources. In the United States, lead-contaminated soil is defined as a hazard if there is 400 ppm of lead in bare soil in children's play areas or an average of 1,200 ppm for bare soil in the rest of the yard (U.S. EPA 2001). Poisoning from lead-contaminated soil is most common among young children who play on the floor and commonly mouth objects, but has also been reported to occur in women who consume lead-contaminated soil. For example, cases of lead poisoning have been reported after the consumption of lead-contaminated soil (Case Study 4-3). Exposure to lead from food grown in lead contaminated soil in urban gardens has also been noted (Finster et al. 2004).

Case Study 4-3. A Case of Lead Poisoning from Soil Ingestion During Pregnancy

S.N. is a 33-year-old woman who was pregnant four times with three living children. She was born in Jamaica, West Indies, and immigrated to the United States during her most recent pregnancy. Her obstetric history included three prior uncomplicated full-term vaginal deliveries. She registered for prenatal care at 19 weeks' gestation with no significant historical problems. On questioning, she revealed a history of pica, eating soil from near her house. Her initial tests included a blood lead level of 26 µg/dL, free erythrocyte protoporphyrin 48 (normal < 35 µg/dL), Hgb 9.5 g/dL, and Ferritin 4.9 ng/dL. She was counseled to stop the pica behavior and referred for genetic and nutritional counseling and to a special lead clinic. Her repeat blood lead level at 23 weeks' gestation was 13 µg/dL. Environmental lead tests of the water were negative. Soil tests were negative, except for areas around the garage door of her house. The patient had no knowledge of lead levels or lead testing during her other pregnancies in Jamaica. She was admitted for induction of labor at 38 weeks' gestation due to preeclampsia. She had a normal spontaneous vaginal delivery of a girl, 3,395 grams. Apgar scores were 9 at 1 minute and 9 at 5 minutes. She was discharged on day 3 and followed postpartum as her blood pressure gradually decreased to normal levels. Her postpartum blood lead level was 13 µg/dL and free erythrocyte protoporphyrin 60. S.N. decided to breastfeed and bottle-feed. At 6 weeks, the baby was noted to have a blood lead level of 20 µg/dL.

From: Hackley B, Katz-Jacobson A. 2003. Lead poisoning in pregnancy: a case study with implications for midwives. J Midwifery Womens Health 48(1):30-8.

Point Sources of Lead

Point sources of lead exposure include active mining and smelting operations, lead contamination at former mining and smelting sites, and industrial emissions, such as those from battery-manufacturing and recycling activities, particularly in international settings where environmental regulations and monitoring programs may not be in place. Studies have documented the impact of lead mining and smelting activities, both in the United States and elsewhere (Baghurst et al. 1987; Benin et al. 1999; Graziano et al. 1990), and women who live near active or former lead mines and smelters may be exposed to high levels of lead contamination.

Leaded Gasoline

Recognition of the toxic effects of lead has prompted interventions that have resulted in reductions in lead exposure in many countries. In the United States, standards to phase out leaded gasoline use were first implemented in 1973 (U.S. Environmental Protection Agency 1973). In 1995, leaded fuel accounted for only 0.6 % of total gasoline sales in the United States and, in 1996, the Clean Air Act banned the sale of leaded fuel for use in on-road vehicles (U.S. Environmental Protection Agency 1996). A worldwide initiative to phase-out lead in gasoline has already stimulated important reductions in ambient air lead levels and population blood lead levels in some countries (Cortez-Lugo et al. 2003; Romieu et al. 1992). A complete phase-out of leaded gasoline was completed throughout the Latin American and Caribbean region by 2005 (Burke 2004; Walsh 2007). However, in some parts of Africa, Asia, and the Middle East, leaded gasoline is still common (Partnership for Clean Fuels and Vehicles 2007). The impact of leaded fuel is more important in urban settings, given their higher vehicular density.

Hobbies and Recreational Activities

Hobbies and recreational activities that may cause exposure to lead include, but are not limited to creating stained glass; enameling copper; casting bronze; making pottery with certain leaded glazes and paints; casting ammunition, fishing weights, or lead figurines; jewelry making and electronics (with lead solder); glassblowing with leaded glass; print-making; refinishing old furniture; distilling liquor; hunting; and target shooting.

Table 4-1. Risk Factors for Lead Exposure in Pregnant and Lactating Women

- **Recent immigration from or residency in areas where ambient lead contamination is high.** Women from countries where leaded gasoline is still being used (or was recently phased out) or where industrial emissions are not well controlled.

- **Living near a point source of lead**, such as lead mines, smelters, or battery recycling plants (even if the establishment is closed).

- **Working with lead or living with someone who does.** Women who work in or who have family members who work in lead-industry (take-home exposures).

- **Using lead-glazed ceramic pottery.** Women who cook, store, or serve food in lead-glazed ceramic pottery made in a traditional process and usually imported by individuals outside the normal commercial channels.

- **Eating nonfood substances (pica).** Women who eat or mouth nonfood items that may be contaminated with lead (such as soil or lead-glazed ceramic pottery).

- **Using alternative or complementary medicines, herbs, or therapies.** Women who use imported home remedies or certain traditional herbs that may be contaminated with lead.

- **Using imported cosmetics or certain food products.** Women who use imported cosmetics, such as kohl or surma, or certain imported foods or spices that may be contaminated with lead.

- **Engaging in certain high-risk hobbies or recreational activities.** Women who engage in high-risk activities or have family members who do.

- **Renovating or remodeling older homes without lead hazard controls in place.** Women who have been disturbing lead paint and/or creating lead dust or spending time in such a home environment.

- **Consumption of lead-contaminated drinking water.** Women whose homes have leaded pipes or source lines with lead.

- **Having a history of previous lead exposure or evidence of elevated body burden of lead.** Women who may have high body burdens of lead from past exposures, particularly those who are deficient in certain key nutrients (calcium, iron).

- **Living with someone identified with an elevated lead level.** Women who may have exposures in common with a child, close friend, or other relative living in same environment.

Table 4-2. Key Recommendations to Prevent or Reduce Lead Exposure in Pregnant and Lactating Women

- Never eat or mouth nonfood items, such as clay, soil, pottery, or paint chips, because they may be contaminated with lead (see Appendix III).

- Avoid jobs or hobbies that may involve lead exposure, and take precautions to avoid take-home lead dust if a household member works with lead. Such work includes construction or home renovation/repair in pre-1978 homes, and lead battery manufacturing or recycling. [See Appendix IV]

- Avoid using imported lead-glazed ceramic pottery produced in cottage industries (described elsewhere in this chapter) and pewter or brass containers or utensils to cook, serve, or store food.

- Avoid using leaded crystal to serve or store beverages.

- Do not use dishes that are chipped or cracked.

- Stay away from repair, repainting, renovation, and remodeling work being done in homes built before 1978 in order to avoid possible exposure to lead-conaiminated dust from old lead-based paint. Avoid exposure to deteriorated lead-based paint in older homes.

- Avoid alternative cosmetics, food additives, and medicines imported from overseas that may contain lead, such as azarcon, kohl, kajal, surma, and many others listed in Appendix V.

- Use caution when consuming candies, spices, and other foods that have been brought into the country by travelers from abroad, especially if they appear to be noncommercial products of unknown safety.

- Eat a balanced diet with adequate intakes of iron and calcium, and avoid the use of cigarettes and alcohol.

Key Recommendations for Initial Blood Lead Testing

- Blood lead testing of all pregnant women in the United States is not recommended.

- State or local public health departments should identify populations at increased risk for lead exposure and provide guidance about community-specific risk factors to assist clinicians in determining the need for blood lead testing for identified populations or for individuals at risk.

- Routine blood lead testing of pregnant women is recommended in clinical settings that serve populations with identified risk factors for lead exposure.

- In clinical settings where routine blood lead testing of pregnant women is not indicated on the basis of community-specific risk factors, health care providers should consider the possibility of lead exposure in individual pregnant women by evaluating risk factors for exposure as part of a comprehensive occupational, environmental, and lifestyle health risk assessment of the pregnant woman [see Table 4-1]. Blood lead testing should be performed if a single risk factor is identified at any point during pregnancy.

- When indicated, blood lead testing should take place at the earliest contact with the patient, ideally pre-conceptionally or at the first prenatal visit, and be conducted using venous blood lead tests only.

- Both maternal and infant blood lead level test results, along with relevant environmental findings, should be incorporated into both the mother's and the infant's medical records in a timely fashion. Even though such records are likely to be maintained separately, these data are necessary for proper medical management of mother and infant.

Key Recommendations for Follow-up Blood Lead Testing

- A toxicological threshold for adverse health effects has not been identified. Thus, follow-up blood lead testing is recommended for pregnant women with BLL ≥5 µg/dL and their newborn infants to inform environmental and clinical decision-making.

- Pregnant women with confirmed BLLs ≥45 µg/dL should be considered as high-risk pregnancies and managed in consultation with experts in lead poisoning and high-risk pregnancy.

INTRODUCTION

This chapter describes considerations for initial and follow-up blood lead testing during pregnancy and early infancy. It provides information for providers, public health agencies, and communities to guide the approach to the testing and follow up of blood lead levels where lead exposure above background levels is either known or thought to be a concern or where there is no information on the epidemiology of blood lead levels among the target groups (pregnant women and infants less than 6 months of age). The tables outlining frequency of follow-up blood lead testing of newborns [Table 5-1] and infants [Table 5-2] exposed *in utero* fill a gap left by the CDC recommendation for the follow-up testing of lead-exposed children, which begins at age 6 months (Centers for Disease Control and Prevention 1991, 2002).

The strategy described in this chapter for secondary prevention of lead toxicity through testing and identification of lead-exposed pregnant women is focused on the individual. However, a primary prevention strategy of community-focused reduction of lead sources is crucial to prevent the adverse consequences of lead exposure. Secondary prevention strategies, such as testing and follow up of lead exposure above background levels in individual women, do not adequately prevent exposure or the resultant adverse health outcomes. An understanding of the community characteristics, ethnicity, cultural practices, local industry and common occupations, and alternative medicine use practices will assist in identifying groups of women at risk for lead exposure. This strategy may be successful in primary prevention of exposure to the developing fetus and infant if it guides health education and outreach activities in high-risk communities.

IDENTIFICATION OF PREGNANT WOMEN WITH ELEVATED BLOOD LEAD LEVELS

Screening for Elevated Blood Lead Levels

The purpose of screening pregnant women is to identify women exposed to lead who can reasonably be expected to benefit from the knowledge of their lead exposures above background levels and subsequent actions to prevent additional lead exposure or adverse effects to themselves or their fetuses. In this report, screening refers to a laboratory test that is performed on a blood sample from an asymptomatic person to determine if that person has evidence of lead exposure above background levels. One goal of identifying pregnant women at risk is to prevent the potential adverse health outcomes for mother and infant associated with lead exposure during pregnancy. As described in Chapter 2, evidence suggests that no threshold exists for the impacts of lead on maternal health or on the birth, growth, and neurodevelopmental outcomes of the offspring. NHANES data on the blood lead levels of U.S. women of childbearing age indicate that a BLL ≥5 µg/dL is higher than the 98th percentile (or 3 standard deviations) for this population (Centers for Disease Control and Prevention 2009, unpublished data). Thus, a BLL ≥5 µg/dL indicates that a pregnant woman has been exposed to lead well above the U.S. average exposure.

The U.S. Preventive Services Task Force (USPSTF) recently completed a review of the evidence for lead screening in pregnancy. USPSTF found no studies examining the effectiveness of screening or interventions on improving health outcomes in asymptomatic pregnant women, and a lack of availability of evidence for interventions to reduce blood lead levels in this population. The potential harms of screening cited include false-positive test results, anxiety, inconvenience, work or school absenteeism, and financial costs associated with repeated testing (Rischitelli et al. 2006; U.S. Preventive Services Task Force 2006). However, the USPSTF review did not assess the health impact on subpopulations exposed to lead prenatally or during breastfeeding or the benefits of screening only such subgroups.

CDC has determined that there is evidence for health effects in asymptomatic pregnant women at the population level and that a threshold for these effects has not been established. However, there is currently a lack of evidence of improved outcomes from interventions provided to pregnant women with a BLL ≥5 µg/dL since no studies on this point exist. Therefore, the traditional model for medical decision-making of a case definition linked directly to a proven clinical treatment is not useful in this context. Until such research data are available, and given the convincing evidence of neurodevelopmental effects of lead in the prenatal period, CDC recommends a precautionary approach, noting that a BLL ≥5 µg/dL in a pregnant woman indicates that she has or has recently had exposure to lead well above that for most women of child bearing age in the U.S. population. Since there are still many potential lead sources that a pregnant woman can encounter, a blood lead test is a simple and inexpensive way to identify pregnant women with lead exposures above background levels, so that lead sources can be identified and further exposure can be prevented in the best interests of the mother and child. In addition, source identification and remediation activities may benefit other household and community members, depending upon the source in question, as well as the mother and fetus/infant in subsequent pregnancies. Finally, in contrast to abstract and generalized anticipatory guidance, blood lead test results above background levels are also concrete and actionable data points that may help focus attention by an expectant woman on the challenge of identifying and reducing lead exposure.

Blood Lead Testing in the General Population and High-risk Subgroups

Universal blood lead testing of all pregnant women in the United States is not warranted (Rischitelli et al. 2006; U.S. Preventive Services Task Force 2006) considering the current estimated prevalence of elevated blood lead levels is less than 1% of women of childbearing age (Centers for Disease Control and Prevention 2009, unpublished data). However, routine blood lead testing may be warranted in specific U.S. subpopulations at increased risk for lead exposure due to local, community-specific factors, such as environmental sources of lead or the demographics of the population. In addition, individual characteristics and behaviors put certain populations of women of childbearing age at increased risk for lead exposure relative to that of the general population.

The presence of risk factors in a subpopulation of pregnant women, for example in a particular clinic population, is an indication for routine blood lead testing among all pregnant women in this subpopulation. [See Case Studies 4-1 and 4-2 for examples from Elmhurst, New York, and California, respectively.] State or local public health departments should provide clinicians with information on community-specific risk factors appropriate for use in determining the need for routine blood lead testing, including data describing the distribution of blood lead levels in the community and local knowledge of immigration patterns and ethnicity, common occupations, alternative medicine use, cultural practices, local industries, and idiosyncratic sources. Routine testing should continue in subpopulations known to be at increased risk until the specific risk factors within that population are better understood and more targeted methods for identifying women at increased risk can be employed.

The presence of a large industry in a community, such as a battery recycling plant or a lead smelter, is also indication for blood lead testing of the local pregnant population. A list of occupations with the potential for lead exposure can be found in Appendix IV. When the prevalence of lead exposure above background levels is known to be high in certain communities, it may benefit the providers to develop a centralized blood lead testing program at a local hospital, clinic, or community center.

Individual Risk Factor Assessments

Blood lead testing of individual pregnant women based on individual risk factors may be warranted even when blood lead testing of population subgroups is not warranted. Identification of women who may be at increased risk for lead exposure consists of a comprehensive occupational, environmental, and lifestyle history to assess individual risk. However, validated risk factor questionnaires do not currently exist to predict who would benefit from blood lead testing. Local variation in lead exposure patterns makes national development of such a tool impractical. Instead, development (or adaptation) and validation of a risk factor questionnaire should occur at the local level, under the leadership of local public health authorities, after local risk factors for lead poisoning in pregnancy have been ascertained.

In general, when risk factor questionnaires are used, a positive answer to any question should prompt the measurement of the patient's blood lead level. The New York City Department of Health and Mental Hygiene developed a short tool consisting of five questions (New York City Department of Health and Mental Hygiene 2006) [see Figure 5-1]. The Minnesota Department of Health recommends a seven-question tool (Minnesota Department of Health 2007) [see Figure 5-2]. At the time of publication of this document, these risk factor questionnaires have not yet been validated. Nevertheless, such questionnaires do have an inherent educational value, as they stimulate dialogue between the health-care provider and patient and create an opportunity to educate families about lead hazards.

Assessments of other risk factor questionnaires primarily for children have been conducted, including one that was adapted for use with pregnant women. Stefanak et al. (1996) assessed the accuracy of the CDC childhood lead poisoning risk questionnaire (Centers for Disease Control and Prevention 1991) for administration as a screening tool to 314 pregnant women. In this study, which included both rural and urban areas, questions associated with elevated blood lead in pregnant women included the following: home built before 1960 with chipping or peeling paint, current smoker, and consumption of more than nine servings of canned food per week. Women who answered "yes" to any one of those questions were five times more likely to have an elevated blood lead level (BLL ≥10 μg/dL) (p<0.001). The authors calculated the sensitivity and negative predictive value of the CDC questionnaire to be 75.7% and 93.1%, respectively, in this population, suggesting a high confidence that a negative response would classify a respondent correctly. However, the positive predictive value was only 46%, suggesting less confidence in a positive response to correctly classify individuals. When a full 19-question survey was administered, the sensitivity and negative predictive value increased to 89.2% and 96.4%, respectively. The performance difference between the questionnaires is most likely because the CDC childhood lead poisoning risk factor questionnaire developed for children does not target the major sources of lead exposure in pregnant women.

Clinical Indicators for Blood Lead Testing

Clinical indications for measuring a blood lead level include the presence of a risk factor for exposure, physical signs or symptoms, or the presence of a household member with known lead exposure above background levels. Most individuals with measurable lead exposure above background levels are asymptomatic. When symptoms or physical findings of lead poisoning are present, they are often difficult to differentiate as they are generally nonspecific and quite common. These include constipation, abdominal pain, anemia, headache, fatigue, myalgias and arthralgias, anorexia, sleep disturbance, difficulty concentrating, and hypertension, among others. Blood lead levels should be measured when these symptoms are present and the suspicion of a source of lead exists. Blood lead levels should also be measured in the work-up of acutely ill pregnant women presenting with severe abdominal colic, seizure, or coma, and considered in the differential diagnosis of consistent constitutional symptoms (e.g., persistent headache, myalgias, fatigue, etc.) and anemia.

Timing of Blood Lead Testing During Pregnancy

Identifying maternal lead exposure prior to conception or early in the pregnancy potentially offers the most benefit to the developing fetus. Unfortunately, lead poisoning is frequently identified late in pregnancy. Klitzman et al. (2002) reports that the median gestational age at diagnosis was 25.4 weeks (range 6 to 39), while Shannon (2003) reports that lead poisoning was discovered in the third trimester in 12 of 15 (86%) subjects after the women presented with subtle but characteristic findings of severe lead poisoning, including malaise, anemia, or basophilic stippling on blood smear. Early blood lead testing may not always identify lead poisoned women sooner in cases where the exposure is first occurring during pregnancy, such as pregnancy-related pica behavior. In these cases, the measurement of a BLL preconception or early in the first trimester may precede the patient's exposure. Earlier testing, however, does have the benefit of early identification in pregnant women with chronic, ongoing, or historical cumulative exposures (Hu 1991; Hu and Hernandez-Avila 2002; Hu et al. 1996). Therefore, it is recommended that blood lead testing of women at increased risk take place at the earliest contact with the patient, ideally preconceptionally or at the first prenatal visit.

Methods to Collect Blood Samples for Testing

Although blood lead levels can be measured from both capillary and venous samples, the preferred method for adults is a venous blood sample in a vacuum tube. Venous samples are more reliable than capillary blood lead levels, which can be inaccurate due to environmental contamination or dilution of the specimen from finger squeezing. Capillary samples can be used if strict protocols are employed to reduce the risk for contamination; however, even if obtained under these conditions, a capillary BLL ≥5 μg/dL requires confirmation with a venous blood lead test.

Methods to Analyze Lead Levels in Blood

Blood lead levels from venous samples should be analyzed by a certified laboratory using one of the approved methods such as: inductively coupled plasma mass spectroscopy (ICP-MS), graphite-furnace atomic absorption spectrophotometry (GFAAS), or anodic-stripping voltammetry (ASV). Specimen tubes for collection should be lead-free and laboratories should be consulted about the preferred specimen tube and collection procedures. For details about laboratory analytic procedures see *Analytical Procedures for the Determination of Lead in Blood and Urine, Approved Guideline* (Parsons et al. 2001); available at http://www.clsi.org/source/orders/free/c40-a.pdf 22.

Using a centralized laboratory ensures the accuracy of testing and enables better compliance with local reporting requirements. Clinical Laboratory Improvement Act (CLIA) certification of laboratories and participation in national proficiency testing programs helps assure that the methods employed for blood lead testing are accurate and precise to within a specified range of BLLs. Regardless of the method employed, CLIA-mandated proficiency testing programs require accuracy to within the range of +/- 4 µg/dL (or +/- 10%). The limits of detection, accuracy, and precision of BLL determination will vary with the type of method used and among laboratories using the same method. Of the three commonly used methods, ICP-MS and GFAAS have limits of detection of about 0.3-1.0 µg/dL with values reported to two significant figures. ASV has a detection limit of 1-3 µg/dL and is less precise usually reporting values as whole numbers, but is adequate for BLL testing above the limit of detection. For medical interpretation and decisions on management, BLLs can be rounded to a whole number.

Measurement of the BLL of patients at risk for lead exposure can also be done at the point-of-care using a portable blood lead analyzer (Pineau et al. 2002; Shannon and Rifai 1997). Although this method offers the benefit of an immediate result and intervention, point-of-care measurements for pregnant women should be limited to situations where sending specimens to a centralized, certified laboratory is not feasible due to logistics, lack of refrigeration, or cost limitations. Any blood lead measurement ≥5 µg/dL obtained by this method should be confirmed by a certified laboratory with a venous blood lead test (as noted in the point-of-care's instrument use guidance).

Interpretation of Blood Lead Test Results

Analytical variability must be considered when interpreting blood lead results. Changes in successive blood lead measurements on an individual can be considered significant only if the net difference of results exceeds the analytic variance of the method. The degree of analytical variability between laboratories that employ different analytic methods usually exceeds that within a single laboratory. Therefore, a single laboratory using one analytical method should be used to best compare multiple blood lead results from an individual or a population (Centers for Disease Control and Prevention 2005). As a practical matter, ACCLPP therefore recommends that trends in blood lead levels for an individual should not be considered clinically significant until the magnitude of the change is ≥5 µg/dL (Binns et al. 2007).

As described above, a BLL ≥5 µg/dL indicates that a pregnant woman has been exposed to lead well above the average U.S. exposure. Separate scientific studies indicate that adverse effects at BLLs ≥5 µg/dL are likely in pregnant women and likely to increase with increasing blood lead levels. Therefore, additional actions on the part of health care providers and public health are indicated for pregnant women with BLLs ≥5 µg/dL and their infants (see Table 6-1).

As described in Chapter 6, occupationally exposed women should be referred to an occupational physician or center treating occupationally exposed adults. Steps to minimize lead exposure should be undertaken if the BLL is ≥5 µg/dL, and medical removal from workplace exposure should be undertaken if the BLL is ≥10 µg/dL.

Transmission of Blood Lead Test Results

Health care providers have two important responsibilities with respect to sharing laboratory reports of blood lead levels. First, blood lead levels of both mother and child should be transmitted and entered into both the mother's and the infant's medical records in a timely fashion. For instance, the infant's initial and sequential

BLLs should be in the mother's chart, and vice versa, as these data should inform decisions about additional blood lead testing, breastfeeding, and environmental interventions, among other actions. In addition, information about identified lead exposure sources can be clinically useful and should be shared.

In jurisdictions where reporting of BLLs is not done by laboratories, health care providers should also notify the Lead Poisoning Prevention Program of the local or state health department of confirmed BLLs ≥10 µg/dL in a pregnant woman to ensure that health department data are complete and that women receive appropriate services from public health. The report should include complete demographic information on the patient, the health care provider's name and phone number, and the method of sample collection (venous or capillary).

FOLLOW-UP TESTING IN THE PREGNANT WOMAN

Once a blood lead level ≥5 µg/dL has been identified, an important component in the management of lead-exposed individuals is follow-up blood lead testing to assess trends. After the source of exposure has been identified and removed, it is expected that the BLL will decline. However, there is no clear formula to estimate the expected rate of decline of BLLs in exposed women or their offspring. Several factors play a role, including duration of the exposure, presence of physiological stressors affecting bone turnover rates, nutritional status, and medical and environmental interventions.

Follow-up blood lead testing is indicated for pregnant women with a BLL ≥5 µg/dL according to the schedules in Table 5-3. At higher BLLs, a follow-up confirmatory BLL might be indicated earlier than on the schedule provided. Even a single BLL ≥5 µg/dL should prompt the asking of certain risk related questions as soon as possible. Depending on the answers, it may be important to take immediate action. For example, if a pregnant woman from India has a BLL of 10 µg/dL and is taking ayurvedic supplements, she should be advised to immediately stop taking the supplements instead of waiting weeks for another BLL.

When the patient's BLL does not fall after several months, the various factors that may impact the rate of decline (i.e., duration of exposure, psychological stressors, nutritional status, and medical and environmental interventions) should be reconsidered. In some cases, further environmental investigation may be needed. A continuing increase in the measured venous BLL during the follow-up period may indicate continuing or possibly increased exposure to lead and indicates a need for further environmental investigation. Potential causes of rising BLLs in pregnant women include the failure to address the source of the lead or inappropriate management of the lead source; continued use of lead-contaminated products such as spices, foods, cosmetic, folk remedies or lead-glazed ceramics that were not revealed during the initial investigation; and increases in mobilization of bone lead stores from past, high-dose exposures. Additionally, prevention of exposure to lead from occupational sources may not be adequate to maintain a BLL below the level of concern. (See Chapter 6 for medical management guidelines for occupationally exposed women.) Measurement of follow-up BLLs is the main method for determining how urgently additional intervention is needed and whether blood lead levels are declining once interventions, such as removal from the source of exposure, have taken place.

As described in Chapter 3, blood lead levels in pregnancy generally follow a U-shaped curve over the course of pregnancy, with peak blood lead level appearing to be at or near delivery. Assuming unchanging lead intake, the combination of hemodilution, increased weight of organs, and enhanced metabolic activity may account for much of the observed decrease in whole blood lead between 12 and 20 weeks gestation. Accelerated absorption of dietary lead, decreased elimination of lead from the body, and release of bone lead, perhaps following the calcium conservation strategies of late pregnancy, may all operate to yield the observed pattern of lead during pregnancy. Bone resorption dynamics change throughout pregnancy, and the implications for follow-up testing are two-fold. Pregnant women who have an initial blood lead level that is ≥5 µg/dL in the first trimester may have a lower BLL on repeat testing during the second trimester, regardless of interventions. This blood lead level may increase prior to delivery and may, in fact, be higher than the initial level. Additionally, the measured BLL of pregnant women in the second and late first trimesters may be an underestimation of the actual body lead burden. However, the magnitude of this change is uncertain and it is unclear whether the change is clinically significant for determining whether a follow-up BLL <5 µg/dL measured in the first or second trimester should be repeated again at or near delivery. In addition, a single blood lead level cannot be used to establish a woman's risk during her entire pregnancy.

FOLLOW-UP TESTING IN THE NEWBORNS AND INFANTS <6 MONTHS OF AGE

Maternal and umbilical cord lead levels at delivery are, in most cases, highly correlated. However, in a woman with a known BLL ≥5 µg/dL during pregnancy, umbilical cord or neonatal lead levels should be measured to establish a baseline for clinical management. Follow-up blood lead testing is indicated for neonates and infants with a BLL ≥5 µg/dL according to the schedules in Tables 5-1 and 5-2. After the child is 6 months of age, recommendations from *Managing Elevated Blood Lead Levels Among Young Children: Recommendations from the Advisory Committee on Childhood Lead Poisoning Prevention* (Centers for Disease Control and Prevention 2002) should be followed.

Potential causes of rising BLLs in newborns and infants under the age of 6 months include environmental sources of lead exposure, such as environmental contamination from lead dust and lead in the diet. Not enough is known about the kinetics of lead in the prenatally exposed newborn to make reliable projections about the rate of change of infant BLLs after birth.

FOLLOW-UP TESTING IN THE LACTATING MOTHER AND NURSING INFANT

Postpartum maternal blood lead levels are expected to increase during the first month after delivery (Osterloh and Kelly 1999; Rothenberg et al. 2000). This increase is thought to be due partially to postpartum hemoconcentration due to fluid loss and is also greater in lactating women than in women who bottle-feed their infants, suggesting that lactation stimulates the release of lead from bone (Tellez-Rojo et al., 2002) and that bone lead mobilization may actually be higher during lactation than in pregnancy (Gulson et al., 1998). These findings illustrate the importance of understanding that an increase in maternal blood lead level after delivery may not necessarily be associated with a new source of exogenous exposure and may, in fact, result from endogenous release of cumulative bone lead stores. However, it is difficult to draw a conclusion from the scientific literature about the magnitude of the change warranting concern. [See Chapter 9 for information on breastfeeding and Table 9-1 for information on follow-up of blood lead levels during lactation.]

Table 5-1. Follow-up of Initial Blood Lead Testing of the Neonate (<1 Month of Age)

Initial Venous Blood Lead Level[a] (BLL; µg/dL)	Perform follow-up test(s)[b]
<5	According to local lead screening guidelines for children.
5-24	Within 1 month (at first newborn visit).[c]
25-44	Within 2 weeks. Consultation with a clinician experienced in the management of children with BLLs in this range is strongly advised.[d]
≥45	Within 24 hours and then at frequent intervals depending on clinical interventions and trend in BLLs. Prompt consultation with a clinician experienced in the management of children with BLLs in this range is strongly advised.[d]

[a]The initial blood lead level may be either from an umbilical cord sample at the time of delivery or an infant venous BLL. A venous blood sample is preferred over a capillary sample. Decisions to initiate or stop breastfeeding or initiate chelation therapy should be based on venous blood lead test results only.

[b]If infants are breastfeeding, also follow recommendations in Chapter 9.

[c]According to pediatric health supervision guidelines (well-baby visit schedule) or as clinically indicated based on trends in blood lead levels.

[d]The higher the BLL on the initial test, the more urgent the need for confirmatory testing.

Table 5-2. Schedule for Follow-up Blood Lead Testing in Infants <6 Months of Age[a,b]

Venous blood lead level (BLL; µg/dL)	Early follow up (first 2-4 tests after identification or until BLL begins to decline)	Later follow up (after BLL begins to decline)
<10	According to local lead screening guidelines for children	According to local lead screening guidelines for children
10-14	3 months[c]	Within 6-9 months
15-19	1-3 months[c]	Within 3-6 months
20-24	1-3 months[c]	Within 1-3 months
25-44	2 weeks-1 month[d]	Within 1 month
≥45	Within 24 hours[d]	As directed by clinician managing chelation treatment

Adapted from Centers for Disease Control and Prevention. 2002. Managing elevated blood lead levels among young children: recommendations from the Advisory Committee on Childhood Lead Poisoning Prevention. Atlanta: U.S. Department of Health and Human Services.

[a]After 6 months of age, recommendations from Managing Elevated Blood Lead Levels Among Young Children: Recommendations from the Advisory Committee on Childhood Lead Poisoning Prevention (Centers for Disease Control and Prevention 2002) should be followed.

[b]If infants are breastfeeding, also follow recommendations in Chapter 9.

[c]Some case managers or primary care providers may choose to repeat blood lead tests on all new patients within a month to ensure that their BLL levels are not rising more quickly than anticipated. Seasonal variation of BLLs exists and may be more apparent in colder climate areas. Greater exposure in the summer months may necessitate more frequent follow ups.

[d]Consultation with a clinician experienced in the management of children with BLLs in this range is strongly advised.

Table 5-3. Frequency of Maternal Blood Lead Follow-up Testing During Pregnancy

Venous[a] Blood Lead Level (BLL; µg/dL)	Perform follow-up test(s)[b]
<5	None (no follow-up testing is indicated).
5-14	Within 1 month. Obtain a maternal BLL[c] or cord BLL at delivery.
15-24	Within 1 month and then every 2-3 months. Obtain a maternal BLL[c] or cord BLL at delivery. More-frequent testing may be indicated based on risk factor history.
25-44	Within 1-4 weeks and then every month. Obtain a maternal BLL[c] or cord BLL at delivery.
≥45	Within 24 hours and then at frequent intervals depending on clinical interventions and trend in BLLs. Consultation with a clinician experienced in the management of pregnant women with BLLs in this range is strongly advised. Obtain a maternal BLL or cord BLL at delivery.

[a]Venous blood sample is recommended for maternal blood lead testing.

[b]The higher the BLL on the screening test, the more urgent the need for confirmatory testing.

[c]If possible, obtain a maternal BLL prior to delivery since BLLs tend to rise over the course of pregnancy.

Figure 5-1. New York City Department of Health and Mental Hygiene: Recommended Lead Risk Assessment Questions for Pregnant Women

Health-care providers should use a blood lead test to screen pregnant women if they answer "yes" to any of the following questions:

1. Were you born, or have you spent any time, outside of the United States?
   In NYC, approximately 95% of identified lead-poisoned pregnant women are foreign born. Countries of birth in descending order of frequency include Mexico, India, Bangladesh, Russia, Pakistan, Ecuador, Haiti, Jamaica, Morocco, Dominican Republic, Guatemala, Guyana, El Salvador, Gambia, Ghana, Honduras, Israel, Ivory Coast, Korea, Nepal, Sierra Leone, and Trinidad.

2. During the past 12 months, did you use any imported health remedies, spices, foods, ceramics, or cosmetics?

3. At any time during your pregnancy, did you eat, chew on, or mouth nonfood items such as clay, crushed pottery, soil, or paint chips?

4. In the last 12 months, has there been any renovation or repair work in your home or apartment building?

5. Have you ever had a job or hobby that involved possible lead exposure, such as home renovation or working with glass, ceramics, or jewelry?

Figure 5-2. Minnesota Department of Health: Recommended Lead Risk Assessment Questions for Pregnant Women

Health-care providers should use a blood lead test to screen pregnant women if they answer "yes" or "don't know" to any of the following questions, or if they have moved to Minnesota from a major metropolitan area or another country within the last 12 months:

1. Do you or others in your household have an occupation that involves lead exposure?

2. Sometimes pregnant women have the urge to eat things that are not food, such as clay, soil, plaster, or paint chips. Do you ever eat any of these things—even accidentally?

3. Do you live in a house built before 1978 with ongoing renovations that generate a lot of dust (for example, sanding and scraping)?

4. To your knowledge, has your home been tested for lead in the water and if so, were you told that the level was high?

5. Do you use any traditional folk remedies or cosmetics that are not sold in a regular drug store or are homemade?

6. Do you or others in your household have any hobbies or activities likely to cause lead exposure?

7. Do you use non-commercially prepared pottery or leaded crystal?

Key Recommendations for Health Care Providers for the Management of Pregnant and Lactating Women with Blood Lead Levels ≥5 µg/dL

For women with prenatal **blood lead levels ≥5 µg/dL**,

- Attempt to determine source(s) of lead exposure and counsel patients on avoiding further exposure, including identification and assessment of pica behavior (see Chapter 4).

- Assess nutritional adequacy and counsel on eating a balanced diet with adequate intakes of iron and calcium (see Chapter 7).

- Perform confirmatory and follow-up blood lead testing according to the recommended schedules (see Chapter 5 [and Chapter 9 if breastfeeding]).

- For occupationally exposed women, review the proper use of personal protective equipment and consider contacting the employer to encourage reducing exposure.

- Encourage breastfeeding consistent with the provisos in Chapter 9.

For women with prenatal **blood lead levels of 10-14 µg/dL**, ALL OF THE ABOVE, PLUS:

- Notify Lead Poisoning Prevention Program of local health department if BLLs ≥10 µg/dL are not reported by laboratory.

- Refer occupationally exposed women to occupational medicine specialists and remove from workplace lead exposure.

For women with prenatal **blood lead levels of 15-44 µg/dL**, ALL OF THE ABOVE, PLUS:

- Support environmental risk assessment by the corresponding local or state health department with subsequent source reduction and case management.

For women with prenatal **blood lead levels ≥45 µg/dL**, ALL OF THE ABOVE, PLUS:

- Treat as high-risk pregnancy and consult with an expert in lead poisoning on chelation and other treatment decisions (see Chapter 8).

Note: Women of childbearing age with BLLs ≥5 µg/dL who are not currently pregnant or breastfeeding should be followed according to the OSHA medical surveillance guidelines in Appendix C.

INTRODUCTION

This chapter summarizes actions to be undertaken by health care providers, in coordination with local and state health departments, in providing clinical and environmental services to pregnant and lactating women with BLLs ≥5 µg/dL. Both the health department and health care provider have roles to play in keeping pregnant and lactating women and their offspring safe from further lead exposure. The chapter also describes how public health case management can work to coordinate actions between health departments and health care providers to optimize the health of and prevent lead exposure for both the affected mother and fetus or infant.

This report recommends follow-up activities and interventions beginning at BLLs ≥5 µg/dL in pregnant women; Table 6-1 presents specific CDC recommendations for medical and public health actions according to blood lead levels of the pregnant/lactating woman receiving intervention. Because the prevalence of BLLs ≥5 µg/dL, and especially ≥15 µg/dL, is low in the United States, the frequency of follow-up testing recommended herein should not be an undue burden on the health care system. Although the BLL at which particular elements of case management will be initiated is variable by jurisdiction, education and follow-up BLL monitoring should be available for any pregnant woman who has a confirmed BLL ≥5 µg/dL. More intense management, including home environmental and source investigation, should be available to any pregnant woman with a BLL ≥15 µg/dL.

Unlike the blood lead level of concern of 10 µg/dL for children, which is a communitywide action level, a BLL of 5 µg/dL in pregnant women serves a different purpose: it flags the occurrence of prior (or ongoing) lead exposure above background levels, which may not otherwise be recognized. Given the vulnerability of a developing fetus to adverse effects and the possibility of preventing additional exposures, and despite the lack of proven interventions linked to improved outcomes, CDC feels it is prudent to initiate prevention and screening activities for pregnant women showing any evidence of lead exposure above background levels. And, as noted earlier, in contrast to abstract and generalized anticipatory guidance, blood lead test results above background levels are also concrete and actionable data points that may help focus attention by an expectant woman on the challenge of identifying and reducing lead exposure.

This chapter describes the role of clinicians in medical management of pregnant and lactating women with BLLs ≥5 µg/dL, including both **clinical interventions**, with reference to detailed chapters, and **environmental counseling to reduce lead exposures**. This chapter also reviews the role of public health agencies in providing **environmental investigations** and **case management**. These essential activities complement those provided by health care providers to ensure that pregnant women receive the full spectrum of appropriate services to identify and reduce exposures to lead.

MEDICAL MANAGEMENT: ROLE OF THE HEALTH CARE PROVIDER

Medical management of pregnant women with BLL ≥5 µg/dL consists of two parallel tracks: environmental management and clinical services. The mainstay of management for pregnant women with blood lead levels ≥5 µg/dL is removal of the source, disruption of the route of exposure, or avoidance of the lead containing substance or activity. Recommendations for reducing lead exposure are presented below.

Recommended clinical care is described throughout this report in the chapters presenting the research base on blood lead testing, nutrition, chelation, breastfeeding, and other issues. For the convenience of readers, a brief overview of important aspects of clinical care to accompany environmental risk reduction is provided in Box 6-1. Each topic presented is discussed in detail in separate chapters, as noted.

Reducing lead exposure can be a complex challenge, which does not always lend itself to straightforward interventions. Lead exposure can occur in the home, community, or workplace, so identifying specific sources of lead and exposure pathway(s) for an individual is essential to reducing exposure for a particular woman. Any or all of the following strategies may need to be applied depending on a woman's residence, lifestyle, or occupation. This section describes the essential actions recommended for health care providers to assess lead exposure and counsel on its reduction.

Source identification beyond obtaining a thorough environmental and occupational history should be conducted in collaboration with the local health department when BLLs are ≥15 µg/dL. During this process, local or state health departments will visit the home to conduct in-person interviews and collect samples that allow for more-thorough understanding of the risk factors and lead sources and pathways of exposure. In some jurisdictions, an investigation of the workplace may take place as well. This information should be shared with the health care providers for both the mother and infant. Health care providers can assist in the investigation by providing information to health departments on suspected sources that are identified during the care of the patient. In identifying the source or risk factors, testing of all family and household members of the patient for blood lead levels will reveal whether the source is common to everyone or unique to the patient.

Evaluate Occupational Exposure and Make Appropriate Notifications

While blood lead levels in occupationally exposed individuals have fallen dramatically since lead industry standards were revised in 1978 (Anderson and Islam 2006), occupational exposures are still a source of lead exposure in women (Centers for Disease Control and Prevention 2007; Fletcher et al. 1999). Public health departments and health care providers should evaluate occupation as a possible source of lead exposure in pregnant or lactating women with BLLs ≥5 µg/dL and, if occupational exposure exists, refer these women to an occupational physician or occupational medicine center that treats occupationally exposed adults. Appendix IV lists major lead-using industries.

Under current OSHA standards, workplace protections to reduce lead exposure include medical surveillance, periodic air monitoring, and provision of change and shower facilities to reduce take-home exposure. Medical removal is required by OSHA only when blood lead concentrations exceed 50 µg/dL (for construction) or 60 µg/dL (for general industry). BLLs of 40 µg/dL trigger a medical evaluation. However, the OSHA standards are out of date and are inadequate for protecting the health of lead-exposed workers, especially pregnant women and their offspring. Adverse health effects have been associated with much lower blood lead levels currently set as benchmarks for OSHA enforcement.

New evidence has emerged over the last 20 years showing that both cumulative as well as acute lead exposures pose significant health risks (Kosnett et al. 2007). As discussed in Chapter 2 of this document, lead exposure during pregnancy has been associated with an increased risk for spontaneous abortion and adverse effects on fetal growth and neurodevelopment. In response to current research findings, recent recommendations by Kosnett et al. (2007) and by the Association of Occupational and Environmental Clinics (2007) call for setting the general lead industry blood lead level of concern to 10 µg/dL; for occupationally exposed women who are or may become pregnant, the goal is to maintain a BLL <5 µg/dL.

From a clinical perspective, it is important to note that the OSHA Medical Surveillance Guidelines included as Appendix C to the 1977 Lead Standard (www.osha.gov/pls/oshaweb/owadisp.show_document?p_table=STANDARDS&p_id=10033) explicitly states:

> "Recommendations [regarding medical removal protection] may be more stringent than the specific provisions of the standard. The examining physician, therefore, is given broad flexibility to tailor special protective procedures to the needs of individual employees. This flexibility extends to the evaluation and management of pregnant workers and male and female workers who are planning to raise children. Based on the history, physical examination, and laboratory studies, the physician might recommend special protective measures or medical removal for an employee who is pregnant or who is planning to conceive a child when, in the physician's judgment, continued exposure to lead at the current job would pose a significant risk."

The appendix goes on to state: "The adverse effects of lead on reproduction are being actively researched and OSHA encourages the physician to remain abreast of recent developments in the area to best advise pregnant workers or workers planning to conceive children."

Since substantial research developments have occurred since the 1970s when the OSHA standards were developed, occupationally exposed women who are or may become pregnant should be removed from lead exposure if their blood lead level is ≥10 µg/dL. If the blood lead level is in the range of 5 to 9 µg/dL, the health care provider should ask about potential sources of lead exposure on the job and review appropriate use of personal protective equipment in an effort to reduce exposure. Workplace hygiene should be emphasized in order to keep exposure as low as possible and to prevent take-home exposures for other household members. Specifically, patients should be advised to

- Wear a respirator and keep it clean.

- Use wet cleaning methods and HEPA vacuums to clean work areas. Never dry sweep or use compressed air.

- Wash hands and face before eating and drinking. Never eat or drink in the work area.

- Normal handwashing and cleaning of eating surfaces may not remove all surface lead, 'lead visualization' wipes are available can help determine if lead has been removed to an adequate degree.

- When possible, wash or shower and change clothes and shoes before leaving work. Keep all work items away from family areas in the home, and wash and dry work clothes separately from other laundry.

Where feasible, the occupational medicine provider should consider contacting the woman's employer with recommended best practices to monitor and reduce lead exposure in their workplace. An example of such a letter is provided in Appendix XIV. Appendix XV contains the California Department of Public Health Workplace Hazard Alert. Prior to issuing such a letter, the healthcare provider should discuss the contents with the affected employee, and obtain her authorization. Although the letter in Appendix XIV refers to the medical removal protection provisions of the OSHA lead standards, the provider and the employee should be aware that some patients (e.g., employees of government agencies, mines, railroads and airlines) may work for a business that does not necessarily fall under OSHA jurisdiction. For these employees, the reference to the OSHA standard should be omitted and the employee should give explicit consent for release of medical information to her employer.

Identify and Discourage Pica Behavior

As discussed in Chapter 4, the behavior common to all definitions of pica is a pattern of deliberate ingestion of nonfood items, which can cause lead exposure if the substances consumed are contaminated with lead. All pregnant women, but especially those with blood lead levels ≥ 5 µg/dL, should be counseled to never eat nonfood items that may contain lead, such as clay, soil, pottery, or paint chips. Appendix III lists commonly reported pica substances.

Once pica is identified, the specific behavior must be characterized in order to determine how best to intervene. Clinicians are encouraged to follow a standardized history outline to obtain a more complete picture of pica behavior for an individual woman. Table 6-2 provides suggested factors to assess and characterize pica behavior, including such issues as the reason(s) for the behavior (if known) and the substance(s) being consumed. Only a few studies are available that evaluate the effectiveness of interventions designed to reduce or eliminate pica behavior. Most of these studies evaluated the impact of interventions on pica behavior in developmentally delayed individuals or those with obsessive-compulsive disorders (Goh et al., 1999; McAdam, et al. 2004; Piazza et al. 1998). Other studies have attempted to reduce pica behavior by providing vitamin supplements and improving the quality of the diet. While this approach appears to be effective in some case reports (Bugle and Rubin 1993; Pace and Toyer 2000), a randomized, double blind, placebo-controlled, two-by-two factorial study found that micronutrient supplementation did not affect geophagy (eating earth) in 220 school-aged children in Zambia (Nchito et al. 2004). They concluded that the results supported the premise that geophagy is a learned activity and that nutritional deficiencies associated with geophagy are more likely to be a result, not a cause, of this practice. No intervention studies were found that included pregnant women.

Therefore, until further research is available that can guide clinical practice, interventions should promote alternative, healthier strategies in response to the patient's apparent reasons for pica. The approach depends upon eliciting accurate information from the patient about the behavior. In the clinical setting, it may be useful to ask women specifically about the discomforts of pregnancy and the techniques being used to minimize them. Pica has been commonly reported to be used in pregnancy to help relieve abdominal pain, diarrhea, and nausea; to assuage cravings and to improve appetite; and to impart a sense of well-being. Obstetrical providers also should inquire about cravings. Ice pica is particularly common and is often accompanied by pica associated with less benign substances. Inquiring first about general cravings in pregnancy, then about specific cravings for ice, and finally cravings for other less-commonly ingested nonfood items may be more likely to uncover pica behavior. Follow-up questions inquiring about the ingestion of other substances commonly used by members of a woman's community may also help elicit a history of pica.

If the substance is consumed due to cravings, then substitution with a similar, but uncontaminated, substance could be suggested. If a woman is experiencing stomach upset, nausea, or lack of appetite, more appropriate interventions should be followed. Current recommendations of the American College of Obstetricians and Gynecologists (ACOG) for the effective management of nausea and vomiting in pregnancy include vitamin B6 supplementation, use of antiemetic medications, and nonpharmacological approaches such as use of "sea-bands" which use pressure points on the wrist to suppress nausea. These interventions can reduce the discomfort associated with nausea and vomiting of pregnancy by 70% (American College of Obstetricians and Gynecologists 2004). When associated with a psychiatric disorder, appropriate referrals for counseling and behavior modification are warranted.

Descriptive studies have found associations between nutritional deficiencies and pica. Several studies reported lower serum ferritin levels (Edwards et al. 1994; Geissler et al. 1998), lower hemoglobin or hematocrit levels (Corbett et al. 2003; Edwards et al. 1994; Geissler et al. 1998; Rainville 1998), or higher rates of anemia (Kettaneh et al. 2005) in those who engage in pica, while others have found no health effects associated with pica (Smulian et al. 1995). Therefore, women who engage in pica behavior, regardless of the substance consumed, require nutritional counseling.

Counsel Women About Avoiding Sources of Lead Exposure

Avoid alternative products that may contain lead and stay informed of new risks

As discussed in Chapter 4, certain products have been found to be contaminated with lead. Some products have been associated clearly with lead poisoning cases and women should be counseled to avoid these products. These include alternative cosmetics, food additives, and medicines imported from overseas that may contain lead, such as azarcon, kohl, kajal, surma, and many others listed in Appendix V. Pregnant women should be informed that herbal medicines and alternative remedies imported personally or ordered from other countries by mail or online are not subject to FDA premarket approval and therefore their safety cannot be assured, even if the product is professionally packaged and labeled. Pregnant women should be cautioned against consuming candies, spices, and other foods that have been brought into the country from travelers abroad, especially if they appear to be noncommercial products, since their safety is unknown.

Obstetrical providers should advise pregnant women not to expose their fetuses to the risks of herbal medicines and supplements (Marcus and Snodgrass 2005). Herbal medicines and supplements are often regarded as safe by the public and some health care providers, but there is no scientific basis for that belief. In addition, certain herbal medicines and supplements are known to be contaminated with lead and, therefore, should be avoided. There are no rigorous scientific studies of the safety of herbal medicines and supplements during pregnancy, and the Teratology Society has stated that it should not be assumed that they are safe for the embryo or fetus (Friedman 2000).

The literature also contains numerous reports of excessive lead intake associated with the use of lead-glazed ceramic pottery produced by artisans or small manufacturers overseas. As noted earlier, pregnant women should be warned that lead leaches out of these products if they are used for food preparation or storage, especially if used to store acidic liquids such as wine or juice. Leaded crystal glassware is another potential lead source, but one that has not been linked with lead poisoning cases.

On occasion, products available through domestic channels of commerce are found to cause lead exposures to consumers. Recent exposures of concern reported by the media have included jewelry, toys, and other products. In some cases, federal agencies have authority to issue recalls of contaminated products, but sometimes they can only issue warnings. For instance, dietary supplements sold in the United States are not subject to FDA premarket approval, but FDA has authority to act if products are adulterated (e.g., lead contaminated) or misbranded. In either instance, consumer education is essential to avoiding these exposures. Consumers and health care providers can monitor FDA and CPSC recalls and CDC alerts in order to be apprised of newly recognized products of concern. Local health departments can also communicate this information to communities and medical providers. Pregnant women should be given an updated list of products found to be contaminated with lead at their prenatal visits. [For more information, see Chapter 4 and American Academy of Pediatrics (2005); Binns et al. (2007);Centers for Disease Control and Prevention (2002)]. The Consumer Product Safety Improvement Act (CPSIA), which took effect in February 2009, lowered the allowable lead content of consumer products intended for children 12 and younger, setting the standard at 600 ppm of lead in any accessible part. Beginning in August 2009, the allowable concentration declined to 300 ppm, and in August 2011 it will decline to 100 ppm. Starting in 2010, manufacturers must test their products and certify that they meet CPSIA standards. In the meantime, products exceeding the new standard remain prohibited and are subject to recall.

Avoid using lead-contaminated drinking water

Lead found in drinking water is usually due to corrosion that causes lead to leach out of plumbing pipes. The Safe Drinking Water Act (1991) prohibited the sale of lead-containing pipe for residential use (U.S. Environmental Protection Agency 1991). Homes built before 1986 are more likely to have lead in pipes, fittings, solder, fixtures, or faucets. Therefore, owners of older homes may want to test their water for lead. Certain attributes of the water, such as its temperature and pH, as well as the presence of additives, can all affect lead levels. Families with private wells as a water source will need to test their water to determine if lead contamination is a problem, as this is not regulated by EPA.

The EPA's community action level for lead in tap water is 15 ppb. If test results exceed this level, public water systems must comply with public education requirements, as well as conduct additional testing. Such public water systems may also be required to conduct source water treatment and/or lead service line replacement. Reducing lead levels in water may also require replacing internal plumbing such as pipes or fixtures or both. Until the source(s) of lead is removed, homeowners should employ several strategies to minimize their exposure to lead in tap water. Flushing the system for several minutes after nonuse discards water that has been standing in the system and is more likely to contain lead. All tap water used for consumption—whether for drinking, cooking, or particularly for preparation of infant formula—should be flushed before use. Use of bottled or filtered water are other alternatives, although not all filtration systems remove lead and not all bottled water is guaranteed to be lead-free. For detailed instructions for flushing water, along with testing information and federal regulations, see the EPA Lead in Drinking Water Web page (http://www.epa.gov/safewater/lead/index.html).

Avoid exposure to lead hazards in housing (paint, dust, soil)

As noted in Chapter 4, lead-based paint hazards are a major source of exposure for young children. In contrast, the research literature suggests that pregnant women are more likely to be exposed to lead-based paint hazards associated with renovations in older homes. Nevertheless, pregnant women should be educated about the potential risks associated with lead-based paint in older housing for several important reasons. First, pregnant women should understand the importance of using lead-safe work practices in older homes during repair, renovation, repainting, or remodeling work. Failing to minimize and contain dust generated by any activity that disturbs paint can increase or create exposure risk. Dangerous paint removal and repair techniques that generate lead dust or fumes such as dry scraping, sanding, burning of paint with a torch, or using a high-temperature heat gun should be avoided—and may be illegal in some jurisdictions or in federally subsidized housing. Without appropriate education, there is a risk that families (or renovation workers) will inadvertently create or worsen lead-based paint hazards as they work diligently to prepare the baby's room or make other home improvements, thereby exposing the pregnant woman and fetus to lead during the pregnancy or afterward when the baby comes home.

Federal law requires that property owners disclose known lead-based paint and lead hazards to prospective buyers and renters of older homes and that remodeling contractors give lead information to residents before renovating homes built before 1978. A new EPA regulation (promulgated April 2008; effective April 2010) requires lead-safe work practices during renovation/repainting projects, and includes strict controls on disturbance of lead paint by a contractor performing renovation in a residence where a pregnant woman resides (see http://www.epa.gov/lead/pubs/renovation.htm). Pregnant women and their families should be encouraged to inquire whether painters or other contractors scheduled to perform work in their homes have received training in lead-safe work practices.

Families should also understand the importance of maintaining painted surfaces in older homes. While intact lead-based paint poses little risk, peeling paint or other signs of paint deterioration in a pre-1978 home can result in lead exposure hazards. If there is peeling paint (or any other indication of a problem) in the home of a family that is expecting or has young children, and lead-based paint is suspected to be present, the homeowner or tenant should contact the local health department for advice on options such as testing and remediation.

Appropriate remediation strategies vary according to the location and condition of the lead-based paint and the extent of the contamination. Interventions can include a range of activities such as professional cleaning; thorough repair or replacement of components (e.g., entire windows, window sashes, trim/molding, or door jambs), paint stabilization, complete repainting, or complete paint removal. All of these interventions have been found to significantly reduce lead dust levels for at least 3 years postintervention, with the more intensive treatments found to be associated with greater post-intervention reductions (Dixon et al. 2005). In cases where heavy soil contamination has occurred, the soil may need to be removed. However, when less contamination is present, techniques such as planting with ground covers or installing gravel pathways, drip line boxes, or raised planting beds and play areas may be sufficient (Binns et al. 2004; Dixon et al. 2006).

After interventions have been completed in the home, the home should not be reoccupied until it has passed lead dust clearance testing, indicating that the home has been adequately cleaned and that invisible lead dust has not been left behind. Numerous resources are available for the general public. For more information, see Chapter 11, Resources and Referral Information.

Minimize lead exposure from point sources

Women who live close to active lead mines, smelters, or battery recycling plants should take precautions to avoid exposure to lead via inhalation exposures or ingestion of hazardous waste (e.g., mine tailings, acid mine drainage) through contamination of the home environment from industrial lead dust or fumes.

Avoid hobbies and recreational activities that may involve lead exposure

Numerous recreational activities can result in exposure to lead. These activities include crafts (print making, stained glass, ceramics), outdoor sports (hunting and fishing), and liquor distillation, among others. [See Appendix IV for a detailed list.] Since women may not know that these activities carry a risk for lead exposure, consumer education is critical. General safety procedures such as performing these activities in well-ventilated spaces, frequent hand washing, and the use of jacketed ammunition at shooting ranges, can all minimize the risk of lead exposures from recreational activities. Under some circumstances, consumption of game meat (e.g., venison, wild fowl) harvested with lead ammunition may pose a risk for excess lead exposure (Kosnett 2009). Health care facilities providing care to pregnant women should provide informational brochures to pregnant women on the risks associated with these activities.

ENVIRONMENTAL AND CASE MANAGEMENT: ROLE OF PUBLIC HEALTH AGENCIES

This section describes the essential role of public health agencies in assuring appropriate services for pregnant women needing intervention for lead exposure above background levels. Such public health services are recommended at various blood lead levels to complement ongoing medical management being provided by the woman's health care provider (see Table 6-1). Specifically, public health agencies ensure that lead hazards in the home environment are assessed and remediated. Public health agencies also provide case management services to ensure that all appropriate services are provided. Public health agencies can also provide guidance about reimbursement issues regarding environmental investigation or case management and make referrals to private providers, such as lead risk assessors, if necessary.

Environmental Investigation and Management

As previously noted, the critical element in the prevention of lead exposure is the control or elimination of all sources of lead, which must include the home environment to be effective. The goal of environmental management is to ensure a lead-safe home for mothers and babies. To this end, it is recommended that an investigation of the home environment, which is variously called an environmental investigation, exposure assessment, or risk assessment, be conducted for all women and newborn infants with BLLs of ≥15 µg/dL in order to identify potential sources of lead and pathways of exposure and to identify appropriate activities to reduce or prevent further lead exposure. This investigation and subsequent control activities should be carried out by the local or state health department, or under its supervision, as part of case management activities for pregnant and lactating women identified with blood lead levels ≥15 µg/dL.

The investigation should include questions about potential lead exposure pathways, a visual inspection of the home and other relevant environments, and testing of specific media for the presence of lead (such as water, household dust, soil, paint chips, foods, ethnic remedies, spices, ceramic ware, or other suspected sources of lead), as indicated. Examples of environmental management protocols for pregnant women are found in Appendix VIII (New York City Department of Health [NYC DOH] Pregnancy Risk Assessment Form), which is used for all women with prenatal BLLs of ≥15 µg/dL); Appendix IX (Minnesota DOH Assessment Interview Form); and Appendix X (Minnesota DOH Lead-Based Paint Risk Assessment Form), which is used for both pregnant women and for children with elevated blood lead levels). An example of an environmental management protocol for infants of mothers with elevated prenatal blood lead levels who do not have elevated BLLs is found in Appendix XI (NYC DOH Primary Prevention Information Form). An example of a protocol for environmental risk assessment for case management of young infants and children with blood lead levels of 15 µg/dL or higher is provided in Appendix XII (NYC DOH Child Risk Assessment Form).

At a minimum, environmental management should include isolating the expectant mother from known exposure sources, by workplace removal for occupational exposures and through temporary relocation until hazard remediation has been completed and clearance achieved for lead-based paint hazards in the home. Local and state health departments may also utilize information and resources provided by the Centers for Disease Control and Prevention's National Center for Environmental Health (NCEH) and other agencies and organizations [see Chapter 11 for resources and referral information] to provide the most current and updated case management services to their constituents (Centers for Disease Control and Prevention 2002).

Case Management

This section is intended to facilitate the management of pregnant and lactating women and newborn infants with lead exposure above background levels by providing information and guidance to health department personnel who provide or oversee care coordination and follow-up activities.

Case management of pregnant women with lead exposure involves coordinating, providing, and overseeing the services required to reduce their BLLs to prevent harm to the developing fetus. It is based on the efforts of an organized team that includes the pregnant woman and newborn infant's health care providers. A hallmark of effective case management is ongoing communication with the health care and other service providers and a cooperative approach to solving any problems that may arise during efforts to decrease the mother-infant pair's BLLs and eliminate lead hazards in the their environment.

CDC recommends that public health agencies provide case management services for pregnant women with blood lead levels ≥15 µg/dL (See Table 6-1). These services are adapted from the current model of case management adopted by CDC for young children, which has eight components: a) client identification and outreach, b) individual assessment and diagnosis, c) service planning and resource identification, d) the linking of clients to needed services, e) service implementation and coordination, f) the monitoring of service delivery, g) advocacy, and h) evaluation (Centers for Disease Control and Prevention 2002). Typical case management activities could include the following, depending upon the patient's needs and local resources:

- Assess factors that may impact the woman's BLL (including sources of lead, nutritional status, access to services, family interaction, and understanding).

- Visit the woman's residence and other sites where the woman spends significant amounts of time, such as a job site, to conduct a visual investigation of the site and identify sources of environmental lead exposure. Such visits may be made by a case manager and/or by certified environmental investigators or risk assessors.

- Develop a written plan for intervention.

- Oversee the activities of the case management team.

- Coordinate implementation of the plan, including collaboration with the primary health care provider(s) and other specialists.

- Evaluate compliance with the plan and the success of the plan.

- Ensure that a woman receives services in a timely fashion consistent with guidance.

Another variable, the duration of management, will depend on when the blood lead level ≥5 µg/dL is identified—during the prenatal period, at birth, or while the mother-infant pair is nursing. The interventions recommended in this report are for the secondary prevention of adverse health effects from lead exposure; that is, to prevent further lead exposure and to reduce BLLs in pregnant women who have been identified as having lead exposure. However, the ultimate goal is primary prevention of any lead exposure of the developing fetus or newborn infant. Of course, primary prevention is also indicated for women of reproductive age who may become pregnant, not only those who are already pregnant. The importance of primary prevention should not be overlooked, since the behavioral and cognitive effects of lead exposure in young children may be irreversible.

Practices and resources for case management of lead exposure vary markedly among states, cities, and jurisdictions. (In some communities, case management is called care coordination.) The sources of exposure and prevalence of blood lead levels above background levels among pregnant and lactating women and newborn infants also vary by geographic location and community-specific risk factors and may not be readily identifiable. Therefore, users of these guidelines may need to modify them to meet the needs unique to their specific communities. CDC provides technical assistance for the development and implementation of case management protocols.

Box 6-1: Medical Management of Pregnant Women With BLL ≥5 µg/dL

This box provides clinicians with a concise reference on general considerations in medical management of their patients with confirmed lead exposure above background levels. Readers are encouraged to refer to the relevant chapters for additional information.

Counseling patients on identifying and avoiding lead sources (Chapter 4)

For all patients, but especially those with known lead exposures, health care providers should provide guidance regarding sources of lead and help identify potential sources of lead in patients' environments. Public health agencies may have additional information on community-specific risk factors based on geographic location, occupation, or ethnic background. If not completed prior to determination of initial blood lead level, providers should take a complete occupational and environmental history, including questions that may identify the presence of risk factors for lead exposure.

Identification and counseling regarding pica behavior (Chapters 4 and 6)

Many studies agree that pica behavior is likely to be underreported. Identifying pica in a clinical setting may best be accomplished by treating it as a sensitive issue: proceeding from general to more-specific questions and from less-intrusive to more-intrusive questions. A recommended approach is to ask women specifically about techniques being used to minimize the discomforts of pregnancy and about cravings, inquiring first about general cravings in pregnancy, then about specific cravings for ice, and finally cravings for other less commonly ingested nonfood items. Follow-up questions inquiring about the ingestion of other substances commonly used by members of a woman's community may also help elicit a history of pica. If a substance is consumed due to cravings, then substitution with a similar, but uncontaminated, substance could be suggested. When associated with a psychiatric disorder, appropriate referrals for counseling and behavior modification are warranted. Women who engage in pica behavior, regardless of the substance consumed, may benefit from nutritional counseling due to the documented associations between nutritional deficiencies and pica.

Nutritional assessment and referrals (Chapter 7)

Pregnant and lactating women with a current or past BLL ≥5 µg/dL should be assessed for the adequacy of their diet and provided with prenatal vitamins and nutritional advice emphasizing calcium and iron intake. A balanced diet with a dietary calcium intake of 2,000 milligrams daily should be maintained, either through diet or by supplementation or by a combination of both. Additionally, iron status should be evaluated and supplementation provided in order to correct and prevent any iron deficiency. Women with anemia (defined in pregnancy as a hemoglobin level <11 g/dL in the first trimester and third trimester and <10.5 g/dL in the second trimester), requires higher dosing (Institute of Medicine 1990). Generally, pregnant women with iron deficiency anemia should be prescribed 60 to 120 mg of iron daily in divided doses. Dosage can be reduced to 30 mg daily once anemia is corrected. Women receiving supplemental iron or calcium should be encouraged to split the dose, taking no more than 500 mg of calcium or 60 mg of iron at one time, as only small amounts of these nutrients can be absorbed at any one time. Obstetrical providers should advise pregnant women not to expose their fetuses to the risks of herbal medicines, since there is no evidence of their safety and some are known to be lead-contaminated.

Interpretation and follow-up of blood lead tests (Chapter 5)

Pregnant women identified with blood lead levels ≥5 µg/dL should be tested per Table 5-3. Follow-up blood lead testing should be performed according to schedules provided in Table 5-1 for newborns and Table 5-2 for infants under 6 months of age. Adjust the frequency of follow-up tests according to the chronicity of exposure; risk factors for continued, repeat, or future exposure; and types of clinical interventions. Occupationally exposed women should be referred to an occupational physician or center treating occupationally exposed adults and removed from the workplace lead exposure at BLL ≥10 µg/dL. If not reported directly by the clinical laboratory, the health care provider should notify the Lead Poisoning Prevention Program of the local or state health department of BLLs ≥10 µg/dL. Communication with the local or state health department and the pediatric health care provider is crucial in ensuring appropriate follow-up care and developmental monitoring and referrals. Pregnant women identified with blood lead levels ≥5 µg/dL should be tested at the time of birth to establish a baseline to guide postnatal care for mother and child, and followed up according to the testing schedule in Table 9-1. If past exposure to lead was higher than for most people, maternal blood lead levels may increase slightly during lactation due to the liberation of lead from bone stores.

Assisting with identification of lead sources in the environment (Chapters 4 and 6)

The essential activity in management of pregnant women with blood lead levels ≥5 µg/dL is removal of the lead source, disruption of the route of exposure, or avoidance of the lead-containing substance or activity. Source identification beyond obtaining a thorough environmental and occupational history should be conducted in collaboration with the local health department when BLLs ≥15 µg/dL, which will conduct an environmental investigation of the home environment in most jurisdictions. This process usually includes in-home interviews and collection of environmental samples to confirm lead sources and pathways of exposure. Health care providers can assist by providing information to health departments on suspected sources identified during patient care. Findings should be shared with the health care providers of the mother and infant.

Chelation therapy (Chapter 8)

In consultation with a lead poisoning expert, pregnant women with confirmed BLLs ≥45 µg/dL may be considered for chelation therapy and should be considered as high risk pregnancies. Immediate removal from the lead source is still the first priority. In some cases, women may need hospitalization. Reserving the use of chelating agents for later in pregnancy is consistent with the general concern about the use of unusual drugs during the period of organogenesis (National Research Council, 2000). However, BLLs ≥70 µg/dL may result in significant maternal toxicity and chelation therapy should be considered, regardless of trimester, in consultation with experts in lead poisoning and high-risk pregnancies. Chelation therapy should also be considered in neonates and infants less than 6 months of age for a confirmed BLL ≥45 µg/dL.

Counseling on breastfeeding (Chapter 9)

Initiation of breastfeeding should be encouraged for mothers with BLLs <40 µg/dL. At maternal blood lead levels between 20-39 µg/dL, breastfeeding should be intiated accompanied by sequential infant BLLs to monitor trends. A woman with a confirmed BLL ≥40 µg/dL should not initiate breastfeeding. She should be advised to pump and discard her breast milk until her blood lead has declined to <40 µg/dL. Breastfeeding should continue for all infants with BLLs <5 µg/dL or trending downward. For breastfed infants whose blood lead levels are rising or failing to decline by 5 µg/dL or more, environmental and other sources of lead exposure should be evaluated. If no external source is identified, and maternal BLLs >20 µg/dL and infant BLLs ≥5 µg/dL, then breast milk should be suspected as the source, and temporary interruption of breastfeeding until maternal blood lead levels decline should be considered.

Table 6-1. Recommended Actions by Blood Lead Level in Pregnancy

BLL	Health Care Providers	Public Health Providers
<5	• Provide anticipatory guidance routinely and health education materials to all pregnant and lactating women	• Collect all blood lead test results • Develop and disseminate guidelines and health education materials to providers • Provide community-specific risk factors and population-based blood lead testing guidance to clinicians
5-9	Above actions plus • Attempt to determine source(s) of lead exposure and counsel patients on strategies to reduce exposure • For occupationally exposed women, review proper use of personal protective equipment and consider contacting the employer • Assess nutritional adequacy • Confirmatory and follow-up testing (see Table 5-3)	As above
10-14	Above actions plus • Notify lead poisoning prevention program of local health department if not reported by laboratory • Refer occupationally exposed women to occupational medicine specialists • For occupationally exposed women, recommend removal from exposure	Above actions plus • Send out health education materials to patient • For occupationally exposed women, remove from exposure
15–44[a]	Above actions plus • Assist local health department with complete exposure source assessment	Above actions plus • Perform or refer for environmental investigation, source reduction/lead hazard control, case management
≥45[b]	Above actions plus • Treat as high-risk pregnancy • Consider chelation (inpatient) (see Chapter 8) in consultation with lead poisoning expert	Above actions plus • Facilitate consultation with an identified lead poisoning expert experienced in managing chelation in pregnant women

[a]Environmental interventions to control lead exposures at blood lead levels below those in this chart support the goal of lead-safe housing for all children and are appropriate in jurisdictions with resources available to provide such services.

[b]Blood lead levels ≥70 μg/dL may result in significant maternal toxicity; therefore, chelation should be considered regardless of trimester of pregnancy and in consultation with an identified lead poisoning expert (see Chapter 8 for more details).

Table 6-2. Suggested Factors to Assess and Characterize Pica Behavior

Topic	Reason Why Information Is Important	Specific Questions to Ask
Demographics	Context, identify populations at risk	Age, race, ethnicity, country, and region of origin
Substance(s) consumed	Determine if substance(s) are harmful and if extent of use likely to pose health risks, identify source of pica substance(s) for public health interventions if needed	What substance(s) consumed? Dose consumed (amount and frequency)? Substance consumed throughout pregnancy? Where obtained? (Be as specific as possible in case a sample needs to be obtained for testing for contamination)
Reason for use	Useful in being able to elicit a pica history in women of similar background or experiencing similar symptoms, helpful in developing an appropriate plan to help individual woman stop the intake of harmful substances	Reason(s) for use: treatment for specific symptom, general health, or spiritual or emotional well-being
Pica behavior	Understanding of the persistence of the behavior and a clue to how difficult it will be to eradicate	Age at onset? Use affected by hormonal changes (menses, pregnancy, lactation) or stress? Substitution if usual pica substance not available? Is it truly "pica" behavior or a manifestation of an obsessive-compulsive disorder?
Pregnancy history	Improve the understanding of how pica behavior affects pregnancy outcomes	Current pregnancy: gestational age at delivery, birth weight of child, preeclampsia, gestational diabetes Previous pregnancy history: spontaneous abortions, preterm births, low birth weight or macrosomia
Community context	Information will be useful in identifying communities at risk and in planning public health interventions if needed	Current community? Who else consumes substance in community (family, neighbors)? What quality(ies) about the substance is/are important? What problems are thought to be associated with its use?

Key Points for Nutrition and Lead

- The human body's nutritional status affects the absorption, deposition, and excretion of lead and may also affect lead toxicity.

- Lead exposure can also modify the body's ability to utilize nutrients.

- Avoidance of lead exposure remains the primary preventive strategy for reducing adverse health effects. However, the existence of nutrient-lead interactions suggests that optimizing nutritional status during pregnancy and lactation may assist in preventing the adverse consequences of lead exposure.

General Nutritional Recommendations for Pregnant and Lactating Women

- All pregnant and lactating women should eat a balanced diet in order to maintain adequate amounts of vitamins, nutrients, and minerals.

- All pregnant and lactating women should be evaluated for iron status and be provided with supplementation in order to correct iron deficiency.

- All pregnant and lactating women should be evaluated for the adequacy of their diets and be provided with appropriate nutritional advice and prenatal vitamins.

- Women in need of assistance should be referred to programs, such as WIC or the Supplemental Nutrition Assistance Program (SNAP) (formerly food stamps).

- All pregnant and lactating women should avoid the use of alcohol, cigarettes, herbal medicines, and any other substance that may adversely affect the developing fetus or infant.

Recommendations for Pregnant and Lactating Women with Blood Lead Levels ≥5 µg/dL

- In pregnant and lactating women with BLLs ≥5 µg/dL or with a history of lead exposure, a dietary calcium intake of 2,000 milligrams daily should be maintained, either through diet or in combination with supplementation.

OVERVIEW OF THE RELATION BETWEEN NUTRITION AND LEAD

Pregnancy and the first 2 years of life are exceptionally important intervals with respect to adequate maternal and child nutrition (Horton 2008). Pregnancy and lactation are also critically important periods from a toxicological perspective because of the special significance of the potential for adverse effects of toxic exposures on early human development. If inadequate nutritional status increases susceptibility to the toxic effects of lead, lifelong adverse effects are more likely. In addition, lead exposure can interfere with the metabolism of nutrients—an especially important consideration when nutritional status is marginal. This chapter provides an overview of the information on dietary intake and lead levels in pregnant women. These data are limited. Any beneficial effects of dietary supplementation must be demonstrated in well-designed (randomized, placebo-controlled) clinical trials. However, given the importance of basic nutrition in normal pregnancy and lactation, this chapter provides practical recommendations based on the limited suggestive data available for primary and secondary prevention of lead exposure. Recommended dietary intakes (dietary reference intakes [DRIs]—formerly called RDAs) are from the Institute of Medicine, Food and Nutrition Board, unless specifically noted otherwise, and are provided for reference as Appendix XIII (Institute of Medicine 1997, 2001).

Decades of laboratory and clinical investigation have confirmed that the body's nutritional condition affects lead absorption, deposition, metabolism, and excretion (for reviews see Ahamed and Siddiqui 2007; Bogden et al. 2001; Mahaffey 1980, 1985; Mahaffey et al. 1992; Ros and Mwanri 2003). The physiological mechanisms that are the basis for nutrition/lead interactions are multiple and include nutrients: binding lead in the gut, competing with lead for absorption, altering intestinal cell avidity for lead, or altering affinity of target tissues for lead (Ballew and Bowman 2001). Lead can modify the metabolism of nutrients (Pounds, 1991; Sauk and Somerman 1991). For example, changes in iron metabolism and changes in the formation of the metabolically active forms of vitamin D occur with lead exposure. As understanding of cellular biology has advanced, the mechanisms through which nutritional status (at least for the divalent cations, calcium and iron) alter the metabolic response to lead are becoming clarified (Godwin 2001).

Avoidance of lead exposure remains the primary preventive strategy for reducing adverse effects of lead exposure. However, the existence of nutrient-lead interactions suggests that optimizing nutritional status during pregnancy and lactation may reduce the adverse consequences once lead exposure has occurred. Although the lead-nutrient interaction data are limited and somewhat inconsistent, ensuring adequate intakes of minerals such as calcium; iron; selenium; and zinc, and vitamins C, D, and E is a strategy that is generally health promoting, is associated with few risks, and may confer additional benefits to lead-exposed pregnant and lactating women.

Whether there are benefits for lead poisoned pregnant and lactating women resulting from ingestion of dietary supplements in excess of nutritional requirements is not clear and super-supplementation is not recommended. Differences in response between marginally adequate and super-nutritional status may be physiological. For example, the physiological mechanisms that foster adaptation to low dietary intakes (e.g., increased production of binding proteins in the gastrointestinal tract that can transport lead, as well as calcium or iron) may differ significantly from those that occur when nutrient intakes are higher than required. Dietary supplementation with nutrients at levels higher than those required by nonexposed women may constitute a secondary prevention effort aimed at reducing circulating levels of lead in the mother and at reducing lead exposure to the developing fetus and nursing infant.

Studies of the effects of nutrition and blood lead levels are complicated by a number of different factors. A general problem is that variability in the nutritional status of subjects can impact whether there is a response to changes in the nutrient level. For example, iron absorption is increased when the body is deficient in iron, but when the body is iron-replete absorption of additional iron is inhibited (Finch 1994). These same mechanisms also influence the percent of lead that is absorbed. Specific problems related to observational studies are discussed below.

OBSERVATIONAL STUDIES OF ASSOCIATIONS BETWEEN BLOOD LEAD AND MATERNAL DIET

The majority of the research on the influence of nutrition on lead status during pregnancy and lactation has been observational. Such studies can only determine the associations between nutritional status and lead poisoning, not whether these associations are causal. Observational studes are further complicated because the intercorrelations between nutrients in the diet limit the identification of the effects of specific dietary components Observational studies on the association of maternal diet and lead have shown varying results.

In an observational study of maternal diet during pregnancy, higher intakes of calcium, iron, and vitamin D were associated with lower neonatal blood lead levels (Schell et al. 2003). Before treatment, more than 50% of the mothers had dietary intakes below the recommended dietary allowances for zinc, calcium, iron, vitamin D, and kilocalories. Maternal and neonatal blood lead levels were correlated and all of the neonatal blood lead levels were low (geometric mean = 1.58 µg/dL).

West (1994) investigated the relationship between prenatal vitamin supplement use and maternal blood lead levels and pregnancy outcomes in 349 African American women. Supplement users had significantly lower blood lead levels than those who did not use supplements (p = 0.0001). This study did not describe the content of the supplements consumed or provide adherence data, but levels of calcium and vitamins C and E were confirmed by blood analysis and were higher among the reported supplement-users, suggesting that the self-reports were accurate.

Among postpartum women in Mexico City, lower levels of bone lead were associated with higher intakes of calcium, vitamin D, phosphorus, magnesium iron, zinc, and vitamin C, though these relationships showed inconsistent trends (Ettinger et al. 2004). Gulson et al. (2006) measured daily intakes of the micronutrients calcium, magnesium, sodium, potassium, barium, strontium, phosphorus, zinc, iron, and copper from 6-day duplicate diets (2-13 collections per individual) and blood lead concentrations in a small number of mother-child pairs (total of 21 pregnant and 15 nonpregnant subjects in one cohort, nine pregnant subjects in a second cohort, and one group of ten 6- to 11-year-old-children) to evaluate the association of dietary intakes of selected micronutrients and blood lead. They found no statistically significant relationship between blood lead concentration and intake of specific micronutrients (Gulson et al. 2006).

ROLE OF SPECIFIC NUTRIENTS WITH RESPECT TO LEAD

Calcium

Association of dietary calcium intake and lead

Increased lead absorption and tissue retention among overtly calcium-deficient experimental animals have been confirmed in multiple species. As shown in experimental animal studies reported in the 1970s, a diet clearly deficient in only calcium when fed to rats for several months produced much higher tissue stores of lead than occurred in animals fed comparable amounts of lead plus a calcium-adequate diet (Mahaffey et al. 1973; Mahaffey-Six and Goyer 1972). Unusually high deposition of lead in nonosseous tissues (including the kidneys) occurred in contrast with less dramatic elevations of bone lead (Mahaffey et al. 1973). This difference likely reflects impaired bone formation and deposition of lead into bones of the high-lead, low-calcium animals (Mahaffey et al. 1973). The increased absorption and retention of lead by calcium-deficient animals has been confirmed in other species (among others, see information for dogs (Hamir et al. 1982; Stowe and Vandevelde 1979) and horses (Willoughby et al. 1972). Generally, the major calcium effects on lead absorption and distribution occur when dietary calcium is deficient (Hertz-Picciotto et al. 2000). Little influence of calcium on lead metabolism is observed by increasing calcium intake above required levels in animal studies, i.e., the equivalent of super supplementation (e.g., Barton et al. 1978; Mahaffey et al. 1973).

Confirmation of the impact of low dietary calcium intakes has also been found among human subjects who were also shown to have increased lead absorption when their diets were low in calcium (Heard and Chamberlain 1982). Several cross-sectional studies of calcium intake and blood lead levels in women of childbearing age and pregnant women have shown an inverse relationship between calcium-rich foods or calcium intake and blood lead levels. Lacasana-Navarro et al (1996) observed a statistically significant association among women of reproductive age between increased calcium intake and reduced risk of blood lead levels >10 µg/dL. Farias et al. (1996) showed that consumption of foods providing calcium (corn tortillas and milk products) was associated with reduced blood lead levels. Researchers also observed a statistically significant trend among women of reproductive age between decreased risk of elevated blood lead levels (>10 µg/dL) with increasing calcium intake (Lacasana-Navarro et al. 1996). Higher milk intake during pregnancy has also been associated with lower maternal and umbilical cord lead levels in postpartum women in Mexico (Hernandez-Avila et al. 1997).

Dietary calcium supplementation and lead levels

During pregnancy and lactation, lead accumulated in the maternal skeleton is released (Gulson et al. 1999; Manton et al. 2003; Osterloh and Kelly 1999), with greater mobilization of lead during lactation than during pregnancy (Gulson et al. 1998). Calcium supplements have been suggested as a means of reducing mobilization of skeletal mineral. Observations of the variability in release of skeletal lead reinforced the suggestion that low calcium intake may contribute to mobilization of skeletal lead during pregnancy (Gulson et al. 1999). Use of calcium supplements to meet fetal demand for calcium and thereby reduce maternal bone mobilization has been described. Results from Gulson et al. (2004) indicated that calcium supplements were ineffective in minimizing the mobilization of lead from the skeleton during lactation; however, this small observational study lacked a control group and was not designed to properly account for other potential confounding factors.

Calcium supplementation (1,200 mg at bedtime) during the third trimester of pregnancy has been shown, in a randomized crossover trial design, to reduce maternal bone resorption by 14% on average in comparison to placebo (Janakiraman et al. 2003), suggesting that calcium supplements may reduce maternal bone lead mobilization during the third trimester of pregnancy.

Two large randomized clinical trials have been conducted to assess whether calcium supplements reduce blood lead levels during pregnancy and lactation. In a randomized, double-blind, placebo-control trial of calcium supplementation during lactation, Hernandez-Avila et al. (2003) showed that 1,200-mg daily dietary supplementation with calcium carbonate among lactating women reduced maternal BLLs 15%-20% over the course of lactation. Compared with women who received the placebo, those who took supplements had a modest decrease in their blood lead levels of -0.12 µg/dL at 3 months (95% CI = -0.71 to 0.46 µg/dL) and -0.22 µg/dL at 6 months (95% CI = -0.77 to 0.34 µg/dL). The effect was more apparent among women who were most compliant with supplement use and had patella bone lead >5 µg/g bone (-1.16 µg/dL; 95% CI = -0.23 to -2.08). During the second and third trimesters of pregnancy, calcium supplementation (1,200 mg) was associated with an average reduction of 19% in blood lead concentration in relation to placebo (p<0.001) (Ettinger et al. 2009). In another randomized control trial, calcium supplementation (1,200 mg) was associated with modest reductions in blood lead when administered during pregnancy. These effects were strongest in the most-compliant women, including those who: consumed >75% pills (-24%, p<0.001); or had baseline blood lead greater than 5 µg/dL (-17%, p<0.01); or reported use of lead-glazed ceramics and high bone lead (-31%, p<0.01). In the subset of most-compliant women with high patella bone lead (>5 µg/g) and reported use of lead-glazed ceramics, the reduction in blood lead of 31% corresponds to an average reduction of 1.95 µg/dL (95% CI = -0.78 to -2.87). Bone resorption was also reduced by 13% in the supplement group compared with the placebo group (p = 0.002) (Tellez-Rojo et al. 2006). Calcium supplementation was also associated with 5%-10% lower breast milk lead levels among these women over the course of lactation (Ettinger et al. 2006), suggesting that calcium supplementation may also be an intervention strategy to reduce lead in breast milk from both current and previously accumulated sources. Such data support the role of calcium supplementation in decreasing bone resorption, which can release bone lead stores. Calcium supplementation may also decrease intestinal absorption of lead.

Overall, calcium supplementation has been associated with modest reductions in blood lead levels both when administered during pregnancy and lactation. Suppression of bone resorption appears to be the most likely mechanism, although reduced absorption of lead from the gastrointestinal tract may also contribute to this change. It has been suggested that high levels of calcium are needed to supply the nutritional needs of the developing fetus (Johnson 2001).

Calcium status in U.S. women

Calcium requirements during pregnancy and lactation have been investigated extensively. The increased fetal/infant demand for calcium is met by increasing maternal gastrointestinal absorption, decreasing renal excretion, and increasing bone mineral mobilization (Kovacs and Kronenberg 1997). Physiological adaptations (including endocrine responses) are part of why there is no simple relationship between dietary calcium intake and calcium availability to mother, fetus, or infant (Prentice 2000a). In general, however, Americans do not meet dietary recommendations for calcium (Ma et al. 2007), with ethnic minorities and socially disadvantaged groups more likely not meeting dietary calcium recommendations (Affenito et al. 2007). The recommended intakes for calcium are 1,300 mg for pregnant and lactating women 18 years and younger and 1,000 mg for pregnant and lactating women 19 years of age and older.

Estimated calcium intake during pregnancy in the United States varies substantially. Based on data from 1999-2000 NHANES, average calcium consumption for women of childbearing age was between 820 and 940 grams from both diet and supplements. Earlier data from NHANES II showed that for white women in the 18-through-39 year age group mean calcium intake from food was 642 mg/day, contrasted with 467 mg/day among black, non-Hispanic women (Looker et al. 1993). African Americans in all age groups have been shown to consume fewer mean servings of total dairy, milk, cheese, and yogurt than non-African-Americans and have lower calcium intakes (Fulgoni et al. 2007; Weinberg et al. 2004). Meeting dietary recommendations for calcium on a dairy-free diet is difficult (Gao et al. 2006), but can be made easier through the use of calcium-fortified foods such as citrus juices (Gao et al. 2006) and consumption of ready-to-eat cereals, which facilitate milk intake (Song et al. 2006). In contrast to several of the studies cited above, the assessment by Harville et al. (2004) evaluated total oral calcium intake including both food and antacids. Although median oral calcium intake exceeded 1,200 mg/day, more than 10% of the youngest women consumed <600 mg calcium/day. Within the overall group, 10% of African-American women and 6% of white women reported being either lactose intolerant or allergic to milk. However, there was no difference in calcium intake (both approximately 1,200 mg/day) for women reporting lactose intolerance and not being intolerant. It should be noted that in this particular study, many of the women were enrolled in the Women, Infants, and Children (WIC) program which supplies milk and cheese. In this study racial differences in calcium intake were not significant.

Calcium requirements are increased substantially during pregnancy and lactation to meet the demands of the developing fetus and nursing infant (Prentice 2000b). Approximately 25 to 30 grams of calcium are transferred to the fetus during pregnancy, with the majority of this transfer occurring during the third trimester (Institute of Medicine 1990). The major physiological adaptation of the mother to meet this increased calcium requirement is increased efficiency in intestinal absorption of calcium. Decreased renal excretion of calcium and increased bone mineral mobilization are other maternal mechanisms used to meet the needs of the fetus. The Institute of Medicine (IOM) currently recommends 1,000 mg calcium per day for pregnant and lactating women 19-50 years (and 1,300 mg per day for pregnant and lactating women <19 years) (Institute of Medicine 1997). Optimal calcium intake may be achieved through diet, calcium-fortified foods, calcium supplements, or various combinations of these.

NIH has articulated several challenges to optimate calcium intake (National Institutes of Health 1994). High oxalate and phytate in a limited number of foods can reduce the availability of calcium in these foods. Other factors, such as drugs (glucocorticoids), can decrease calcium absorption. There are also genetic factors that may significantly influence many aspects of calcium metabolism. Vitamin D metabolites enhance calcium absorption. Sources of vitamin D, besides supplements, include sunlight, vitamin D-fortified liquid dairy products, cod liver oil, and fatty fish. Calcium and vitamin D need not be taken together to be effective. Excessive doses of vitamin D may introduce risks such as hypercalciuria and hypercalcemia and should be avoided. In addition, high levels of calcium intake have several potential adverse effects but there are adaptive mechanisms that protect from calcium intoxication at calcium intakes less than approximately 4 g/day. Even at intake levels less than 4 g/day, people may be more susceptible to developing hypercalcemia or hypercalciuria and high blood calcium levels may produce renal damage. There is also some concern that increased calcium intake might interfere with absorption of other nutrients, such as iron, or medications. Ingestion of some forms of calcium supplements or milk may reduce iron absorption by as much as 50%. However, calcium formations that contain citrate and ascorbic acid enhance iron absorption.

There are two randomized placebo-controlled trials that aimed to decrease lead exposure to fetus and nursing infant by providing 1,200 milligrams of daily calcium supplementation to maternal diet during pregnancy (Ettinger et al. 2008) and lactation (Hernandez-Avila et al. 2003). Both studies found that, on average, women in the calcium supplement group had 20% lower maternal blood lead levels than the placebo group at the end of follow up, suggesting decreased potential for exposure to the fetus and nursing infant. These studies were carried out in Mexico City, Mexico where the estimated average dietary calcium intake was about 800 milligrams per day, similar to estimates in the United States. NHANES data on dietary intake of selected minerals in 1999-2000 indicate that for women aged 20-39, the average dietary intake of calcium is 797 mg (Ervin et al. 2004). In pregnant women with exposure to lead, high calcium intake (2,000 mg/day) may diminish pregnancy-induced increases in blood lead levels by decreasing intestinal absorption of lead or by decreasing maternal bone resorption (mobilization), thereby reducing exposures to the fetus (Johnson 2001). Thus, the amount of calcium supplement should be adjusted by combining estimated average dietary intake and supplementation in order to achieve the recommended calcium intake of 2,000 mg per day. Care should be taken as some calcium supplements, particularly those derived from natural sources (bonemeal, dolomite, or oyster shell), have been found to contain high levels of lead (Bourgoin et al. 1993; Ross et al. 2000; Scelfo and Flegal 2000).

Summary

In summary, calcium supplementation in pregnant women with elevated blood lead levels may be beneficial in reducing blood lead levels. For pregnant and lactating women with BLLs ≥5 µg/dL or a history of lead exposure above background levels, a dietary calcium intake of 2,000 mg daily should be maintained either through diet or in combination with supplements.

Iron

Association of dietary iron intake and iron status with lead levels

Both low iron status and elevated lead exposure impair hematopoiesis and intellectual development during gestation and infancy (Black et al. 2008). Exposure to lead and reduced iron status result in greater impairment than the lead-associated impairment in heme biosynthesis alone (Kwong et al. 2004; Mahaffey-Six and Goyer 1973). Such findings were confirmed in humans, as well as experimental animals (Barton et al., 1978; Mahaffey 1983).

Iron absorption is highly regulated physiologically and iron absorption is reduced when iron stores are enlarged (Finch 1994). Overall, variation of iron stores in a normal range do not increase lead absorption, but iron deficiency raises the level of divalent metal transporter proteins which carry lead as well as iron (Morgan and Oates 2002). The ability to control iron absorption through regulation of the molecular mechanisms of iron absorption appears during late infancy (Leong et al. 2003).

Iron deficiency is associated with increases in absorption and deposition of lead (Barton et al. 1978). Several cross-sectional studies in children showed an inverse relationship between iron status and blood lead (Bradman et al. 2003; Choi and Kim 2003; Hammad et al. 1996). Consistent with pediatric studies, cross-sectional studies of lead-exposed adults have found that lower serum iron and dietary intake, as well as increased rates of iron deficiency anemia, were associated with higher blood lead levels and better iron status was associated with lower blood lead levels (Baghurst et al. 1987; Graziano et al. 1990; Kim et al. 2003). These studies have generally used dietary intake or laboratory tests (e.g., serum iron or ferritin) to determine iron status.

There are few studies that have investigated the association between iron intake or iron status and blood lead levels. These studies do not provide consistent findings. Schell et al. (2003) studied the effect of maternal diet during pregnancy on neonatal blood lead levels. Among the nutrients studied, iron had the largest impact on newborn lead levels: a two standard-deviation decrease in maternal iron intake (from 30.2 to 11.8 mg/day) was associated with a 0.51 µg/dL increase in newborn lead (29% of the mean newborn lead level of 1.72 µg/dL). More than 50% of mothers in this study had intakes below the recommended dietary allowance for iron in pregnancy. However, data from a nationally representative population survey that included reproductive-aged women (N = 4,394 women aged 20-49 years) found a positive association between dietary iron intake and blood lead levels (Lee et al. 2005).

Dietary iron supplementation and lead

Studies of the association between iron status and blood lead levels found that children with iron-deficiency had higher blood lead levels than iron-replete children (Markowitz et al. 1990; Wright et al. 1999, 2003). Consequently, many experts recommend that iron supplementation be prescribed only to iron-deficient children, irrespective of lead exposure, and do not recommend universal iron supplementation for the prevention or treatment of lead poisoning in children (Wright et al. 1999).

Iron supplementation has been shown to prevent lead-induced disruption of the blood-brain barrier during rat development (Wang et al. 2007a). The supplemental iron protected the blood brain barrier from changes in permeability caused by lead (Wang et al. 2007a) and was also protective against lead-induced apoptosis (Wang et al. 2007b). A prospective study of the effects of prenatal lead exposure on child development was carried out in Yugoslavia with outcomes assessed at age 4 years (Wasserman et al. 1994). Because 34% of the cohort was iron deficient (hemoglobin concentrations <10.5 g/dL at age 2 years and serum ferritin concentrations <12 ng/dL), iron supplements were provided when children were 18 to 38 months of age. Treatment of iron deficiency improved the hematological profile. Low-iron status and elevated lead exposure both affect infants' intellectual development. Lead exposure was associated with cumulative losses in cognitive function during the preschool years. Deficits attributable to iron-deficiency anemia at age 2 (Wasserman et al. 1992) appear to have been reversed by age 4 in response to iron supplementation.

Effectiveness and strategies for iron supplementation during pregnancy have been evaluated, indicating that the efficacy of the supplement intervention is dependent on the following: composition of the diet; presence of a condition, such as pregnancy, that would alter iron absorption or loss; composition of the supplement; severity of the iron deficiency at baseline; and the duration of the intervention (Beard 2000). There have been no supplementation trials addressing the effects of iron on lead levels in pregnancy and the research data are too scanty to determine the relationship between maternal iron intake and maternal or neonatal blood lead levels. However, given that iron deficiency is common among pregnant women (Kraemer and Zimmermann 2007), until further data are available, all women should be evaluated for the adequacy of their iron status and intake and be provided with appropriate nutritional advice and supplements if deficiencies exist.

Iron status in U.S. women

Pregnancy is the most at-risk period for developing iron-deficiency anemia (American College of Obstetrics and Gynecology 2008; Beard 2000). The current recommended intakes for iron are 27 mg in pregnant women and 10 mg in lactating women (Institute of Medicine 2001). While there is some uncertainty regarding the most useful indicators of iron status during pregnancy, cell indices (including mean cell volume, percent hypochromic red blood cells, percent reticulocytes, and cellular hemoglobin in reticulocytes) have been recommended as indicators of iron status (Ervasti et al. 2007), but their usefulness in diagnosing iron deficiency longitudinally needs to be confirmed.

Based on NHANES III data, 9% to 11% of adolescent girls and women of childbearing age were iron deficient [defined as having an abnormal value for at least two of three laboratory tests for iron status that included erythrocyte protoporphyrin, transferrin saturation, or serum ferritin] (Looker et al. 1997). Iron-deficiency anemia was found in 5% of women, which corresponds to an estimated 3.3 million U.S. women. Iron deficiency was more common among women who were from minority, low-income, and multiparous groups (Looker et al. 1997, 1999). Among women ages 19 through 50 years who participated in NHANES during the years 1988 through 1994, $72 \pm 4\%$ of pregnant women and $60 \pm 4\%$ of lactating women (Cogswell et al. 2003) were iron deficient. Use of supplements containing iron was associated with a significant reduction in the prevalence of iron deficiency among women ages 19-through-50 years, but the study lacked statistical power to make this assessment for pregnant and lactating women (Cogswell et al. 2003). Low-income women and minority women were less likely to consume supplements (Cogswell et al. 2003). Analyses of data from the Special

Supplemental Nutrition Program for Women, Infants, and Children in 12 U.S. states indicated that the prevalence of post-partum anemia was 27%, reaching 48% among non-Hispanic black women (Bodnar et al. 2001). Using NHANES III data, Bodnar et al. (2001) estimated that, among women with a poverty index ratio >130%, postpartum women (up to 12 months postpartum) had the highest rates of iron deficiency of between 12% and 13%. Mexican-American females have a higher prevalence of iron-deficiency anemia than did non-Hispanic white females (Frith-Terhune et al. 2000).

Summary

Studies of the effect of iron supplementation in lead poisoned women are not available. Thus, iron supplementation in pregnant and lactating women should be consistent with those given for pregnancy and lactation. No additional iron supplementation is recommended for women with elevated BLLs. However, the iron status of all pregnant women should be evaluated and supplementation should be provided to correct any deficiency.

Zinc

Deficiencies of other trace elements, such as zinc, may increase both lead absorption and lead toxicity (Cerklewski and Forbes 1976). Although of substantial importance worldwide (Black et al. 2008), zinc deficiency is not common in the United States (Hotz et al. 2003). Suboptimal zinc status may be caused by lack of zinc in the diet, but more likely is caused by inhibition of zinc absorption by factors such as other trace metals (e.g. iron, copper, lead, cadmium) (Lonnerdal 2000). Serum zinc concentration is influenced by multiple covariables and declines during pregnancy, presumably reflecting hemodilution that occurs during pregnancy (Hotz et al. 2003). In general, dietary protein is associated with increased zinc absorption and the U.S. population generally receives sufficient protein from dietary sources. Hence, zinc deficiency is not considered of major importance in altering susceptibility to lead toxicity in the U.S. population.

Ascorbic Acid (Vitamin C)

Another category of nutrient-lead interactions involve nutrients noted for their antioxidant properties (e.g., ascorbic acid [vitamin C], vitamin E, selenium, thiamine). Antioxidants are involved in the prevention of cellular damage that occurs from free radicals (atoms or groups of atoms that can be formed when oxygen interacts with certain molecules). The role of the antioxidant nutrients in altering the outcomes of lead exposure is not well established. Supplementation with vitamin C and other antioxidants (such as vitamin E and selenium) may prevent lead-induced oxidative damage due to lead exposure and bolster the body's antioxidant defense system. Unfortunately, the research conducted to date is insufficient in either quality or quantity to evaluate many of these hypotheses.

In addition to its antioxidant properties, vitamin C has been suggested as acting as a natural chelating agent that enhances the urinary elimination of lead from the body (Simon and Hudes 1999). Two large cross-sectional studies in adults have found associations between blood lead levels and dietary intake or serum levels of vitamin C (Lee et al. 2005; Simon and Hudes 1999). In an analysis of nutritional data provided by over 15,000 adult participants in NHANES III, Simon and Hudes (1999) found that adults in the highest two serum vitamin C tertiles had a 65% to 68% lower prevalence of elevated blood lead levels compared to adults in the lowest tertile (p = 0.03). In another analysis of NHANES III data, Lee et al. (2005) described the relationship between serum vitamin C and blood lead levels in over 4,000 reproductive-aged women (20-49 years). Women with high serum vitamin C levels had a 2.5 lower odds of having blood lead levels in the highest decile (>4 µg/dL). Among postpartum women in Mexico City, higher intakes of vitamin C were associated with lower levels of breast milk lead (Ettinger et al. 2004).

Studies with human subjects have also found that supplementation with vitamin C reduced lead levels (Dawson et al. 1999). One study randomly assigned nonoccupationally exposed male smokers into three treatment groups (placebo N = 25, Vitamin C 200 mg daily N = 25, and vitamin C 1,000 mg daily N = 25). Baseline blood lead levels were low and similar to that reported by other studies of the general population. Supplementation with 1,000 mg of vitamin C (but not 200 mg) reduced blood lead levels by 81% (Dawson et al. 1999). However, according to a literature review by Hsu and Guo (2002), the benefit of vitamin C supplementation seems to be found most consistently in studies with subjects with lower lead levels. Human and animal studies with higher blood lead levels in general tend to show minimal to no improvement with vitamin C supplementation.

Determining the dose of vitamin C needed to lower blood lead levels is unclear in that dose-response was not typically observed in these studies. Blood lead levels were lowered only in those studies which the vitamin C intake exceeded nutritionally recommended intakes. The safety of exceeding these levels is unclear. In summary, the research to date suggests that vitamin C may lower blood lead levels. However, further research is needed to confirm these conclusions, since the studies conducted to date have relatively small numbers of subjects and do not include pregnant or lactating women.

Vitamin D

A final category of nutritional interactions with lead is interference by lead with formation of metabolites of the nutrient. The primary example of this is the severe compromise found in formation of the metabolites of vitamin D (i.e., the endocrine function of vitamin D) as lead exposure increases (Mahaffey et al. 1983; Rosen et al. 1980; Smith et al. 1981). Lead is well established as inhibiting the renal synthesis of 1,25-dihydroxyvitamin D in rats (Smith et al. 1981), chicks (Fullmer 1995), and young children (Rosen et al. 1980). As the body burden of lead increases (exposures associated with children's blood across blood lead concentrations of 12 to 120 μg/dL), there is a linear decline in 1,25-dihydroxyvitamin D (Mahaffey et al. 1983). To date, this interaction has not been evaluated among pregnant or lactating women.

Important sources of vitamin D are from synthesis of vitamin D through sunlight activation of pro-vitamin D present in skin and dietary intake (Holick 2007). Many factors influence the efficiency of cutaneous production of vitamin D. In winter months, ultraviolet B rays, needed to promote cutaneous vitamin D production, are absent at latitudes above 35° N (i.e., north of Memphis, Tennessee). Dark-skinned individuals require exposures about 5-10 times as long as light-skinned individuals to achieve similar levels of cutaneous vitamin D production. (Holick 2004). Even in summer months, sun exposures outside the peak sun hours of 10:00 AM to 3:00 PM have limited impact on cutaneous vitamin D synthesis (Holick 2003). Application of sunscreen blocks production of vitamin D (Holick 2007). Higher prepregnancy body mass index is associated with lower vitamin D status (Bodnar 2007a). Additionally, women who wear concealing clothing or are house-bound may have low vitamin D. Clinicians should therefore be aware of the potential for multiple risk factors for inadequate vitamin D status among certain recent immigrants who may not receive adequate exposure to sunlight.

Vitamin D status in U.S. women

The recommended adequate intake of vitamin D in both pregnant and lactating women is 200 IU. However, only about half of U.S. women ages 19-50 years get this amount of vitamin D daily from diet or supplement sources (Moore et al. 2004). The lowest mean dietary intakes of vitamin D in the U.S. population (based on data from food consumption patterns identified in the NHANES III and multiple years of the Continuing Survey of Food Intakes by Individuals [http://www.ars.usda.gov/Services/docs.htm?docid=14392]) were among teenage girls and women (Moore et al. 2004). The American Academy of Pediatrics (AAP) recommends that all children and adolescents receiving <400 IU/day from foods receive a supplement of 400 IU vitamin D daily (Wagner et al. 2008). In adults, daily supplementation with 400 IU vitamin D increases 25(OH)D by 7.0 nmol/L (Heaney 2003). Supplementation of a pregnant woman with 400 IU vitamin D, as in prenatal vitamins, has little effect on her 25(OH)D concentration (Wagner 2008).

Inadequate vitamin D status is common among women in the United States (Bodnar et al. 2007a,b; Hollis 2005; Hollis and Wagner 2004; Looker et al. 2008; Specker 2004; Specker et al. 1994). There is no universal consensus on adequate levels of 25-hydroxyvitamin D, but 75-80 nmol/L (Calvo and Whiting 2006) is a common benchmark. The AAP recommends that pregnant women maintain a 25(OH)D level of [3]80 nmol/L (32 ng/mL) (Wagner et al. 2008).

Based on NHANES 2000-2004 data, lower-than-optimal serum 25-hydroxyvitamin D levels were frequent (Looker et al. 2008); 49.1% of non-Hispanic white pregnant women, 76.4% of Mexican-American pregnant women, and 92.2% of non-Hispanic black pregnant women had serum 25-hydroxyvitamin D <75 nmol/L and 8.5%, 74.6%, and 41.6%, respectively, had serum 25-hydroxyvitamin D <50 nmol/L (Looker et al. 2008). Among a sample of pregnant women residing in northern United States, 25(OH) vitamin D levels were considered ≤ 80 nmol/L in 83.3% of black women and 47.1% of white women; more than 90% of these women used prenatal vitamins (Bodnar et al. 2007b).

Summary

Because data on the association of lead and Vitamin D are limited, no specific recommendation is made for supplementation of vitamin D in lead poisoned pregnant or lactating women. Adequate levels of vitamin D should be maintained.

NUTRITIONAL ASSESSMENT AND REFERRALS

All pregnant women should be assessed for the adequacy of their diets and be provided with appropriate nutritional advice and prenatal vitamins. This should be reinforced and maintained throughout pregnancy and lactation. General nutritional guidance is readily available; for example, see Dunlop et al. (2008) and Gardiner et al. (2008). Nutritional assessment of pregnant and lactating women with blood lead levels ≥5 µg/dL should be, at a minimum, consistent with anticipatory guidance, evaluation, and nutritional recommendations for all pregnant and lactating women. However, in pregnant and lactating women with a current or past BLL ≥5 µg/dL, certain nutritional recommendations should particularly be reinforced. Calcium and iron are of particular focus here for reasons that are related to how calcium and iron influence blood lead levels and pregnancy outcomes. A balanced diet with a dietary calcium intake of 2,000 milligrams daily should be maintained through diet, supplementation, or a combination of both. Additionally, iron status should be evaluated and supplementation provided in order to correct and prevent any iron deficiency. Anemia is the most easily identifiable indicator of functional iron deficiency. The Institute of Medicine (IOM) recommends starting iron supplementation after 12 weeks of pregnancy with the lowest dose needed. Women with anemia (defined in pregnancy as a hemoglobin level less than 11 g/dL in the first trimester and third trimester, and less than 10.5 g/dL in the second trimester), require higher dosing (Institute of Medicine 1990). Generally, pregnant women with iron deficiency anemia should be prescribed 60 to 120 mg of iron daily in divided doses. Dosage can be reduced to 30 mg daily once anemia is corrected. Women receiving supplemental iron or calcium should be encouraged to split the dose, taking no more than 500 mg of calcium or 60 mg of iron at one time, as only small amounts of these nutrients can be absorbed at any one time.

Referrals and Resources

Practitioners who interact with pregnant or lactating women should routinely screen for the presence of nutrient deficiencies like iron deficiency. Although comprehensive assessment of dietary adequacy is not routinely conducted in medical office visits, all pregnant and lactating women should be screened for the adequacy of their diets. If the presence of dietary inadequacy is suspected, women should be provided appropriate nutritional advice and should be referred to resources designed to improve knowledge and/or access. Appendix XIII contains nutritional reference information, including dietary reference intakes: recommended vitamin and elements intakes for individuals, tolerable upper intake levels, food sources for key nutrients, dietary assessment tools, and other background information. Resources that might be useful for referrals or interactions with patients are summarized in this section.

Registered dietitian

A registered dietitian (RD) is a health professional who has received specialty training in food and nutrition. Using various dietary assessment tools, an RD can conduct a thorough assessment of an individual's dietary intake and can identify dietary inadequacies. Local RDs can be located by contacting local health care facilities, such as hospitals or health centers, or by using the Find A Nutrition Professional link of the American Dietetic Association Web site (http://www.eatright.org).

WIC

The Special Supplemental Nutrition Program for Women, Infants, and Children (WIC) is a federal grant program that provides nutritious foods, nutrition education, and referrals to low-income (at or below 185% of the U.S. poverty income guidelines) pregnant and lactating women (in addition to infants and children) who are at nutritional risk. The two major types of nutrition risk recognized for WIC eligibility are medically based risks—such as anemia, underweight, overweight, history of pregnancy complications, or poor pregnancy outcomes—and dietary risks—such as failure to meet the dietary guidelines or inappropriate nutrition practices.

In most WIC state agencies, WIC participants receive checks or vouchers to purchase specific foods each month that are designed to supplement their diets. The foods provided are high in one or more of the following nutrients: protein, calcium, iron, and vitamins A and C. These are the nutrients frequently lacking in the diets of the program's target population. Detailed information about WIC including eligibility criteria, contact information, and instructions for applying can be found on the WIC Web site (http://www.fns.usda.gov/wic/).

Supplemental Nutrition Assistance Program (formerly the Food Stamp Program)

The Supplemental Nutrition Assistance Program (SNAP) is a federal program that provides low-income households with subsidies they can use like cash at most grocery stores. The assistance can be used to buy breads and cereals; fruits and vegetables; protein foods like meat, fish, and poultry; and dairy products. For additional information, call 1-800-221-5689 or visit the SNAP Web site (http://www.fns.usda.gov/snap/).

MyPyramid

The USDA Center for Nutrition Policy and Promotion launched the MyPyramid for Pregnancy and Breastfeeding Web site in May 2008 (http://www.mypyramid.gov/mypyramidmoms/). This Web site allows pregnant and lactating women to create a personalized MyPyramid Plan for Moms that shows what and how much to eat from each food group during each trimester of pregnancy and each stage of breastfeeding. The site also provides additional information on nutritional needs during pregnancy and breastfeeding, weight gain during pregnancy and weight loss during breastfeeding, dietary supplements, food safety, and special health needs.

Key Recommendations for Chelation Therapy

- Chelation therapy should be considered for pregnant women with confirmed blood lead levels ≥45 µg/dL on a case-by-case basis, in consultation with an expert in lead poisoning.

- Pregnant women with confirmed BLLs ≥45 µg/dL should be considered as having high-risk pregnancies and managed in consultation with an expert in high-risk pregnancy.

- Pregnant women with life-threatening lead encephalopathy should be chelated regardless of trimester.

- Insufficient data exist regarding the advisability of chelation for pregnant women with BLLs <45 µg/dL.

- Infants (0-6 months of age) with a confirmed BLL of ≥45 µg/dL should be considered as candidates for chelation in consultation with an expert in pediatric lead chelation therapy.

- Before considering chelation therapy for a pregnant woman (or infant), blood lead levels should be repeated and confirmed using an additional venous blood lead sample collected within 24 hours.

- Chelation therapy must occur in a lead-safe environment; therefore, prior to initiating chelation therapy, the patient should be removed from further lead exposure (see Chapter 6).

INTRODUCTION

There is a potential role for chelation therapy to treat pregnant woman and newborns, and, in some cases, chelation may be life-saving. However, the scientific evidence to support its use is very limited, and chelation during pregnancy and in the early postpartum period should be initiated only in consultation with an expert in treatment for lead poisoning.

OVERVIEW OF CHELATION

Chelation therapy utilzes the chemical characterstics of a chelating agent to remove lead from participation in biological reactions in the body, by binding the agent with the metal (lead) to form a chelate. A chelate is defined as a "complex formation involving a metal ion and two or more polar groupings of a single molecule" (Stedman's 2008). Notice that this definition does not indicate the fate of the chelated metal. Possibilities include excretion of the chelate, persistence in the tissue where the bonding occurred, or redistribution to other tissues. Ideally, the drug should effectively increase lead excretion, be easily administered, be affordable, and be safe. The consequences of lead removal should be to halt further toxicity and to reverse previous lead effects (Markowitz 2000).

DRUGS AVAILABLE IN THE UNITED STATES

There are four drugs ($CaNa_2EDTA$, DMSA, BAL, PCA) in use for lead chelation in the United States (Table 8-1) and others are in use elsewhere. None of these drugs specifically bind only lead and, thus, some loss of essential elements also occurs. The toxicity profiles of these drugs differ. Two of the drugs are administered orally (DMSA, PCA) and two must be given parenterally (BAL im only; $CaNa_2EDTA$ im or iv). The latter two require expert nursing care and are always used in the hospital. The former two are used in both inpatient and outpatient settings. All of these drugs increase lead excretion, primarily through the kidneys (Aposhian 1982; Graziano et al. 1999). There may also be tissue redistribution during or as a consequence of chelation.

The introduction of chelating agents for the treatment of severe lead poisoning (blood lead ≥70 µg/dL) was associated with a marked decline in lead-related mortality in children, from 30% to <1% (Chisolm 1968). Chelation treatment at lower blood lead levels, where mortality is not a major concern, is associated with a fall in blood lead levels and an improvement in biochemical markers of lead toxicity, such as erythrocyte proto-porphyrin (EP) levels and delta-aminolevulinic acid dehydratase (ALAD) activity (Graziano et al. 1991; Piomelli 1996). Depending on the amount of lead in the body prior to chelation, the effect of treatment on blood lead is generally temporary, with levels increasing within 2 weeks after the conclusion of a course of treatment in many patients. The effect on the biochemical markers of toxicity is disparate. ALAD activity declines as blood lead rebounds, whereas EP levels tend to fall if no further lead absorption occurs, despite the rebound in blood lead. All of the drugs increase the excretion of essential metals, but to differing degrees. DMSA appears to be the most specific for binding heavy metals such as lead and mercury. The excessive loss of essential metals has been postulated to account for the observed teratogenicity associated with all of the agents tested in animal studies.

Utility of These Drugs in Other Populations

Candidates for chelation therapy differ by age group. Previous CDC guidelines (1991) established a blood lead level of ≥45 µg/dL as the indication for treatment of children regardless of symptoms. At these levels, gastro-intestinal symptoms may occur in a a large number of children; biochemical toxicity is demonstrable in the majority of children (elevated EP level, decreased ALAD activity); and, subclinically, cognitive scores are likely lower. Additionally, and of importance, such children are very likely to excrete large amounts of lead in re-sponse to chelation treatment—much greater amounts than they would spontaneously excrete over periods of time comparable to a course of chelation. However, the amount excreted is only a small fraction of the total lead in the body. Though symptoms and biochemical markers of toxicity may improve post chelation, there is no documentation of cognitive improvements in nonencephalopathic children. For blood lead levels of <45 µg/dL, chelation treatment can also lower blood lead levels and improve biochemical markers of toxicity tem-porarily. However, there is no evidence that lead excretion is substantially increased for the majority of chil-dren. A randomized placebo-controlled trial of succimer for children with initial BLLs of 20–44 µg/dL also failed to demonstrate any difference in mean cognitive scores when tested 2 years later (Rogan et al. 2001). There are no published guidelines identifying a specific blood lead level as requiring chelation therapy in adults nor is there a universal protocol for which agents to use, dose, or duration of treatment.

CONCERNS ABOUT CHELATION THERAPY DURING PREGNANCY

Consideration of chelation therapy during pregnancy requires identification of the targeted beneficiary and estimation of the anticipated benefits and risks. Limited availability of research findings on comparable pa-tients means that extrapolation from data on other types of patients are necessary to make treatment deci-sions. Since the correlation between maternal and newborn blood lead levels is high as measured by cord and maternal blood lead levels determined at delivery, maternal blood lead level can be used as a proxy for the fetus' blood lead level. Therefore, if the known risks and benefits of chelation treatment for lead poisoned children are extrapolated to fetuses, then a blood lead level ≥45 µg/dL in the mother's blood would trigger chelation treatment of the fetus in situations where the fetus is the intended beneficiary of the treatment. If the intended beneficiary of chelation therapy is the pregnant woman, then there is insufficient clinical data to guide decisions about treatment by blood lead level in the absence of symptoms.

No chelation-attributable toxicities have been reported in the existing published case reports. However, very limited information is available to understand any potential short- or long-term effects. Use of chelat-ing agents should therefore only be considered in consultation with experts in lead poisoning and high risk pregnancies.

CLINICAL EVIDENCE IN PREGNANCY AND IN THE NEWBORN

The literature search identified only case reports of chelation therapy during pregnancy (see Table 8-2) and early postpartum (see Table 8-3). In general, maternal blood lead levels decline after a course of chelation and neonatal blood lead levels at birth were also lower than peak maternal levels during the pregnancy. However, very limited information is available to determine if any long term benefit is derived from *in utero* treatment or whether adverse effects occur from chelation. In the few case reports, babies did not appear to have gross developmental delays.

The women in the case reports were selected for chelation therapy based on their blood lead levels with the lowest pretreatment level reported as 44 μg/dL, although in that case a prior blood lead of 62 μg/dL was observed. All women appeared to have been treated during the second half of pregnancy. All but one of the women were treated with varying amounts and for varying durations with $CaNa_2EDTA$. A single patient also received BAL in addition to $CaNa_2EDTA$. A single case reported the exclusive use of DMSA. In all cases, $CaNa_2EDTA$ therapy was associated with a decline in maternal blood lead levels. There was no change in maternal blood lead after the one case of treatment with DMSA (18-day course). However, she was treated as outpatient without apparent oversight for either compliance or ongoing lead exposure. In all but one case a healthy newborn was delivered. The exception occurred in a case where maternal blood lead pretreatment was 104 μg/dL. The woman received $CaNa_2EDTA$ and BAL. The 1.6 kg infant was born prematurely after antepartum hemorrhage 36 hours into treatment. This baby was later noted to have developmental delay and hearing deficit. No consistent pattern in cord blood lead levels was apparent in the few cases where they were reported. The interval between chelation and delivery also varied from months to minutes. Cord blood lead levels were higher than maternal blood lead in the case treated with DMSA and in that of the sick premature infant described. In the other cases cord blood lead levels were lower than maternal prechelation levels. In several reports, chelation treatment was not initiated until shortly before or soon after delivery and was directed toward the newborns. Various drugs at full dosages have been used singly or in combination: $CaNa_2EDTA$ alone, $CaNa_2EDTA$ and BAL, $CaNa_2EDTA$ and DMSA, and DMSA alone. In general, chelation therapy was well tolerated by the infants.

Exchange transfusion has been used, in combination with chelation therapy, to successfully lower blood lead levels in neonates (Hamilton et al. 2001; Mycyk and Leikin 2004). In one case report, after a single-volume exchange transfusion, the infant with a cord blood lead level of 100 μg/dL was chelated on day 2 with a combination of BAL and $CaNa_2EDTA$ for 5 days, at the end of which the blood lead was 37 μg/dL (Mycyk and Leikin 2004). Chelation was continued for 19 days with DMSA, at the end of which the infant's blood lead was 38 μg/dL. Both the exchange and chelation treatments were described as "well tolerated." Of particular interest in this case is that maternal blood lead at preconception was 117 μg/dL and declined to 72 μg/dL by the third trimester. The mother was not chelated during her pregnancy. The baby was delivered at 40 weeks with a blood lead level of 100 μg/dL, weighed 3.7 kg, and achieved normal developmental milestones at 1 month of age. Another case report (Hamilton et al. 2001) describes a double-volume exchange transfusion plus 5 days intravenous $CaNa_2EDTA$ where the infant blood lead of 114 μg/dL fell to 12.8 μg/dL immediately following the exchange transfusion. Caution is advised, however, as Bearer et al. (2000, 2003) report on blood transfusions in newborn premature infants as an unexpected source of lead exposure. The relative benefits/risks of chelation versus exchange transfusion have not been investigated.

SUMMARY AND RECOMMENDATIONS REGARDING CHELATION THERAPY

While chelation may be beneficial especially in protecting the mother with very elevated blood lead levels, given the lack of controlled studies and the paucity of even published case reports or series, chelation therapy should be undertaken only with advice from experts in this field. Such decision making should weigh the lack of definitive evidence of safety for the fetus (especially in the first trimester) against the extensive safety profile and experience with these drugs in children and adults. Recommendations for chelation therapy prenatally and postnatally are presented below:

Prenatal Chelation of the Mother

BLLs ≥70 µg/dL may result in significant maternal toxicity and chelation therapy should be considered, regardless of trimester, in consultation with an expert in the management of lead poisoning, high-risk pregnancies, and neonatology. Lead poisoning may be life threatening at levels greater than 100 µg/dL, though many cases have been described where patients with such levels were asymptomatic. Encephalopathic pregnant women should be chelated regardless of trimester.

Pregnant women with confirmed BLLs ≥45 µg/dL (repeated on at least two venous blood samples collected within 24 hours) may be considered for chelation therapy and should be managed in conjunction with experts in high-risk pregnancy and lead poisoning. Immediate removal from the lead source is still the first priority and, in some cases, pregnant women may require hospitalization. When chelation is being considered, it should be performed in an inpatient setting only with close monitoring of the patient and in consultation with a physician with expertise in the field of lead chelation therapy. Data regarding the reproductive risk associated with chelation during pregnancy are sparse. Most case reports of infant outcomes report on the use of chelating agents after the first trimester (see Table 8-2). Reserving the use of chelating agents for later in pregnancy is consistent with the general concern about the use of unusual drugs during the period of organogenesis (National Research Council, 2000). However, severe maternal lead intoxication, such as encephalopathy, will warrant chelation regardless of the stage of pregnancy. (Contact the CDC Healthy Homes and Lead Poisoning Prevention branch [http://www.cdc.gov/nceh/lead] or the American College of Medical Toxicology [http://www.acmt.net] for a list of experts).

Neonatal Chelation of the Infant

Chelation should be considered in neonates and infants less than 6 months of age for a confirmed BLL ≥45 µg/dL in consultation with a pediatric expert in lead chelation therapy. The limited data published suggest that toxicities for 0- to 6-month-olds are no different than those of 6- to 12-month-olds. Chelation treatment must occur in an environment free of lead hazards; therefore, prior to initiating chelation therapy, the patient should be removed from further lead exposure. Very limited data are available on the use of exchange transfusion as an alternative in this age group.

Chelating Agents

Three of the four available chelating agents ($CaNa_2EDTA$, BAL, DMSA) have been used during pregnancy and may be considered. Data for penicillamine used in pregnancy are unavailable. (This drug is FDA-approved for use in children, but its use in pregnancy is not approved.) The most experience, little as it is, has been with $CaNa_2EDTA$. This drug may be used intravenously at regular doses for 5 days. [Important Note: Calcium edetate ($CaNa_2EDTA$) must not be confused with edetate disodium (Na_2EDTA). From 2003 to 2005, three individuals— including two children—died of cardiac arrest caused by hypocalcemia during chelation therapy, as a result of inadvertent treatment with edetate disodium (Na_2EDTA) (Brown et al. 2006).]

Table 8-1. Chelating Agents Used to Treat Lead Poisoning

Name	Synonym(s)	Chemical Name	Number of Reported Cases[a] Used in Pregnancy
Calcium Edetate[b]	Calcium disodium versenate, versenate, edetate disodium calcium (CaNa$_2$EDTA)	Calcium disodium ethylene diamine tetraacetate	6
Succimer[c]	Chemet™, meso-2,3-dimercaptosuccinic acid (DMSA)	Meso 2,3-dimercaptosuccinic acid	1
BAL[d]	Dimercaprol, British anti-Lewisite, BAL in Oil (BAL)	2,3-dimercapto-L-propanol	1
D-penicillamine	Penicillamine, PCA, cuprimine (D-pen)	3-mercapto-D-valine	0

[a]See Tables 8-2 and 8-3 for details of the case reports

[b]Never use edetate disodium (Na^{2}EDTA) alone without calcium (Brown et al. 2006)

[c]Succimer did not lower BLL after 1 course of treatment (Horowitz et al. 2001)

[d]Used together with Calcium Edetate (CaNa^{2}EDTA) (Tait et al. 2002)

Table 8-2. Published Experience with Chelating Agents During Pregnancy in Humans

Authors/Location/Year Published	Blood Lead (µg/dL)	Timing of Chelation	Drug Used Dose/Route	Biochemical Outcome	Chronic vs Acute	Clinical History/ Reported Outcomes
Abendroth et al./ Germany/1971	80	5th month	CaNa$_2$EDTA 0.5 g/ day iv 3x/wk wkly for 4wks	BLL 30 µg/dL at end of chelation	Acute (3 wks)	"Good health" at 4 years of age
Angle and McIntyre/ Nebraska/1964	240	8th month	CaNa$_2$EDTA 75 mg/ kg/d, iv/7d	At delivery 4 wks post Rx: urinary copropor. negative in mother and baby	Chronic	4 wks post-treatment, cord BLL <60 µg/dL; "normal neurological and developmental assessment at 4 years of age"
Timpo et al./ New York/1979	86	8th month	CaNa$_2$EDTA 1g/iv bid/ 3d	BLL >41 µg/dL 2d post Rx; 26 µg/dL 1 wk postpartum	Chronic	8 days post-treatment, cord BLL 60 µg/dL; BLL 72 at 2 wks postpartum. 38 wks gestation, wt 2,665 g, length 45 cm, hc 32 cm (all within normal limits), "normal developmental evaluation at 1 8 months of age"
Horowitz and Mirkin/ Oregon/2001	44	7th month	DMSA 30mg/kg/po/ for 5d and 20 mg/kg/ po for 13d - all outpatient	BLL 44 µg/dL at end of chelation	Chronic	Cord BLL 126 µg/dL; healthy appearing at birth, 37 week gestation, wt 3,040 g, lt 48 cm, hc 35 cm, "described by pediatrician as appearing normal at 6 months of age"
Olmedo et al./ New York/1999 (abstract only)	130	8th month	CaNa$_2$EDTA 1g/iv/d/ for 2d; baby delivered after 2d	BLL 48 µg/dL after 2d	Acute (1 wk)	Cord BLL 78 µg/dL; healthy appearing 2.4 kg baby
Tait et al./ Australia/2002	104	7th month	CaNa$_2$EDTA iv/dose not reported/2d, and BAL im/dose not reported/2d	BLL 46 µg/dL 12 hr before delivery	Chronic	Cord BLL 152 µg/dL; antepartum hemorrhage immediately prior to delivery; wt 1.6 kg (75%), diaphragmatic palsy at birth, developmental delay, unilateral deafness
Klitzman et al./ New York/2002	53	8th month	CaNa$_2$EDTA 1 g/ iv/d/5d	BLL 20 µg/dL at delivery	Chronic	Cord BLL 20 µg/dL; healthy appearing newborn

Table 8-3. Published Experience with Chelating Agents during Early Postpartum in Humans

Authors/Location/Year Published	Blood Lead (µg/dL)	Prescribed Treatment	Drug Used Dose/Route	Biochemical Outcome	Chronic vs Acute	Clinical History/Reported Outcomes
Singh et al./Boston/1978	50 @ birth; 50 @ 3 wks	Chelation @ 3 wks CaNa$_2$EDTA	CaNa$_2$EDTA	1 month postchelation Pb 27; recurrent rebound Pb 46 for 9 mos. without further chelation	Chronic (>6 wks)	Apgar 9/10, birth weight 3,200 g, 40 wks, normal birth exam; normal Denver @ 10 months
Timpo et al./New York/1979	Cord 60; 72 @ 14 days	Chelation @ 2 weeks CaNa$_2$EDTA	CaNa$_2$EDTA 150 mg/d x 5d iv	post chelation Pb 49; repeat chelation at 5 mos for Pb 49	Chronic	Apgar 6/8, birthweight 2,665g, 38 wks; normal EEG and developmental evaluation @18 mos.
Sensirivatana et al./Bangkok/1983	113 @ 2 mos.	Chelation @ 2 mos. CaNa$_2$EDTA/BAL, then PCA	CaNa$_2$EDTA 50 mg/kg/day x 5d (3 courses); BAL 15 mg/kg/day x 5d; PCA 40 mg/kg/day x 5d	post CaNa$_2$EDTA/BAL chelation 62	Chronic	Birth weight 3,250g; seizures @ presentation; Gesell Devl.Test: @3 mos-mental age 1.5 mos., @9 mos.- mental age 8.5 mos., @16 mos.- mental age 18.5 mos.
Ghafour et al./Kuwait/1984	66 @ 12 days; 81 @ 17 days	Chelation @ 17 days CaNa$_2$EDTA/BAL	CaNa$_2$EDTA 40 mg/kg/ im q12h; BAL 4 mg/kg/im q8h; 5d	Day 23: Pb 57; day 32: Pb 29	Chronic	Apgar 7/9, birthweight 2,300g, 37 wks, neonatal seizures; poor language development @2 yrs
Adamovich/Hungary/1987	4 @ birth day; 76 @ 1 day post-exchange for Rh incompatibility	Observation	None	Day 7 Pb 42	Acute	Not reported
Rothenberg et al. /Los Angeles/1992	Cord 70; 100 @ 6 wks	Clinic refused to chelate	None	Pb <40 @12 wks	Acute (<4 wks)	"Healthy newborn"; hypertonic @2, 15, 30 days, EEG normal @12 mos.; Psychometric tests "normal" to 3 yrs; short attention span @ all ages
Walsh et al./California/1999 (abstract only)	Newborn Pb 84	Chelation DMSA	DMSA 10 mg/kg/dose q8 x 5d, then bid x 12d	Pb 34 @end chelation day 35	Acute	"Seemed developing normally @ 296 days"
Guzman/Dallas, TX/2000 (abstract only)	37 @ 3 weeks	Chelation CaNa$_2$EDTA, DMSA	CaNa$_2$EDTA 50 mg/kg/d x 5 days continuous iv	Pb 17 @end chelation; Pb 26 @7 wks and succimer begun (3 courses over 3 months)	Chronic	Not reported

Authors/Location/Year Published	Blood Lead (µg/dL)	Prescribed Treatment	Drug Used Dose/Route	Biochemical Outcome	Chronic vs Acute	Clinical History/Reported Outcomes
Olmeda et al./New York/1999	Cord 78	Chelation CaNa₂EDTA/BAL	BAL 300 mg/m2/d im x 1d; CaNa₂EDTA 1,000 mg/m2/d iv x7d	Pb 21 @postchelation	Acute	32 wks, 2.4 kg;
Olmeda et al./New York/1999	Cord 78; 44 pre-chelation day 3	Chelation @3 days CaNa₂EDTA	CaNa₂EDTA 1,500 mg/m2/day iv x 5d	Unknown	Chronic	Not reported
Hamilton et al. Los Angeles/2001	Cord 114	Exchange transfusion (double volume) day 2; chelation CaNa₂EDTA	CaNa₂EDTA iv; 5d	Pb 13 postexchange; <5 post chelation	Chronic	Apgar 9/9, birthweight 3,870g, 41 wks; hypotonic neonate; BAEP normal
Horowitz/Portland, OR/2001	Cord 126 (mom 57); 75 @ 4 days	Chelation @4 days; CaNa₂EDTA/BAL; DMSA	CaNa₂EDTA 1,000 mg/m2/d iv x 3d; BAL 50 mg/m2/q4h im x 3d; DMSA 350 mg/m2/q8h x5d, q12h x 14d	Pb 31 @ 6wks; Pb 39 @11 wks and DMSA begun; Pb 21 @ 5 mos.	Chronic	Apgar 8/9, birthweight 3,040g, 37 wks; 6 mos f/u "normal appearing"
Tait et al /Australia/2002	Cord 152	Chelation @2 days CaNa₂EDTA/BAL; DMSA @10 days	CaNa₂EDTA 50 mg/kg/d iv;BAL 4 mg/kg/dose q4h im; DMSA 30mg/kg/day beginning day 10 x 3wks	Pb transient increase to 236 day 2 of chelation; required 5 courses CaNa₂EDTA, 2 of DMSA in first 2 mos. postpartum	Chronic	Apgar 4/6, birthweight 1,600g, 3 0 wks; flaccid nonresponsive neonate, hypoventilation diaphragmatic palsy; extubated day 42; neurodevelopment @ 5 mos. showed 2 mos. delay
Mycyk and Leiken/Chicago/2004	Cord 100	Exchange transfusion (single volume) @day 1; BAL/CaNa₂EDTA day 2, DMSA @7 days	CaNa₂EDTA 50mg/kg/d continuous iv x 5d; BAL 20 mg/kg/day divided q4h im; DMSA 10 mg/kg/dose q8h x 5d, then q12h x 14d	Post exchange Pb 28; Pb post-parenteral chelation 38; post oral chelation 38 @1 mo. age	Chronic	Apgar 8/9, birthweight 3,700g, 40 wks; normal PE @birth; "normal development" @1 mo.
Powell et al./Australia/2006	Cord 80	Chelation @11 days DMSA	DMSA 10 mg/kg/dose q8h x 5d, then q12h x14d	Pb ~30 post-chelation, no rebound @ 4 mos.	Chronic (years)	Apgar 9/9, birthweight 2,280g, 35 wks; poor suck, sleepiness as neonate; @ 12 months global delay of 5-6 mos.

Key Considerations for Breastfeeding

- Human breast milk is specific to the needs of the infant and is the most complete and ideal source for infant nourishment in the first year of life.

Key Recommendations for Initiation of Breastfeeding

- Measurement of levels of lead in breast milk is not recommended.

- Mothers with BLLs <40 µg/dL should breastfeed.

- Mothers with confirmed BLLs ≥40 µg/dL should begin breastfeeding when their blood lead levels drop below 40 µg/dL. Until then, they should pump and discard their breast milk.

- These reccomendations are not appropriate in countries where infant mortality from infectious diseases is high (World Health Organization Collaborative Study Team on the Role of Breastfeeding on the Prevention of Infant Mortality 2000).

Key Recommendations for Continuation of Breastfeeding

- Breastfeeding should continue for all infants with BLLs below 5 µg/dL.

- Infants born to mothers with BLL ≥5 µg/dL can continue to breastfeed unless there are indications that the breast milk is contributing to elevating BLLs. These infants should have blood lead tests at birth and be followed according to the schedule in Chapter 5.

- For infants whose blood lead levels are rising or failing to decline by 5 µg/dL or more, environmental and other sources of lead exposure should be evaluated. If no external source is identified, and maternal BLLs are >20 µg/dL and infant BLL ≥5 µg/dL, then breast milk should be suspected as the source, and temporary interruption of breastfeeding until maternal blood lead levels decline should be considered.

Key Recommendations for Use of Reconstituted Infant Formula

- Infant formula requiring reconstitution should be made only with water from the cold water tap. Flush the tap for at least 3 minutes before use and then heat the water or use bottled or filtered tap water known to be free of lead.

Breastfeeding is an optimal infant feeding practice compared with other infant feeding practices which carry risks. With regard to short-term risks, lack of breastfeeding is associated with increases in common childhood infections, such as diarrhea (Chien and Howie 2001) and ear infections (Ip et al. 2007), with potentially serious complications such as meningitis, dehydration, and hearing impairment. Lack of breastfeeding also increases the risk for some relatively rare but severe infections and diseases, such as severe lower respiratory infections (Bachrach et al. 2003; Ip et al. 2007), leukemia (Ip et al. 2007; Kwan et al. 2004), and—especially important for preterm infants—necrotizing enterocolitis (Ip et al. 2007). The risk of hospitalization for lower respiratory tract disease in the first year of life is more than 250% higher among babies who are formula fed compared with those who were exclusively breastfed at least 4 months (Bachrach et al. 2003). Furthermore, the risk for Sudden Infant Death Syndrome is 56% higher among formula-fed versus breastfed infants (Ip et al. 2007). The Agency for Healthcare Research and Quality (2007) report also concludes that formula feeding has long-term health effects related to increased risks for certain chronic diseases and conditions, such as type 2 diabetes (Owen 2006) and childhood obesity (Arenz et al. 2004), both of which have increased among U.S. children over time.

Decisions made with regard to breastfeeding by a mother whose blood lead levels exceed background levels should be based on scientific evidence suggesting undue risk for the child. Scientific observations have consistently shown that biologically significant elevations in milk lead concentration do not occur in lactating women at the blood lead concentrations typical of women with long-term residence in developed countries. Only a small number of American women will meet the crieteria to defer breastfeeding, though more will be subject to additional follow up out of an abundance of caution. Transfer of lead can occur from maternal plasma to breast milk in roughly the same concentrations. This chapter describes recommendations for breastfeeding by women with blood lead levels above background levels and summarizes the scientific evidence supporting these recommendations.

INTRODUCTION

The overall goal in counseling a woman whether or not to breastfeed is to provide the best possible nutritional and nurturing environment for the infant. Any decision either not to initiate or to discontinue breastfeeding must be made only after careful consideration of all the factors involved. The basis of the initial decision-making process should include a thorough discussion between the mother and her health care provider of the factors to be considered. This discussion should ideally take place before the baby is born. Many factors have an impact on whether or not a woman with a blood lead level ≥5 µg/dL chooses to breastfeed her child. Many of these factors are poorly quantified and others are not readily quantifiable. Thus, a detailed and balanced discussion is essential.

THE IMPORTANCE OF BREASTFEEDING

Due to the unique nutritional characteristics of human milk, breastfeeding is understood to be the optimal mode of nutrient delivery to term infants. The U.S. Department of Health and Human Services' Blueprint for Action on Breastfeeding (U.S. Department of Health and Human Services 2000) emphasizes the value of breastfeeding, as does AAP (American Academy of Pediatrics 2005). Human breast milk is specific to the needs of the human infant. It provides the ideal nutrients for human growth and development in the first year of life, in a form that is readily transferred into the infant's bloodstream. Human milk also protects the breastfed infant against certain common infections and reduces the incidence of certain chronic diseases as well as symptoms of allergy (U.S. Department of Health and Human Services 2000). Women who breastfeed experience less postpartum bleeding, earlier return to prepregnancy weight and a reduced risk for ovarian cancer and premenopausal breast cancer (U.S. Department of Health and Human Services 2000). Breastfeeding also provides the added benefit of the mother-child bonding that takes place during nursing sessions.

The decision to breastfeed in the presence of a possible contraindication should be made on an individual basis, considering the risk of the complication to the infant and mother versus the tremendous benefits of breastfeeding (Lawrence 1997; Lawrence and Lawrence 2005).

The current AAP statement on breastfeeding does not address the issue of breastfeeding by mothers with lead exposure above background levels (American Academy of Pediatrics 2005). An earlier statement specifically addressing the transfer of toxic environmental agents through breast milk and the risk of infant exposure to environmental toxicants by this route suggests that before advising against breastfeeding, the practitioner should weigh the benefits of breastfeeding against the risks of not receiving human milk (American Academy of Pediatrics 2001).

Specifically with regard to lead, a technical information bulletin published by the Health Resources and Services Administration in 1997 held that breastfeeding is not contraindicated unless the concentration of lead in maternal blood exceeds 40 µg/dL (Lawrence 1997). This recommendation was one small section of a larger review of the evidence then available on breastfeeding benefits and contraindications. It has not been updated since publication.

LEAD IN BREAST MILK

Since maternal blood is the medium from which lead is transferred to breast milk and ultimately to the nursing infant, the relationship of lead in maternal blood to lead in breast milk is of key importance. Early studies supported the belief that milk lead levels were one-tenth to one-fifth the levels of lead in maternal whole blood (for a review, see Abadin et al. 1997). These high values were due in part to contamination and analytical inaccuracies in the laboratory measurement of lead in breast milk. (See Chapter 3 for discussion of issues associated with laboratory analysis of lead in human milk.)

Recent carefully conducted studies of lead in breast milk consistently show breast milk lead to maternal blood lead ratios of approximately 3% or less; that is, a milk lead concentration of 3 µg/dL (or 30 µg/L) would be associated with a maternal blood lead concentration of 100 µg/dL, or a milk lead concentration of 0.3 µg/dL (3 µg/L) would be associated with a maternal blood lead concentration of 10 µg/dL. Gulson et al. (1998) found that the breast milk lead to blood lead ratio was less than 3% in 15 adult female immigrants to Australia with blood lead concentrations up to 34 µg/dL. Li et al. (2000) evaluated 119 nonoccupationally exposed women in Shanghai, reporting a mean maternal blood lead concentration of 14.3 µg/dL and a mean milk lead to blood lead ratio of 3.9%. Counter et al. (2004) reported ratios of milk lead concentration to maternal blood lead concentration in 13 nursing mothers from Ecuadorian Andean villages. The ratios ranged from 0.4% to 3.3% in 12 of the subjects, appearing to increase with increasing blood lead level. The thirteenth subject, with a blood lead concentration of 27.4 µg/dL, had a milk lead to blood lead ratio of 7.5%. Ettinger et al. (2004a) showed that breast milk lead was significantly correlated with maternal blood lead at one month postpartum in 310 lactating women in Mexico City. The ratio of the geometric mean milk lead concentration to the geometric mean maternal blood lead concentration was 0.013, or 1.3%, and the highest observed blood lead concentration was 29.9 µg/dL.

There is limited evidence that with closely spaced multiple pregnancies, baseline maternal blood lead concentrations are lower and the increases in maternal blood lead concentrations occurring during late pregnancy and lactation are reduced relative to those in the first pregnancy (Manton et al. 2003; Rothenberg et al. 1994). However, for most women in the United States, more than 98% of whom have blood lead levels <5 µg/dL, this has no practical implications.

INFANT LEAD EXPOSURE FROM BREAST MILK

Limited experimental observations suggest that breast milk lead has a relatively small impact on infant blood lead. It is generally agreed that biologically significant elevations in milk lead concentration do not occur in lactating women at the blood lead concentrations typical of women with long-term residence in developed countries (Gulson et al. 2003; Manton et al. 2003; Sowers et al. 2002). Other sources of lead also contribute to the nursing infant's blood lead level. Manton et al. (2000) concluded from lead isotope analyses that the principal source of lead exposure in very young children, irrespective of whether they are breast- or bottle-fed, is hand-to-mouth activity. However, the relative importance of early hand-to-mouth activity depends on the child's environment. Neonatal bone turnover is another potential source of lead in infant blood (Gulson et al. 2001) that should be factored into expectations about infant blood lead levels. Bone turnover is very high in the newborn because both bone accretion and bone loss during reshaping of the growing bone are high. The rapid turnover of bone lead is reflected in a short blood lead half-life in very young children compared to older children, with bone turnover varying by age, rather than to the length of the exposure (Manton et al. 2000; O'Flaherty 1995).

Although levels of lead in breast milk are generally low, they can influence infant blood lead levels over and above the influence of maternal blood to which the infant was exposed *in utero*. In a large-scale study of breast milk and infant blood lead levels, milk lead was found to account for 10% of the variance in 6-month blood lead and there was a linear dose–response relationship between breast milk lead and infant blood lead at age 6 months (Rabinowitz et al. 1985). In another study, breast milk lead accounted for 12% of the variance of infant blood lead levels at 1 month of age and levels of breast milk lead were significantly correlated with infant blood lead (Ettinger et al. 2004[b]).

It is possible to estimate milk lead concentrations associated with various maternal blood lead concentrations. As discussed above, the most probable value of the maternal milk lead to blood lead ratio is substantially less than 3%. Table 9-2 illustrates calculated milk lead concentrations at various maternal blood lead concentrations assuming breast milk lead concentration to be 3% of maternal blood lead concentration. Employing a tenfold larger percentage, this calculation might be thought of as providing an upper limit on the milk lead associated with a given maternal blood lead. It partly offsets the effect of binding of lead to milk casein at very low concentrations.

From the breast milk lead, that portion of the nursing infant's blood lead originating from maternal milk can be estimated. Ettinger et al. (2004b) reported that an increase of about 2 μg/L in breast milk lead was associated with a 0.82 μg/dL increase in the blood lead of breast-fed infants at 1 month of age, adjusting for cord blood lead, infant weight change, and reported breastfeeding status. Calculated based on this observed relationship, the increase in infant blood lead concentration associated with different maternal blood lead concentrations can be estimated (Table 9-3). Based on this calculation, the predicted contribution of breast milk lead to infant blood lead at 1 month of age would be about 3.7 μg/dL at a maternal blood lead concentration of 30 μg/dL, 2.5 μg/dL at a maternal blood lead concentration of 20 μg/dL, or 0.25-0.5 μg/dL at maternal blood lead concentrations of 2-4 μg/dL. This calculation is based on a data set whose values did not exceed 30 μg/dL. Its application outside this range represents an extrapolation and becomes progressively less certain as maternal blood lead increases above 30 μg/dL. These calculations are supported by observational data only in infants about 1 month old, but they do not suggest undue concern for lead exposure of nursing infants at maternal blood lead and breast milk lead concentrations typical of those found in the United States.

Evidence also suggests that the breast milk lead to maternal blood lead ratio may increase in a nonlinear fashion when maternal blood lead concentrations exceed about 40 μg/dL. This hypothesis is supported both by observational data on women with very high breast milk lead concentrations (Li et al. 2000; Namihara et al. 1993) and by studies on the components of the blood (e.g., plasma) and breast milk as they relate to maternal lead exposure (Hernandez-Avila et al. 1998; Manton and Cook 1984; Manton et al. 2001; O'Flaherty 1993; Schutz et al. 1996). A finding that breast milk contains proportionally more maternal lead at higher blood lead levels suggests possible risk associated with breastfeeding at maternal blood lead levels above 40 μg/dL. Epidemiological evidence is not entirely consistent about the extent to which maternal blood lead concentrations increase during lactation (Ettinger et al. 2006; Manton et al. 2003; Tellez-Rojo et al. 2002).

The breastfeeding recommendations developed herein are intended for women living in the United States. Insufficient data are available to guide clinical decisions regarding women with extremely high breast milk lead concentrations or in women living or working in lead-polluted areas outside the United States. Some evidence suggests different rates of transfer of lead into breast milk for maternal blood lead concentrations less than and greater than about 40 μg/dL (Li et al. 2000), but available human data are insufficient to make reliable estimates.

RECOMMENDATIONS FOR BREASTFEEDING

On the basis of the health and developmental benefits to infants of breastfeeding and consideration of the available research on the contribution of breast milk lead to infant blood lead, CDC has developed clinical guidance for breastfeeding by women exposed to lead. Initial criteria for breastfeeding are maternal blood lead levels, but ongoing monitoring of infant blood lead levels (described in Chapter 5) provides the additional feedback loop needed for clinical decision making about continuing breastfeeding. Specifically, a rise in infant BLL of 5 µg/dL or more is regarded as clinically significant and affects breastfeeding recommendations. Testing recommendations for women with BLL ≥5 µg/dL identified during pregnancy or at delivery are presented in Table 9-1 and for infants in Tables 5-1 and 5-2. Measurement of breast milk lead is not recommended given current laboratory methods and the availability of maternal blood lead as a proxy.

An important practical challenge to clinicians in implementing these recommendations is ensuring that the recommended laboratory and other findings are entered into both the mother's and the infant's medical records in a timely fashion, as noted in Chapter 5. For instance, the mother's initial and sequential blood lead levels should be in the infant's chart. Without this data, clinicians lack the information needed to provide appropriate and real-time guidance about breastfeeding.

Initiating Breastfeeding

Initiation of breastfeeding should be encouraged for all mothers with blood lead levels <40 µg/dL, with follow-up recommendations varying by blood lead levels. Initial maternal BLLs <20 µg/dL are unlikely to be associated with a detectable increase in infant blood lead, even using a ratio of breast milk to maternal blood ten times the most likely value, as in the above calculations. In women with BLLs between 5-19 µg/dL, an initial infant blood lead level is warranted to establish a baseline.

At maternal blood lead levels between 20-39 µg/dL, data do not exist to weigh accurately the risks of lead exposure from breast milk against the benefits of breastfeeding. Thus, a prudent course of action is for these women to initiate breastfeeding accompanied by sequential mother and infant blood lead levels to monitor trends, so that adjustments can be made if indicated. Mothers with BLL between 20-39 µg/dL should be retested 2 weeks postpartum and then at 1- to 3-month intervals, depending on the direction and magnitude of trend in infant blood lead levels (Table 9-1).

CDC considered the adverse health and developmental effects associated with lead exposure compared to those associated with not breastfeeding and, based on the available information, determined that at maternal blood lead levels ≥40 µg/dL the adverse developmental effects of ≥5 µg/dL increase in an infant's blood lead level was of greater concern than the risks of not breastfeeding until maternal blood lead level dropped <40 µg/dL. Mothers with blood lead levels ≥40 µg/dL should not initiate breastfeeding immediately. They should be advised to pump and discard their breast milk until their blood lead levels drop below 40 µg/dL. In such cases, infants' blood lead levels should be monitored after the initiation of breastfeeding. This recommendation reaffirms the prevailing guidance about deferring breastfeeding at maternal BLL ≥40 µg/dL.

Continuing Breastfeeding

All infants born to mothers with BLL ≥5 µg/dL should have blood lead tests at birth and be followed according to the schedule in Chapter 5. Breastfeeding should continue for all infants with BLLs below 5 µg/dL or trending downward.

For breastfed infants whose blood lead levels are rising or failing to decline by 5 µg/dL or more, environmental and other sources of lead exposure should be evaluated. If no external source is identified, and maternal BLLs are >20 µg/dL and infant BLL ≥5 µg/dL, then breast milk should be suspected as the source, and temporary interruption of breastfeeding until maternal blood lead levels decline should be considered. There are insufficient data to estimate how many mother-child pairs would meet these criteria, but anecdotal evidence suggests that it would apply to a very small number in the United States.

Follow-up testing of women with BLL ≥5 μg/dL identified during pregnancy or at delivery should follow the schedule outline in Table 9-1. This should include women with known risk factors that are not controlled, regardless of the BLL of the women or their infants.

Lead in Infant Formula

Since breast milk may not be provided exclusively, for an extended period of time, or even at all, many infants are likely to be nourished, at least in part, by commercially available infant formula. Therefore, it is important to characterize the contribution of non-breast milk sources to total potential lead exposure from dietary intake in infants and young children.

Over the past several decades, the FDA and other federal agencies have worked to reduce dietary and other lead exposures of the general population, and in particular of vulnerable subpopulations such as infants, children, and pregnant women (Bolger et al. 1996). Lead-lined and lead-soldered cans are no longer used for commercial infant formula produced in the United States, and the most recent Total Diet Study confirms that currently marketed milk-based ready-to-feed infant formulas in the United States contain no appreciable amounts of lead. Only one sample (in the high-iron category) of 88 samples of high- and low-iron infant formula contained any measurable lead (trace lead detected in 1 sample = 0.007 mg/kg) (U.S. Food and Drug Administration 2007).

To the extent that lead can be found in infant formula, the relative bioavailability of such lead may be less than that of lead in breast milk. For example, it has been documented that iron is more readily absorbed from breast milk than from infant formula (Lonnerdal 1985). Rabinowitz et al. (1985) found breast milk to be the strongest correlate of 6-month blood lead levels while formula lead correlated poorly with infant blood lead levels. However, Gulson et al. (1998) showed that the contribution of formula to infant blood lead varied from 24% to 68% in exclusively formula-fed infants. They later estimated average daily intake of lead at age 6 months for infants in their Australian study group fed exclusively by breast milk to be 0.73 μg (subjects = 17; observations = 78), and for infants fed exclusively by infant formula to be 1.8 μg (subjects = 11; observations = 42) (Gulson et al. 2001). Ettinger et al. (2004b) also found that infants fed exclusively with breast milk had lower blood lead levels than those fed partially with breast milk, suggesting that formula or other dietary sources may contribute more lead to infant diets than breast milk does. In that study, an interquartile range increase in breast milk lead (~2 ppb) increased infant blood lead by 25%, or approximately 1 μg/dL.

There are published reports of lead entering formula through lead in tap water used to prepare infant formula (Shannon and Graef 1989) or the use of leaded storage containers (Shannon 1998). For instance, in a convenience sample of home-prepared reconstituted infant formula collected in a pediatrics department in metropolitan Boston, two of forty samples were found to have lead concentrations above 15 μg/L (Baum and Shannon 1997), which is the EPA lead action level for water. It is recommended that infant formula requiring reconstitution be made only with bottled or filtered tap water, or with cold water after flushing the tap for at least 3 minutes before use. Water authorities, in conjunction with state and local public health authorities, should consider issuing recommendations for the use of tap water in preparing infant formula based on lead levels in local tap water.

Table 9-1. Frequency of Maternal Blood Lead Follow-up Testing During Lactation[a] to Assess Risk for Infant Lead Exposure[b] from Maternal Breast Milk

Initial[c] Venous[d] Blood Lead Level (BLL; µg/dL)	Perform follow-up blood lead test(s)
5-19	Every 3 months, per guidelines for adult blood lead testing (Appendix VI), unless infant blood lead levels are rising or fail to decline.[e]
20-39	2 weeks postpartum and then at 1- to 3-month intervals depending on direction/magnitude of trend in infant BLLs.
≥40	Within 24 hours postpartum and then at frequent intervals depending on clinical interventions and trend in BLLs. Consultation with a clinician experienced in the management of lead poisoning is advised.

[a]If a woman becomes pregnant while lactating, she should be followed according to the schedule for pregnancy [see Table 5-3].

[b]Need to coordinate care between mother and infant in the postpartum period.

[c]Last blood lead level measured in pregnancy or at delivery (maternal or cord BLL).

[d]Venous blood sample is recommended for maternal blood lead testing.

[e]Infant should be monitored according to schedules in Tables 5-1 and 5-2.

Table 9-2. Estimated Daily Intake of Lead from Breast Milk at Different Maternal Blood Lead Concentrations

Maternal Blood Lead Concentration, μg/dL	Maternal Plasma Lead Concentration, μg/dL[a]	Breast Milk Lead Concentration, μg/L[b]	Infant Lead Intake from Breast Milk at Age 9 Months, μg/day[c]	Infant Lead Intake from Breast Milk at Age 12 Months, μg/day[d]
1	0.03	0.3	0.3	0.27
2	0.06	0.6	0.6	0.54
3	0.09	0.9	0.9	0.81
4	0.12	1.2	1.2	1.1
5	0.15	1.5	1.5	1.4
8	0.24	2.4	2.4	2.2
10	0.3	3	3	2.7
20	0.6	6	6	5.4
30	0.9	9	9	8.1
40	1.2	12	12	11.0

[a]Calculated as 3% of maternal blood lead concentration.

[b]Numerically equal to maternal plasma lead concentration, but expressed per liter rather than per deciliter.

[c]Assuming the upper ingestion limit of 1,000 mL milk per day at these ages (U.S. Environmental Protection Agency 1997).

[d]Assuming the upper ingestion limit of 900 mL milk per day at this age (U.S. Environmental Protection Agency 1997).

Table 9-3. Estimated[a] Increase in Infant Blood Lead Concentration[b] Associated with Different Maternal Blood Lead Concentrations at 1 Month Postpartum

Maternal Blood Lead Concentration, µg/dL	Estimated Breast Milk Lead Concentration, µg/L[c]	Estimated Associated Increase in Infant Blood Lead at Age 1 Month, µg/dL[d]
1	0.3	0.12
2	0.6	0.25
3	0.9	0.37
4	1.2	0.49
5	1.5	0.62
8	2.4	0.98
10	3	1.2
20	6	2.5
30	9	3.7
40[e]	12	4.9

[a]This estimation integrates absorption, distribution, and excretion.

[b]These values are estimations based ICP-MS laboratory analysis and increments of less than 2 µg/dLwould not necessarily be detectable in clinical laboratories.

[c]See Table 9-2.

[d]Calculated based on the observation that a 2 µg/L increase in breast milk lead is associated with an increase of 0.82 µg/dL in the blood lead of the nursing infant (Ettinger et al. 2004b).

[e]Extrapolation beyond the range of observed data from Ettinger et al. 2004b (where maternal BLLs ranged from 1-30 µg/dL).

INTRODUCTION

The clinical and public health recommendations presented throughout these guidelines are based on current research findings where available; however, research has not been published to provide definitive guidance on all issues of interest. On other topics, the research base is clear, but existing policy is not consistent with research findings. For some topics, existing training and continuing education mechanisms are not working to deliver key findings to health professionals in critical fields, like obstetrics, pediatrics, family practice, and nursing. Together, these gaps in research, policy, and health education create an infrastructure that fails to reinforce optimal clinical and public health practice. This chapter presents specific research, policy, and health education needs identified by CDC to improve current service delivery and to inform development of future practice guidelines and policy with respect to lead exposure above background levels in pregnancy and lactation.

RESEARCH NEEDS

Biomedical Research

Long-term prospective studies of the effect of lead exposure during fetal development and disease risks later in life

Given the immaturity of the blood-brain barrier in the developing nervous system, children might be more susceptible to morphologic changes in the nervous system during the prenatal and early postnatal periods. Further research is needed on

- Lead kinetics across the placenta and in breast milk, and their relationship to development and disease risk across the lifespan for children exposed to lead *in utero* or as nurslings.

- Specific health outcomes of interest, other than neurodevelopmental effects, such as pregnancy outcome and cardiovascular disease in adulthood following *in utero* exposure.

Follow-up studies of pregnancy outcomes and infant development in women with a history of lead exposure above background levels during pregnancy

Research is needed to better characterize health outcomes for mothers and infants associated with maternal lead exposure during pregnancy—at low elevations of blood lead typical for the U.S. population of women of childbearing age, as well as in more heavily exposed subgroups. Research is needed on

- Specific health outcomes of interest, including pregnancy-related hypertension, low birth weight, and preterm birth.

- Possible association between maternal lead exposure and spontaneous abortion, particularly at BLLs <30 µg/dL.

- Epidemiology of lead exposure during pregnancy and health outcomes.

- Experimental investigation of the biological mechanisms.

Genetic susceptibility to adverse effects of lead exposure (gene-environment interactions)

Some studies have suggested that specific genes may render certain individuals more vulnerable to the adverse effects of lead exposure. Research is needed to

- Characterize whether and how the bioaccumulation and toxicokinetics of lead are associated with genetic variation, such as ALDA phenotype or the HFE gene variants.

- Investigate other potential gene-environment interactions.

Value of maternal biomarkers to predict later infant and childhood blood lead levels

While research has shown that maternal blood lead level is closely associated with infant/cord blood lead level at birth, the kinetics of lead in the newborn exposed *in utero* are not well understood. In addition, it is not clear whether tissue stores built up during gestation may be a significant source of lead as children age. Studies are needed to determine whether maternal biomarkers (maternal or umbilical blood lead levels) are useful to predict postnatal blood lead levels throughout infancy and childhood.

Biokinetics of lead in breastmilk

More information is needed on the biokinetics and cumulative dose of lead to the breastfeeding infant at various maternal flood lead levels. Research is needed to determine how breast milk lead levels change over the course of lactation, and whether there are factors in breast milk or maternal diet that would enhance or retard the absorption of lead from breast milk by the infant.

Biokinetics of lead with nutritional supplementation or super-supplementation during pregnancy

- Large randomized clinical trials are needed to determine if nutritional supplements, diet modification, or a combination of diet and supplements may be a means of secondary prevention of exposure to lead during pregnancy.

- Research is needed to determine whether the impact of nutritional factors differs for women prepregnancy, during pregnancy, or during lactation, or depending on the woman's lead burden or prior chelation therapy. Extrapolation from animal studies may be necessary.

Pharmacokinetics and effectiveness of chelating agents during pregnancy and lactation

Minimal clinical data are available to inform decisions regarding the use of chelating agents in pregnant women, such as data on toxicity, treatment regimen, and timing of treatment. Studies are needed on

- The effects of prenatal chelation on mothers and infants and on lead kinetics across the placenta; however, since this type of research is often not possible in humans due to ethical concerns about research on human subjects, extrapolation from animal studies may be necessary.

- The effectiveness of chelation therapy on mitigation of adverse health outcomes other than neurodevelopment.

Use of educational and developmental support and intellectual stimulation to improve academic/life performance of children exposed to lead *in utero*

Current research shows that lead exposure is associated with lifelong health and developmental effects in humans; however, questions have been raised from animal studies and clinical experience about whether and the extent to which certain cognitive effects can be mitigated by educational interventions during childhood. Long-term follow-up studies of children exposed to lead *in utero* are needed to evaluate whether specific educational or developmental interventions can improve cognitive outcomes. To be useful, such studies must carefully control for factors that may confound the relationship between educational strategies and cognitive outcomes.

Identification and development of new therapeutic agents or mechanisms to remove lead from breast milk and bone or tissue storage sites in women of childbearing age.

Since bone lead stores persist for decades, women and their infants may be at risk for exposure long after environmental sources have been abated. At present, no interventions are available to remove lead from breast milk or from bone or tissue storage sites in women of childbearing age. Identification and development of prepregnancy interventions that decrease bone lead stores, or render them less mobilizable, may prove beneficial.

Health Services Research

Develop estimates for the number and distribution of pregnant women in the United States who should have blood lead tests, and the costs and benefits associated with testing and follow-up care

Limited data are available on the numbers of pregnant women who meet the criteria for blood lead testing recommended in these guidelines. Research is needed to

- Estimate the number of pregnant women in the US who should be tested for lead exposure, the costs for such testing, and the costs for recommended follow-up care. This research should include an assessment of the ability of high-risk women to access blood lead testing and follow-up services, including environmental intervention, as well as determine who bears the burden of these costs.

- Estimate the societal benefits expected to be derived from testing and treating pregnant women for lead exposure as recommended herein.

Develop guidance for validation of risk questionnaires for pregnant women in specific clinical settings and subpopulations

Only a few communities have developed risk questionnaires to inform decisions about blood lead testing of pregnant women; however, these guidelines recommends their use. Practical methods for adapting and validating risk questionnaires at the local level should be developed and disseminated by CDC and state and local health departments. Such guidance would allow local health agencies and health care providers to develop reliable risk questionnaires that are responsive to local conditions.

Optimal timing for blood lead testing during pregnancy

Identification of lead-exposed pregnant women potentially offers the most benefit to women and their infants; however, there are no studies that identify when in pregnancy blood lead testing should be done. Given the curvilinear trajectory of blood lead levels over the course of pregnancy, blood lead testing done in different trimesters may either over- or underestimate the woman's true lead exposure.

Characterize risk factors for pica and clinical strategies to identify pica in pregnant and lactating women

While pica behavior is relatively uncommon in the general population, pica is observed in some populations of pregnant women in the United States, particularly those who have recently immigrated. Research is needed on how clinicians can more effectively identify pica, particularly those factors (age, race, country of origin, nutritional or health status, etc.) that may predispose a woman to pica.

Effectiveness of interventions to reduce pica among pregnant women

Only a few studies are available that evaluate the effectiveness of interventions designed to reduce or eliminate pica behavior; none of these include pregnant women. Studies are needed on the effectiveness of behavior modification strategies for specific types of pica. Given the frequency of pica among some immigrant populations, culturally specific interventions should be a priority for investigation.

HEALTH POLICY NEEDS

Stronger Occupational Standards for Lead Exposure, Especially for Pregnant Women

Current OSHA policy requires medical evaluations at blood lead levels of 40 µg/dL, and removal from the workplace when blood lead levels exceed 50 µg/dL (for construction) or 60 µg/dL (for general industry). Some industries where workers may be exposed to high levels of lead are not protected by OSHA. Current occupational standards were developed over 30 years ago and have not been updated to reflect research findings that lead exposure during pregnancy is associated with adverse effects on fetal growth and neurodevelopment, maternal health, and an increased risk for spontaneous abortion. Updated standards consistent with the current knowledge about the health effects of lead exposure are needed to provide clear guidance to industry, policy makers, and workers, as well as because medical judgments may be influenced by existing regulations.

- The Occupational Safety and Health Administration Standard for lead exposure should be updated to require that occupationally exposed women who are pregnant be removed from lead exposure if their blood lead level is 10 µg/dL or higher.

- If the blood lead level is in the range of 5 to 9 µg/dL, efforts should be made to identify and reduce lead exposure on the job and review appropriate use of personal protective equipment.

- All lead-exposed workers who have the potential to be exposed by lead ingestion, even in the absence of documented elevations in air lead levels, should be under medical surveillance.

- Lead exposure should be regulated in categories of workers currently not covered by the OSHA standard.

Regulation of Alternative Medicines and Dietary Supplements to Ensure Product Safety and Accuracy in Labeling and Marketing

National policy is needed to establish regulatory mechanisms to control the safety and quality of alternative medicines and dietary supplements sold commercially in the United States.

- Health claims for alternative medicines and dietary supplements should meet the same rigorous criteria as claims by drugs used to prevent or treat disease.

- Regulatory standards for the content, labeling, and marketing of such products should be established and enforced.

- The Federal Trade Commission, in cooperation with FDA, should ensure that advertising for dietary supplements is accurate and not misleading.

Regulatory Authority to Require Lead Safety in Dwellings Occupied by Pregnant Women and Resources to Control Lead Hazards in These Units

State and local health or housing agencies should have the statutory authority to require and enforce lead paint hazard abatement in rental housing where pregnant women reside, to allow parents to bring their babies home to safe housing. Such statutes should also have provisions to protect pregnant tenants from retaliatory eviction by property owners unwilling to comply. Jurisdictions should also have public resources available to control lead hazards in those units where private resources are unattainable. [See Chapter 11 for information on lead safety resources.]

Mandatory Reporting of All Adult Blood Lead Levels

Public health agencies need to be informed of blood lead testing results on adults in order to identify and investigate new community exposure sources, monitor epidemiological trends, and assure appropriate interventions for identified cases, including environmental inspection and case management services. Laboratories should be required to report all blood lead level test results on adults to the health department, preferably in standard electronic form. Such reporting could enable health departments to identify pregnant women with lead exposure above background levels for priority interventions.

Reimbursement for Blood Lead Testing and Follow-Up Care for Uninsured Pregnant and Lactating Women and Their Infants

Blood lead testing and follow up services (including case management, nutritional interventions, chelation therapy, and environmental investigation) are essential to appropriate medical management of pregnant and lactating women with lead exposure above background levels. However, a lack of insurance can be prohibitive to proper care for many women. In addition, such services may not be covered by insurance for documented immigrants during their first 5 years of residence in the United States or at all for undocumented immigrants. The State Children's Health Insurance Program allows the use of federal funds for prenatal services to women regardless of immigration status in order to ensure the health of the fetus. States should use these funds for services necessary to reduce or treat lead exposure above background levels during the woman's pregnancy and lactation.

Sharing of Clinical Data Via Electronic Health Records

Proper medical management of pregnant or lactating women with lead exposure above background levels and their infants requires that the medical records of both mother and child contain relevant data related to lead. For example, the infant's chart should contain information about the mother's blood lead level at birth and about identified environmental sources. Likewise, the mother's chart should contain information about the infant's blood lead level. However, such records are likely to be maintained by diferrent health care providers and complicated by differing records systems, the possibility of different maternal/child surnames, etc. The adoption of electronic medical records would permit an automated linkage of the two charts to ensure that appropriate data can be transmitted to the other chart.

HEALTH EDUCATION NEEDS

Continuing Medical Education on Lead and Pregnancy

Continuing Medical Education (CME) training on lead and pregnancy is needed to familiarize health care providers with this current research base and clinical recommendations. CDC, in consultation and cooperation with medical specialty associations (e.g., ACOG, AAP, American Academy of Family Physicians), nursing associations (e.g., American Nurses' Association, American College of Nurse Midwives), and environmental health associations should develop a training course module on lead and pregnancy or alternatively incorporate a discussion of lead exposure and pregnancy into preexisting educational materials, such as the Agency for Toxic Substances and Disease Registry's *Case Studies in Environmental Medicine*, which can be taken for continuing education credit. The training should include information on evaluating risk factors for lead exposure as part of an occupational, environmental, and lifestyle health risk assessment.

Environmental Health Requirement in Basic Practitioner's Curriculum

Pediatric medical and nursing education currently lacks sufficient environmental health content necessary to prepare pediatric health care professionals to prevent, recognize, manage, and treat environmental exposure related disease including lead exposure during pregnancy. Thus, educational opportunities for physicians, nurses, environmental engineers, and other practitioners during their training are needed. Such courses should also incorporate material on cultural competency and health literacy. The Pediatric Environmental Health Specialty Units (PEHSUs) and CDC's provider education series are appropriate vehicles for these courses. CDC and the PEHSUs should coordinate publications and educational offerings with ACOG, AAP, the American Academy of Family Physicians, and the American College of Nurse Midwives.

Preconceptional Counseling on Lead Exposure for Adults of Childbearing Age

Primary and reproductive health care providers should provide counseling to patients of childbearing age about the effects of lead on fertility, pregnancy, and infant outcomes. They should educate their patients about possible lead exposure sources and how to reduce exposure in advance of conception. Such counseling should include referrals to appropriate sources for further assistance in assessing and reducing environmental or occupational lead expsosures. CDC should collaborate with the national professional health organizations, such as the American College of Obstetricians and Gynecologists, American Medical Association, and The American Academy of Family Physicians, and nonprofit organizations, such as the March of Dimes, to develop and disseminate educational materials to convey these messages.

Expand Resources for National Centralized Data Collection and Management Facility

A comprehensive online system is needed to improve dissemination of data on various sources of lead to medical and public health providers and the community. Such a system would provide real-time product identification information to alert providers and the communities at risk for exposure. It would also allow agencies that are testing products (e.g., CPSC, FDA, State of California) to enter information on tainted products into one easily accessible database.

Evaluate the Effectiveness of Currently Available Personal Protective Equipment

The capacity of available personal protective equipment to keep BLLs below 5 µg/dL is an area of needed research. Such studies should also inform the creation of more sophisticated equipment that can ensure that BLLs of workers remain below 5 µg/dL.

CHAPTER 11. RESOURCES AND REFERRAL INFORMATION

Contact information is provided here for key information sources for topics covered in this report. While not an exhaustive list, these resources provide a useful starting point for readers interested in updates, publications, referrals, or additional information.

For information on lead poisoning prevention, including screening, case management, and referrals to state and local lead poisoning prevention programs:

Centers for Disease Control and Prevention (CDC)
Healthy Homes and Lead Poisoning Prevention Branch
4770 Buford Highway NE, Mailstop F-60
Atlanta, GA 30341
(770) 488-3300
http://www.cdc.gov/nceh/lead/

See especially:

☑ Current statement on children, including literature review on low-level health effects in children

☑ Current recommendations for case management of children with elevated blood lead levels

☑ Reports on lead sources and epidemiology

☑ Links to state and local lead poisoning prevention programs

☑ Links to information about recalls of consumer products with lead (or see http://www.cpsc.gov or http://www.fda.gov)

For information on occupational and environmental health resources, expert contacts, and clinic locations nationwide:

American College of Medical Toxicology
10645 N. Tatum Blvd.
Suite 200-111
Phoenix, AZ 85028
Phone: (623) 533-6340
Fax: (623) 533-6340
E-mail: info@acmt.net
http://www.acmt.net

Association of Occupational and Environmental Clinics (AOEC)
1010 Vermont Ave., NW #513
Washington, DC 20005
(202) 347-4976 or Toll Free 888-347-2632
http://www.aoec.org

National Institute for Occupational Safety and Health (NIOSH)
http://www.cdc.gov/niosh/
Occupational Safety and Health Administration (OSHA), U.S. Department of Labor
http://www.osha.gov/SLTC/lead/

Pediatric Environmental Health Specialty Units (PEHSU)
c/o Association of Occupational and Environmental Clinics
1010 Vermont Ave. NW, #513
Washington, DC 20005
888-347-AOEC (888-347-2632)
http://aoec.org/PEHSU/index.html

For information on nutritional support for eligible women and infants, including state contact information:

The Special Supplemental Nutrition Program for Women, Infants and Children (WIC)
Food and Nutrition Service, U.S. Department of Agriculture
http://www.fns.usda.gov/wic/

For information about lead-safe housing, including lead-based paint, renovation, and repainting:

U.S. EPA brochure titled Reducing Lead Hazards When Remodeling Your Home, available at http://www.epa.gov/lead/pubs/rrpamph.pdf

U.S. Department of Housing and Urban Development publication titled Lead Paint Safety Field Guide, available at http://www.hud.gov/offices/lead/library/lead/LeadGuide_Eng.pdf

National Center for Healthy Housing (formerly the National Center for Lead-Safe Housing)
http://www.centerforhealthyhousing.org/html/resources_page.htm

Alliance for Healthy Homes
http://www.afhh.org/res/res_by_topic_lead.htm

For information on lead and drinking water:

Data on local drinking water

http://www.epa.gov/safewater/dwinfo/index.html

Laboratories certified to test for contaminants in drinking water
http://www.epa.gov/safewater/faq/sco.html

National Ground Water Association (for issues related to water quality from private wells)
http://www.wellowner.org

U.S. EPA fact sheets for lead in water http://www.epa.gov/safewater/lead/leadfactsheet.html
http://www.epa.gov/safewater/lead/pdfs/v2final.pdf

For general information about lead poisoning (for consumers or professionals):

National Lead Information Center (NLIC)
1-800-424-LEAD (5323).
Monday through Friday, 8:00 am to 6:00 pm eastern time (except federal holidays)
http://www.epa.gov/lead/pubs/nlic.htm

Office of Healthy Homes and Lead Hazard Control
U.S. Department of Housing and Urban Development
http://www.hud.gov/offices/lead/healthyhomes/lead.cfm

Office of Pollution Prevention and Toxics
U.S. Environmental Protection Agency
http://www.epa.gov/lead/

U.S. Consumer Product Safety Commission – product recalls and safety alerts
http://www.cpsc.gov/

U.S. Food and Drug Administration – product recalls, market withdrawals, and safety alerts
http:// http://www.fda.gov/opacom/7alerts.html

CHAPTER 1 – INTRODUCTION

Albalak R, Noonan G, Buchanan S, Flanders WD, Gotway-Crawford C, Kim D, et al. 2003. Blood lead levels and risk factors for lead poisoning among children in Jakarta, Indonesia. Sci Total Environ 301(1-3):75-85.

American Community Survey. 2004. United States General Demographic Characteristics: 2004. Washington, DC: U.S. Census Bureau.

Barry PS. 1975. A comparison of concentrations of lead in human tissues. Br J Ind Med 32(2):119-39.

Barry PS, Mossman DB. 1970. Lead concentrations in human tissues. Br J Ind Med 27(4):339-51.

Bellinger DC. 2005. Teratogen update: lead and pregnancy. Birth Defects Res A Clin Mol Teratol 73(6):409-20.

Calvert GM, Roscoe RJ. 2007. Lead exposure among females of childbearing age—United States, 2004. MMWR Morb Mortal Wkly Rep 56(16):397-400.

Canfield RL, Henderson CR Jr, Cory-Slechta DA, Cox C, Jusko TA, Lanphear BP. 2003. Intellectual impairment in children with blood lead concentrations below 10 [micro]g per deciliter. N Engl J Med 348(16): 1517-1526.

Centers for Disease Control and Prevention 2004. Lead poisoning associated with ayurvedic medications—five states, 2000-2003. MMWR Morb Mortal Wkly Rep 53(26);582-4.

Crocetti AF, Mushak P, Schwartz J. 1990. Determination of numbers of lead-exposed women of childbearing age and pregnant women: an integrated summary of a report to the U.S. Congress on childhood lead poisoning. Environ Health Perspect 89:121-4.

Garcia Vargas GG, Rubio Andrade M, Del Razo LM, Borja Aburto V, Vera Aguilar E, Cebrian ME. 2001. Lead exposure in children living in a smelter community in region Lagunera, Mexico. J Toxicol Environ Health 62(6): 417-29.

Graber N, Gabinskaya T, Forman J, Gertner M. 2006. Prenatal lead exposure in New York City immigrant communities [poster]. In: Pediatric Academic Societies (PAS) 2006 Annual Meeting, April 29-May 3, 2006, San Francisco.

Gulson BL, Mizon KJ, Korsch MJ, Palmer JM, Donnelly JB. 2003. Mobilization of lead from human bone tissue during pregnancy and lactation—a summary of long-term research. Sci Total Environ 303(1-2):79-104.

Hackley B, Katz-Jacobson A. 2003. Lead poisoning in pregnancy: a case study with implications for midwives. J Midwifery Womens Health 48(1):30-38.

Jacobs DE, Clickner RP, Zhou JY, Viet SM, Marker DA, Rogers JW, et al. 2002. The prevalence of lead-based paint hazards in U.S. housing. Environ Health Perspect 110(10):A599-606.

Jusko TA, Henderson CR, Lanphear BP, Cory-Slechta DA, Parsons PJ, Canfield RL. 2008. Blood lead concentrations < 10 microg/dL and child intelligence at 6 years of age. Environ Health Perspect 116(2):243-8.

Klitzman S, Sharma A, Nicaj L, Vitkevich R, Leighton J. 2002. Lead poisoning among pregnant women in New York City: risk factors and screening practices. J Urban Health 79(2):225-37.

Lanphear BP, Hornung R, Khoury J, Yolton K, Baghurst P, Bellinger DC, et al. 2005. Low-level environmental lead exposure and children's intellectual function: an international pooled analysis. Environ Health Perspect 113(7):894-9.

Marino PE, Landrigan PJ, Graef J, Nussbaum A, Bayan G, Boch K, et al. 1990. A case report of lead paint poisoning during renovation of a Victorian farmhouse. Am J Public Health 80(10):1183-5.

Menke A, Muntner P, Batuman V, Silbergeld E, Guallar E. 2006. Blood lead below 0.48 μmol/L (10 μg/dL) and mortality among US adults. Circulation (114):1388-94.

Minnesota Department of Health. 2004. Blood lead screening guidelines for pregnant women in Minnesota. St. Paul, Minnesota: Minnesota Department of Health.

Navas-Acien A, Guallar E, Silbergeld EK, Rothenberg, SJ. 2007. Lead exposure and cardiovascular disease—a systematic Review. Environ Health Perspect (115):472–82.

New York City Department of Health and Mental Hygiene. 2006. Guidelines for the identification and management of pregnant women with elevated lead levels in New York City. New York, NY: Lead Poisoning Prevention Program.

Roberts JS, Silbergeld EK. 1995. Pregnancy, lactation, and menopause: how physiology and gender affect the toxicity of chemicals. Mt Sinai J Med 62(5):343-55.

Shannon M. 2003. Severe lead poisoning in pregnancy. Ambul Pediatr 3(1):37-9.

Saper RB, Kales SN, Paquin J, Burns MJ, Eisenberg DM, Davis RB, et al. 2004. Heavy metal content of ayurvedic herbal medicine products. JAMA 292(23):2868-73.

Saper RB, Phillips RS, Sehgal A, Khouri N, Davis RB, Paquin J, et al. 2008. Lead, mercury, and arsenic in US- and Indian-manufactured ayurvedic medicines sold via the Internet. JAMA 300:915-23.

Tellez-Rojo MM, Bellinger DC, Arroyo-Quiroz C, Lamadrid-Figueroa H, Mercado-Garcia A, Schnaas-Arrieta L, et al. 2006. Longitudinal associations between blood lead concentrations lower than 10 microg/dL and neurobehavioral development in environmentally exposed children in Mexico City. Pediatrics 118(2):e323-30.

CHAPTER 2 – ADVERSE HEALTH EFFECTS OF LEAD EXPOSURE IN PREGNANCY

Agency for Toxic Substances and Disease Registry. 2007. Toxicological profile for Lead. Atlanta, GA: U.S. Department of Health and Human Services.

Andrews KW, Savitz DA, Hertz-Picciotto I. 1994. Prenatal lead exposure in relation to gestational age and birth weight: a review of epidemiologic studies. Am J Ind Med 26(1):13-32.

Apostoli P, Kiss P, Porru S, Bonde JP, Vanhoorne M. 1998. Male reproductive toxicity of lead in animals and humans. ASCLEPIOS Study Group. Occup Environ Med 55(6):364-74.

Baghurst PA, McMichael AJ, Wigg NR, Vimpani GV, Robertson EF, Roberts RJ, et al. 1992. Environmental exposure to lead and children's intelligence at the age of seven years: the Port Pirie study. N Engl J Med 327(18):1279-84.

Barker DJ. 1990. The fetal and infant origins of adult disease. Br Med J 17;301(6761):1111.

Barker DJ. 1995. Fetal origins of coronary heart disease. Br Med J 311:171-4.

Bearer CF. 1995. How are children different from adults? Environ Health Perspect 103 Suppl 6:7-12.

Bellinger DC. 2004. Lead. Pediatrics 113(4 Suppl):1016-22.

Bellinger D, Leviton A, Waternaux C, Needleman H, Rabinowitz M. 1987. Longitudinal analysis of prenatal and postnatal lead exposure and early cognitive development. N Engl J Med. 316(17):1037-43.

Bellinger D, Leviton A, Sloman J. 1990. Antecedents and correlates of improved cognitive performance in children exposed *in utero* to low levels of lead. Environ Health Perspect 89:5-11.

Bellinger DC, Needleman HL. 2003. Intellectual impairment and blood lead levels. N Engl J Med 349(5):500-2.

Bellinger DC, Stiles KM, Needleman HL. 1992. Low-level lead exposure, intelligence and academic achievement: a long-term follow-up study. Pediatrics 90(6):855-61.

Borja-Aburto VH, Hertz-Picciotto I, Rojas Lopez M, Farias P, Rios C, Blanco J. 1999. Blood lead levels measured prospectively and risk of spontaneous abortion. Am J Epidemiol 150(6):590-7.

Bound JP, Harvey PW, Francis BJ, Awwad F, Gatrell AC. 1997. Involvement of deprivation and environmental lead in neural tube defects: a matched case-control study. Arch Dis Child 76(2):107-12.

Bressler JP, Goldstein GW. 1991. Mechanisms of lead neurotoxicity. Biochem Pharmacol 41(4):479-84.

Burns JM, Baghurst PA, Sawyer MG, McMichael AJ, Tong SL. 1999. Lifetime low-level exposure to environmental lead and children's emotional and behavioral development at ages 11-13 years. the Port Pirie Cohort Study. Am J Epidemiol 149(8):740-9.

Canfield RL, Henderson CR Jr, Cory-Slechta DA, Cox C, Jusko TA, Lanphear BP. 2003. Intellectual impairment in children with blood lead concentrations below 10 [micro]g per deciliter. N Engl J Med 348(16): 1517-26.

Centers for Disease Control and Prevention. 2004. A review of evidence of health effects of blood lead levels <10 µg/dl in children. Review of evidence for Adverse Effects at Lower Blood Lead Levels Work Group of the Advisory Committee on Childhood Lead Poisoning Prevention (ACCLPP). Atlanta: U.S. Department of Health and Human Services.

Cooney GH, Bell A, McBride W, Carter C. 1989a. Low level exposure to lead: the Sydney lead study. Dev Med Child Neurol 31(5):640-9.

Cooney GH, Bell A, McBride W, Carter C. 1989b. Neurobehavioral consequences of prenatal low level exposure to lead. Neurotox Teratol 11:95-104.

Cory-Slechta DA. 1997. Relationships between Pb-induced changes in neurotransmitter system function and behavioral toxicity. Neurotoxicology 18(3):673-88.

Costa LG, Aschner M, Vitalone A, Syversen T, Soldin OP. 2004. Developmental neuropathology of environmental agents. Annu Rev Pharmacol Toxicol 44:87-110.

Dawson EB, Evans DR, Kelly R, Van Hook JW. 2000. Blood cell lead, calcium, and magnesium levels associated with pregnancy-induced hypertension and preeclampsia. Biol Trace Elem Res 74(2):107-16.

Dietrich KN, Berger OG, Succop PA, Hammond PB, Bornschein RL. 1993. The developmental consequences of low to moderate prenatal and postnatal lead exposure: intellectual attainment in the Cincinnati lead study cohort following school entry. Neurotoxicol Teratol 15:37-44.

Dietrich KN, Krafft KM, Bornschein RL, Hammond PB, Berger O, et al. 1987a. Low-level fetal lead exposure effect on neurobehavioral development in early infancy. Pediatrics 80(5):721-30.

Dietrich KN, Krafft KM, Shukla R, Bornschein RL, Succop PA. 1987b. The neurobehavioral effects of early lead exposure. Monogr Am Assoc Ment Defic 8:71-95.

Dietrich KN, Ris MD, Succop PA, Berger OG, Bornschein RL. 2001. Early exposure to lead and juvenile delinquency. Neurotoxicol Teratol 23(6):511-18.

Dietrich KN, Succop PA, Bornschein RL, Krafft KM, Berger O, Hammond PB, et al. 1990. Lead exposure and neurobehavioral development in later infancy. Environ Health Perspect 89:13-9.

Dietrich KN, Ware JH, Salganik M, Radcliffe J, Rogan WJ, Rhoads GG, et al. 2004. Effect of chelation therapy on the neuropsychological and behavioral development of lead-exposed children after school entry. Pediatrics 114(1):19-26.

Ernhart CB, Morrow-Tlucak M, Marler MR, Wolf AW. 1987. Low level lead exposure in the prenatal and early preschool periods: early preschool development. Neurotoxicol Teratol 9(3):259-70.

Ernhart CB, Morrow-Tlucak M, Wolf AW, Super D, Drotar D. 1989. Low level lead exposure in the prenatal and early preschool periods: Intelligence prior to school entry. Neurotoxicol Teratol 11:161-70.

Fergusson DM, Horwood LJ, Lynskey MT. 1997. Early dentine lead levels and educational outcomes at 18 years. J Child Psychol Psychiatry 38(4):471-8.

Goldstein GW. 1990. Lead poisoning and brain cell function. Environ Health Perspect 89:91-4.

Goldstein GW. 1992. Neurologic concepts of lead poisoning in children. Pediatr Ann 21(6):384-8.

Gomaa A, Hu H, Bellinger D, Schwartz J, Tsaih SW, Gonzalez-Cossio T, et al. 2002. Maternal bone lead as an independent risk factor for fetal neurotoxicity: a prospective study. Pediatrics 110(1 Pt 1):110-8.

Gonzalez-Cossio T, Peterson KE, Sanin LH, Fishbein E, Palazuelos E, Aro A, et al. 1997. Decrease in birth weight in relation to maternal bone-lead burden. Pediatrics 100(5):856-62.

Greene T, Ernhart CB. 1991. Prenatal and preschool age lead exposure: relationship with size. Neurotoxicol Teratol 13(4):417-27.

Guerra-Tamayo JL, Hernandez-Cadena L, Tellez-Rojo MM, Mercado-Garcia Adel S, Solano-Gonzalez M, Hernandez-Avila M, et al. 2003. [Time to pregnancy and lead exposure]. Salud Publica Mex 45 Suppl 2:S189-95.

Guilarte TR, Miceli RC, Jett DA. 1994. Neurochemical aspects of hippocampal and cortical Pb2+ neurotoxicity. Neurotoxicology 15(3):459-66.

Gump BB, Stewart P, Reihman J, Lonky E, Darvill T, Parsons PJ, et al. 2008. Low-level prenatal and postnatal blood lead exposure and adrenocortical responses to acute stress in children. Environ Health Perspect 116(2):249-55.

Hernandez-Avila M, Peterson KE, Gonzalez-Cossio T, Sanin LH, Aro A, Schnaas L, et al. 2002. Effect of maternal bone lead on length and head circumference of newborns and 1-month-old infants. Arch Environ Health 57(5):482-8.

Hertz-Picciotto I. 2000. The evidence that lead increases the risk for spontaneous abortion. Am J Ind Med 38(3):300-9.

Hertz-Picciotto I, Croft J. 1993. Review of the relation between blood lead and blood pressure. Epidemiol Rev 15(2):352-73.

Hu H, Tellez-Rojo MM, Bellinger D, Smith D, Ettinger AS, Lamadrid-Figueroa H, et al. 2006. Fetal lead exposure at each stage of pregnancy as a predictor of infant mental development. Environ Health Perspect 114(11):1730-5.

Ingelfinger JR, Schnaper HW. 2005. Renal endowment: developmental origins of adult disease. J Am Soc Nephrol 16(9):2533-6.

Irgens A, Kruger K, Skorve AH, Irgens LM. 1998. Reproductive outcome in offspring of parents occupationally exposed to lead in Norway. Am J Ind Med 34(5):431-7.

Jackson LW, Correa-Villasenor A, Lees PS, Dominici F, Stewart PA, Breysse PN, et al. 2004. Parental lead exposure and total anomalous pulmonary venous return. Birth Defects Res 70(4):185-93.

Jedrychowski W, Perera F, Jankowski J, Rauh V, Flak E, Caldwell KL, et al. 2008. Prenatal low-level lead exposure and developmental delay of infants at age 6 months (Krakow inner city study). Int J Hyg Environ Health 211(3-4):345-51. Epub 2007 Oct 1.

Jensen TK, Bonde JP, Joffe M. 2006. The influence of occupational exposure on male reproductive function. Occup Med (Lond) 56(8):544-53.

Jusko TA, Henderson CR, Lanphear BP, Cory-Slechta DA, Parsons PJ, Canfield RL. 2008. blood lead concentrations < 10 mug/dl and child intelligence at 6 years of age. Environ Health Perspect 116(2):243-8.

Karumanchi SA, Maynard SE, Stillman IE, Epstein FH, Sukhatme VP. 2005. Preeclampsia: a renal perspective. Kidney Int 67(6):2101-13.

Khan IY, Lakasing L, Poston L, Nicolaides KH. 2003. Fetal programming for adult disease: where next? J Matern Fetal Neonatal Med. 2003 13(5):292-9.

Kordas K, Canfield RL, Lopez P, Rosado JL, Vargas GG, Cebrian ME, et al. 2006. Deficits in cognitive function and achievement in Mexican first-graders with low blood lead concentrations. Environ Res 100(3):371-86.

Kosnett MJ, Wedeen RP, Rothenberg SJ, Hipkins KL, Materna BL, Schwartz BS, et al. 2007. Recommendations for medical management of adult lead exposure. Environ Health Perspect 115(3):463-71.

Lamadrid-Figueroa H, Tellez-Rojo MM, Hernandez-Avila M, Trejo-Valdivia B, Solano-Gonzalez M, Mercado-Garcia A, et al. 2007. Association between the plasma/whole blood lead ratio and history of spontaneous abortion: a nested cross-sectional study. BMC Pregnancy Childbirth 7:22.

Lanphear BP, Dietrich K, Auinger P, Cox C. 2000. Cognitive deficits associated with blood lead concentrations <10 microg/dL in US children and adolescents. Public Health Rep 115(6):521-9.

Lanphear BP, Hornung R, Khoury J, Yolton K, Baghurst P, Bellinger DC, et al. 2005. Low-level environmental lead exposure and children's intellectual function: an international pooled analysis. Environ Health Perspect 113(7):894-9.

Laudanski T, Sipowicz M, Modzelewski P, Bolinski J, Szamatowicz J, Razniewska G, et al. 1991. Influence of high lead and cadmium soil content on human reproductive outcome. Int J Gynaecol Obstet 36(4):309-15.

Lindbohm ML, Taskinen H, Kyyronen P, Sallmen M, Anttila A, Hemminki K. 1992. Effects of parental occupational exposure to solvents and lead on spontaneous abortion. Scand J Work Environ Health 18 Suppl 2:37-9.

Magri J, Sammut M, Savona-Ventura C. 2003. Lead and other metals in gestational hypertension. Int J Gynaecol Obstet 83(1):29-36.

McMichael AJ, Baghurst PA, Wigg NR, Vimpani GV, Robertson EF, Roberts RJ. 1988. Port Pirie Cohort Study: environmental exposure to lead and children's abilities at the age of four years. N Engl J Med 319(8):468-75.

McMichael AJ, Vimpani GV, Robertson EF, Baghurst PA, Clark PD. 1986. The Port Pirie cohort study: maternal blood lead and pregnancy outcome. J Epidemiol Commun Health 40(1):18-25.

Murphy MJ, Graziano JH, Popovac D, Kline JK, Mehmeti A, Factor-Litvak P, et al. 1990. Past pregnancy outcomes among women living in the vicinity of a lead smelter in Kosovo, Yugoslavia. Am J Public Health 80(1):33-5.

National High Blood Pressure Education Program Working Group. 2000. Report of the National High Blood Pressure Education Program Working Group on High Blood Pressure in Pregnancy. Am J Obstet Gynecol 183(1):S1-S22.

Needleman HL, Rabinowitz M, Leviton A, Linn S, Schoenbaum S. 1984. The relationship between prenatal exposure to lead and congenital anomalies. JAMA 251(22):2956-9.

Opler MG, Brown AS, Graziano J, Desai M, Zheng W, Schaefer C, et al. 2004. Prenatal lead exposure, delta-aminolevulinic acid, and schizophrenia. Environ Health Perspect 112(5):548-52.

Opler MG, Buka SL, Groeger J, McKeague I, Wei C, Factor-Litvak P, et al. 2008. Prenatal exposure to lead, delta-aminolevulinic acid, and schizophrenia: further evidence. Environ Health Perspect 116(11):1586-90. Epub 2008 Jul 30.

Rabinowitz M, Bellinger D, Leviton A, Needleman H, Schoenbaum S. 1987. Pregnancy hypertension, blood pressure during labor, and blood lead levels. Hypertension 10(4):447-51.

Ris MD, Dietrich KN, Succop PA, Berger OG, Bornschein RL. 2004. Early exposure to lead and neuropsychological outcome in adolescence. J Int Neuropsychol Soc 10(2):261-70.

Rodier PM. 1995. Developing brain as a target of toxicity. Environ Health Perspect 103(Suppl 6):73-6.

Rodier PM. 2004. Environmental causes of central nervous system maldevelopment. Pediatrics 113 (4 Suppl):1076-83.

Rogan WJ, Dietrich KN, Ware JH, Dockery DW, Salganik M, Radcliffe J, et al. 2001. The effect of chelation therapy with succimer on neuropsychological development in children exposed to lead. N Engl J Med 344(19):1421-6.

Rothenberg SJ, Kondrashov V, Manalo M, Jiang J, Cuellar R, Garcia M, et al. 2002. Increases in hypertension and blood pressure during pregnancy with increased bone lead levels. Am J Epidemiol 156(12):1079-87.

Rothenberg SJ, Manalo M, Jiang J, Cuellar R, Reyes S, Sanchez M, et al. 1999. Blood lead level and blood pressure during pregnancy in South Central Los Angeles. Arch Environ Health 54(6):382-9.

Rothenberg SJ, Poblano A, Garza-Morales S. 1994. Prenatal and perinatal low level lead exposure alters brainstem auditory evoked responses in infants. Neurotoxicology 15(3): 695-699.

Rothenberg SJ, Poblano A, Schnaas L. 2000. Brainstem auditory evoked response at five years and prenatal and postnatal blood lead. Neurotoxicol Teratol 22(4):503-10.

Rothenberg SJ, Schnaas L, Cansino-Ortiz S, Perroni-Hernandez E, de la Torre P, Neri-Mendez C, et al. 1989. Neurobehavioral deficits after low level lead exposure in neonates: the Mexico City pilot study. Neurotoxicol Teratol 11(2): 85-93.

Sallmen M, Anttila A, Lindbohm ML, Kyyronen P, Taskinen H, Hemminki K. 1995. Time to pregnancy among women occupationally exposed to lead. J Occup Environ Med 37(8):931-4.

Sanin LH, Gonzalez-Cossio T, Romieu I, Peterson KE, Ruiz S, Palazuelos E, et al. 2001. Effect of maternal lead burden on infant weight and weight gain at one month of age among breastfed infants. Pediatrics 107(5):1016-23.

Schnaas L, Rothenberg SJ, Flores MF, Martinez S, Hernandez C, Osorio E, et al. 2006. Reduced intellectual development in children with prenatal lead exposure. Environ Health Perspect 114(5):791-7.

Selevan SG, Rice DC, Hogan KA, Euling SY, Pfahles-Hutchens A, Bethel J. 2003. Blood lead concentration and delayed puberty in girls. N Engl J Med 348(16):1527-36.

Shen XM, Yan CH, Guo D, Wu SM, Li RQ, Huang H, et al. 1998. Low-level prenatal lead exposure and neurobehavioral development of children in the first year of life: a prospective study in Shanghai. Environ Res 79(1):1-8.

Shukla R, Bornschein RL, Dietrich KN, Buncher CR, Berger OG, Hammond PB, et al. 1989. Fetal and infant lead exposure: effects on growth in stature. Pediatrics 84(4):604-12.

Sowers M, Jannausch M, Scholl T, Li W, Kemp FW, Bogden JD. 2002. Blood lead concentrations and pregnancy outcomes. Arch Environ Health 57(5):489-95.

Tabacova S, Balabaeva L. 1993. Environmental pollutants in relation to complications of pregnancy. Environ Health Perspect 101(Suppl 2):27-31.

Tabacova S, Little RE, Balabaeva L, Pavlova S, Petrov I. 1994. Complications of pregnancy in relation to maternal lipid peroxides, glutathione, and exposure to metals. Reprod Toxicol 8(3):217-24.

Takser L, Mergler D, Lafond J. 2005. Very low level environmental exposure to lead and prolactin levels during pregnancy. Neurotoxicol Teratol 27(3):505-8.

Tellez-Rojo MM, Bellinger DC, Arroyo-Quiroz C, Lamadrid-Figueroa H, Mercado-Garcia A, Schnaas-Arrieta L, et al. 2006. Longitudinal associations between blood lead concentrations lower than 10 microg/dL and neurobehavioral development in environmentally exposed children in Mexico City. Pediatrics 118(2):e323-30.

Tellez-Rojo MM, Hernandez-Avila M, Lamadrid-Figueroa H, Smith D, Hernandez-Cadena L, Mercado A, et al. 2004. Impact of bone lead and bone resorption on plasma and whole blood lead levels during pregnancy. Am J Epidemiol 160(7):668-78.

Tong S, Baghurst P, McMichael A, Sawyer M, Mudge J. 1996. Lifetime exposure to environmental lead and children's intelligence at 11-13 years: the Port Pirie cohort study. Br Med J 312(7046):1569-75.

Tong S, Baghurst PA, Sawyer MG, Burns J, McMichael AJ. 1998. Declining blood lead levels and changes in cognitive function during childhood: the Port Pirie Cohort Study. JAMA 280(22):1915-9.

Torres-Sanchez LE, Berkowitz G, Lopez-Carrillo L, Torres-Arreola L, Rios C, Lopez-Cervantes M. 1999. Intrauterine lead exposure and preterm birth. Environ Res 81(4):297-301.

U.S. Environmental Protection Agency. 1991. Maximum contaminant level goals and national primary drinking water regulations for lead and copper; final rule. Fed Reg 56(11):26460-4.

U.S. Environmental Protection Agency. 2006. Air quality criteria for lead (2006) final report. Washington, DC: U.S. Environmental Protection Agency. EPA/600/R-05/144aF-bF.

Vaziri ND, Sica DA. 2004. Lead-induced hypertension: role of oxidative stress. Curr Hypertens Rep 6(4):314-20.

Vigeh M, Yokoyama K, Mazaheri M, Beheshti S, Ghazizadeh S, Sakai T, et al. 2004. Relationship between increased blood lead and pregnancy hypertension in women without occupational lead exposure in Tehran, Iran. Arch Environ Health 59(2):70-5.

Vigeh M, Yokoyama K, Ramezanzadeh F, Dahaghin M, Sakai T, Morita Y, et al. 2006. Lead and other trace metals in preeclampsia: a case-control study in Tehran, Iran. Environ Res 100(2):268-75.

Wasserman GA, Liu X, Popovac D, Factor-Litvak P, Kline J, Waternaux C, et al. 2000. The Yugoslavia prospective lead study: contributions of prenatal and postnatal lead exposure to early intelligence. Neurotoxicol Teratol 22(6):811-8.

Weiss B, Landrigan PJ. 2000. The developing brain and the environment: an introduction. Environ Health Perspect 108 (Suppl 3):373-4.

White LD, Cory-Slechta DA, Gilbert ME, Tiffany-Castiglioni E, Zawia NH, Virgolini M, et al. 2007. New and evolving concepts in the neurotoxicology of lead. Toxicol Appl Pharmacol 225(1):1-27.

Wigg NR, Vimpani GV, McMichael AJ, Baghurst PA, Robertson EF, Roberts RJ. 1988. Port Pirie cohort study: Childhood blood lead and neuropsychological development at age two years. J Epidemiol Commun Health 42:213-9.

Wright JP, Dietrich KN, Ris MD, Hornung RW, Wessel SD, Lanphear BP, et al. 2008. Association of Prenatal and Childhood Blood Lead Concentrations with Criminal Arrests in Early Adulthood. PLoS Med 5(5):e101.

Wu T, Buck GM, Mendola P. 2003. Blood lead levels and sexual maturation in U.S. girls: the Third National Health and Nutrition Examination Survey, 1988-1994. Environ Health Perspect 111(5):737-41.

CHAPTER 3 – BIOKINETICS AND BIOMARKERS OF LEAD IN PREGNANCY AND LACTATION

Abadin HG, Hibbs BF, Pohl HR. 1997. Breast-feeding exposure of infants to cadmium, lead, and mercury: a public health viewpoint. Toxicol Ind Health 13(4):495-517.

Alexander FW, Delves HT. 1981. Blood lead levels during pregnancy. Int Arch Occup Environ Health 48(1):35-9.

Anderson HA, Wolff MS. 2000. Environmental contaminants in human milk. J Expos Anal Environ Epidemiol 10(6 Pt 2):755-60.

Baghurst PA, Robertson EF, McMichael AJ, Vimpani GV, Wigg NR, Roberts RR. 1987. The Port Pirie cohort study: lead effects on pregnancy outcome and early childhood development. Neurotoxicology 8(3):395-401.

Baghurst PA, Robertson EF, Oldfield RK, King BM, McMichael AJ, Vimpani GV, et al. 1991. Lead in the placenta, membranes, and umbilical cord in relation to pregnancy outcome in a lead-smelter community. Environ Health Perspect 90: 315-20.

Barbosa Jr. F, Tanus-Santos JE, Gerlach RF, Parsons PJ. 2005. A critical review of biomarkers used for monitoring human exposure to lead: advantages, limitations, and future needs. Environ Health Perspect 113(12):1669-74.

Barltrop D. 1969. Environmental lead and its paediatric significance. Postgrad Med J 45(520):129-34.

Barry PS. 1975. A comparison of concentrations of lead in human tissues. Br J Ind Med 32(2):119-39.

Barry PS, Mossman DB. 1970. Lead concentrations in human tissues. Br J Ind Med 27(4):339-51.

Bonithon-Kopp C, Huel G, Grasmick C, Sarmini H, Moreau T. 1986. Effects of pregnancy on the inter-individual variations in blood levels of lead, cadmium and mercury. Biol Res Pregnancy Perinatol 7(1):37-42.

Carbonne R, Laforgia N, Crollo E, Mautone A, Lolascon A. 1998. Maternal and neonatal lead exposure in southern Italy. Biol Neonate 73(6) :362-366.

Cavalleri A, Minoia C, Pozzoli L, Polatti F, Bolis PF. 1978. Lead in red blood cells and in plasma of pregnant women and their offspring. Environ Res 17(3):403-8.

Chatranon W, Chavalittamrong B, Kritalugsana S, Pringsulaka P. 1978. Lead concentrations in breast milk at various stages of lactation. Southeast Asian J Trop Med Public Health 9(3):420-2.

Chuang HY, Schwartz J, Gonzales-Cossio T, Lugo MC, Palazuelos E, Aro A, et al. 2001. Interrelations of lead levels in bone, venous blood, and umbilical cord blood with exogenous lead exposure through maternal plasma lead in peripartum women. Environ Health Perspect 109(5):527-32.

Coni E, Falconieri P, Ferrante E, Semeraro P, Beccaloni E, Stacchini A, et al. 1990. Reference values for essential and toxic elements in human milk. Ann Ist Super Sanita 26(2):119-30.

deSilva PE. 1981. Determination of lead in plasma and studies on its relationship to lead in erythrocytes. Br J Ind Med 38(3):209-17.

Ettinger AS, Tellez-Rojo MM, Amarasiriwardena C, Gonzalez-Cossio T, Peterson KE, Aro A, et al. 2004a. Levels of lead in breast milk and their relation to maternal blood and bone lead levels at one month postpartum. Environ Health Perspect 112(8):926-31.

Ettinger AS, Tellez-Rojo MM, Amarasiriwardena C, Bellinger D, Peterson K, Schwartz J, et al. 2004b. Effect of breast milk lead on infant blood lead levels at 1 month of age. Environ Health Perspect 112(14):1381-5.

Ettinger AS, Tellez-Rojo MM, Amarasiriwardena C, Peterson KE, Schwartz J, Aro A, et al. 2006. Influence of maternal bone lead burden and calcium intake on levels of lead in breast milk over the course of lactation. Am J Epidemiol 163(1):48-56.

Farias P, Borja-Aburto VH, Rios C, Hertz-Picciotto I, Rojas-Lopez M, Chavez-Ayala R. 1996. Blood lead levels in pregnant women of high and low socioeconomic status in Mexico City. Environ Health Perspect 104(10):1070-4.

Franklin CA, Inskip MJ, Baccanale CL, Edwards CM, Manton WI, Edwards E, et al. 1997. Use of sequentially administered stable lead isotopes to investigate changes in blood lead during pregnancy in a nonhuman primate (Macaca fascicularis). Fundam Appl Toxicol 39(2):109-19.

Friel JK, Mercer C, Andrews WL, Simmons BR, Jackson SE, Longerich HP. 1996. Laboratory gloves as a source of trace element contamination. Biol Trace Elem Res 54(2):135-42.

Gershanik JJ, Brooks GG, Little JA. 1974. Blood lead values in pregnant women and their offspring. Am J Obstet Gynecol 119(4):508-11.

Goyer RA. 1990. Transplacental transport of lead. Environ Health Perspect 89:101-5.

Graziano JH, Popovac D, Factor-Litvak P, Shrout P, Kline J, Murphy MJ, et al. 1990. Determinants of elevated blood lead during pregnancy in a population surrounding a lead smelter in Kosovo, Yugoslavia. Environ Health Perspect 89:95-100.

Gulson BL, Jameson CW, Mahaffey KR, Mizon KJ, Korsch MJ, Vimpani G. 1997. Pregnancy increases mobilization of lead from maternal skeleton. J Lab Clin Med 130(1):51-62.

Gulson BL, Mahaffey KR, Jameson CW, Mizon KJ, Korsch MJ, Cameron MA, et al. 1998a. Mobilization of lead from the skeleton during the postnatal period is larger than during pregnancy. J Lab Clin Med 131(4):324-9.

Gulson BL, Jameson CW, Mahaffey KR, Mizon KJ, Patison N, Law AJ, et al. 1998b. Relationships of lead in breast milk to lead in blood, urine, and diet of the infant and mother. Environ Health Perspect 106(10):667-74.

Hallen IP, Jorhem L, Lagerkvist BJ, Oskarsson A. 1995. Lead and cadmium levels in human milk and blood. Sci Total Environ 166:149-55.

Harville EW, Hertz-Picciotto I, Schramm M, Watt-Morse M, Chantala K, Osterloh J, et al. 2005. Factors influencing the difference between maternal and cord blood lead. Occup Environ Med 62(4):263-9.

Hayslip CC, Klein TA, Wray HL, Duncan WE. 1989. The effects of lactation on bone mineral content in healthy postpartum women. Obstet Gynecol 73(4):588-92.

Hernandez-Avila M, Gonzalez-Cossio T, Palazuelos E, Romieu I, Aro A, Fishbein E, et al. 1996. Dietary and environmental determinants of blood and bone lead levels in lactating postpartum women living in Mexico City. Environ Health Perspect 104(10):1076-82.

Hernandez-Avila M, Smith D, Meneses F, Sanin LH, Hu H. 1998. The influence of bone and blood lead on plasma lead levels in environmentally exposed adults. Environ Health Perspect 106(8):473-7.

Hertz-Picciotto I, Schramm M, Watt-Morse M, Chantala K, Anderson J, Osterloh J. 2000. Patterns and determinants of blood lead during pregnancy. Am J Epidemiol 152(9):829-37.

Hu H. 1998. Bone lead as a new biologic marker of lead dose: recent findings and implications for public health. Environ Health Perspect 106 (Suppl 4):961-7.

Hu H, Hashimoto D, Besser M. 1996. Levels of lead in blood and bone of women giving birth in a Boston hospital. Arch Environ Health 51(1):52-8.

Hu H, Hernandez-Avila M. 2002. Invited commentary: lead, bones, women, and pregnancy—the poison within? Am J Epidemiol 156(12):1088-91.

Hu H, Rabinowitz M, Smith D. 1998. Bone lead as a biological marker in epidemiologic studies of chronic toxicity: conceptual paradigms. Environ Health Perspect 106(1):1-8.

Hu H, Tellez-Rojo MM, Bellinger D, Smith D, Ettinger AS, Lamadrid-Figueroa H, et al. 2006. Fetal lead exposure at each stage of pregnancy as a predictor of infant mental development. Environ Health Perspect 114(11):1730-5.

Kehoe RA, Thaman F, Cholak J. 1933. Lead absorption and excretion in relation to the diagnosis of lead poisoning. J Ind Hygiene 15:320.

Knowles JA. 1974. Breast milk: a source of more than nutrition for the neonate. Clin Toxicol 7(1):69-82.

Lamadrid-Figueroa H, Tellez-Rojo MM, Hernandez-Cadena L, Mercado-Garcia A, Smith D, Solano-Gonzalez M, et al. 2006. Biological markers of fetal lead exposure at each stage of pregnancy. J Toxicol Environ Health 69(19):1781-96.

Larsson B, Slorach SA, Hagman U, Hofvander Y. 1981. WHO collaborative breast feeding study. II. Levels of lead and cadmium in Swedish human milk, 1978-1979. Acta Paediatr Scand 70(3):281-4.

Manton WI. 1985. Total contribution of airborne lead to blood lead. Br J Ind Med 42(3):168-72.

Manton WI, Angle CR, Stanek KL, Kuntzelman D, Reese YR, Kuehnemann TJ. 2003. Release of lead from bone in pregnancy and lactation. Environ Res 92(2):139-51.

Manton WI, Cook JD. 1984. High accuracy (stable isotope dilution) measurements of lead in serum and cerebrospinal fluid. Br J Ind Med 41(3):313-9.

Marcus AH. 1985. Multicompartment kinetic models for lead. I. Bone diffusion models for long-term retention. Environ Res 36(2):441-58.

Markowitz ME, Shen XM. 2001. Assessment of bone lead during pregnancy: a pilot study. Environ Res 85(2): 83-9.

Mayer-Popken O, Denkhaus W, Konietzko H. 1986. Lead content of fetal tissues after maternal intoxication. Arch Toxicol 58(3):203-4.

Mendola P, Selevan SG, Gutter S, Rice D. 2002. Environmental factors associated with a spectrum of neurodevelopmental deficits. Ment Retard Dev Disabil Res Rev 8(3):188-97.

Murthy GK, Rhea US. 1971. Cadmium, copper, iron, lead, manganese, and zinc in evaporated milk, infant products, and human milk. J Dairy Sci 54(7):1001-5.

Namihira D, Saldivar L, Pustilnik N, Carreon GJ, Salinas ME. 1993. Lead in human blood and milk from nursing women living near a smelter in Mexico City. J Toxicol Environ Health 38(3):225-32.

Newman J. 1997. Caution regarding nipple shields. J Hum Lact 13(1):12-3.

Ong CN, Phoon WO, Lee BL, Lim LE, Chua LH. 1986. Lead in plasma and its relationships to other biological indicators. Ann Occup Hyg 30(2):219-28.

Osterloh JD, Kelly TJ. 1999. Study of the effect of lactational bone loss on blood lead concentrations in humans. Environ Health Perspect 107(3):187-94.

Rabinowitz M, Leviton A, Needleman H. 1984. Variability of blood lead concentrations during infancy. Arch Environ Health 39(2):74-7.

Rabinowitz MB. 1991. Toxicokinetics of bone lead. Environ Health Perspect 91:33-7.

Rabinowitz MB, Wetherill GW, Kopple JD. 1976. Kinetic analysis of lead metabolism in healthy humans. J Clin Invest 58(2):260-70.

Riess ML, Halm JK. 2007. Lead poisoning in an adult: lead mobilization by pregnancy? J Gen Intern Med 22(8):1212-5.

Roberts JS, Silbergeld EK. 1995. Pregnancy, lactation, and menopause: how physiology and gender affect the toxicity of chemicals. Mt Sinai J Med 62(5):343-55.

Rothenberg SJ, Karchmer S, Schnaas L, Perroni E, Zea F, Fernandez Alba J. 1994. Changes in serial blood lead levels during pregnancy. Environ Health Perspect 102(10): 876-880.

Rothenberg SJ, Karchmer S, Schnaas L, Perroni E, Zea F, Salinas V, et al. 1996. Maternal influences on cord blood lead levels. J Expo Anal Environ Epidemiol 6(2):211-227.

Rothenberg SJ, Khan F, Manalo M, Jiang J, Cuellar R, Reyes S, et al. 2000. Maternal bone lead contribution to blood lead during and after pregnancy. Environ Res 82(1):81-90.

Rothenberg SJ, Schnaas-Arrieta L, Ugartechea JC, Perroni-Hernandez E, Perez-Guerrero IA, Cansino-Prtiz S, et al. 1992. A documented case of perinatal lead poisoning. Am J Public Health 82(4):613-4.

Ryu JE, Ziegler EE, Fomon SJ. 1978. Maternal lead exposure and blood lead concentration in infancy. J Pediatr 93(3):476-8.

Satin KP, Neutra RR, Guirguis G, Flessel P. 1991. Umbilical cord blood lead levels in California. Arch Environ Health 46(3):167-73.

Scanlon J. 1971. Umbilical cord blood lead concentration. Relationship to urban or suburban residency during gestation. Am J Dis Child 121(4):325-6.

Schell LM, Czerwinski S, Stark AD, Parsons PJ, Gomez M, Samelson R. 2000. Variation in blood lead and hematocrit levels during pregnancy in a socioeconomically disadvantaged population. Arch Environ Health 55(2): 134-40.

Schnaas L, Rothenberg SJ, Flores MF, Martinez S, Hernandez C, Osorio E, et al. 2006. Reduced intellectual development in children with prenatal lead exposure. Environ Health Perspect 114(5):791-7.

Shannon M. 2003. Severe lead poisoning in pregnancy. Ambul Pediatr 3(1):37-9.

Silbergeld EK. 1986. Maternally mediated exposure of the fetus: *in utero* exposure to lead and other toxins. Neurotoxicology 7(2):557-68.

Sim MR, McNeil JJ. 1992. Monitoring chemical exposure using breast milk: a methodological review. Am J Epidemiol 136(1):1-11.

Smith DR, Ilustre RP, Osterloh JD. 1998. Methodological considerations for the accurate determination of lead in human plasma and serum. Am J Ind Med 33(5):430-8.

Smith DR, Osterloh JD, Flegal AR. 1996. Use of endogenous, stable lead isotopes to determine release of lead from the skeleton. Environ Health Perspect 104(1):60-6.

Solomon GM, Weiss PM. 2002. Chemical contaminants in breast milk: time trends and regional variability. Environ Health Perspect 110(6):A339-47.

Sowers M. 1996. Pregnancy and lactation as risk factors for subsequent bone loss and osteoporosis. J Bone Miner Res 11(8):1052-60.

Sowers M, Jannausch M, Scholl T, Li W, Kemp FW, Bogden JD. 2002. Blood lead concentrations and pregnancy outcomes. Arch Environ Health 57(5):489-95.

Stacchini A, Coni E, Beccaloni E, Fornarelli L, Alimonti A, Bolis GB, et al. 1989. Criteria for reference value assessment of elements in human tissues. Ann Ist Super Sanita. 25(3):379-84.

Tellez-Rojo MM, Hernandez-Avila M, Gonzalez-Cossio T, Romieu I, Aro A, Palazuelos E, et al. 2002. Impact of breastfeeding on the mobilization of lead from bone. Am J Epidemiol 155(5):420-8.

Tellez-Rojo MM, Hernandez-Avila M, Lamadrid-Figueroa H, Smith D, Hernandez-Cadena L, Mercado A, et al. 2004. Impact of bone lead and bone resorption on plasma and whole blood lead levels during pregnancy. Am J Epidemiol 160(7):668-78.

Thompson GN, Robertson EF, Fitzgerald S. 1985. Lead mobilization during pregnancy. Med J Aust 143(3):131.

Tompsett SL, Anderson AB. 1935. The lead content of human tissues and excreta. Biochem J 29(8):1851-64.

Tsaih SW, Schwartz J, Lee ML, Amarasiriwardena C, Aro A, Sparrow D, et al. 1999. The independent contribution of bone and erythrocyte lead to urinary lead among middle-aged and elderly men: the normative aging study. Environ Health Perspect 107(5):391-6.

CHAPTER 4 – RISK FACTORS AND SOURCES OF LEAD EXPOSURE IN PREGNANT AND LACTATING WOMEN

Abrahams P, Parsons J. 1996. Geophagy in the tropics: a literature review. Geograph J 162:63-72

American Psychiatric Association. 1994. Diagnostic and statistical manual of mental disorders 4th revision: DSM-IV. Washington, DC: American Psychiatric Press.

Anderson H, Islam K. 2006. Trends in occupational and adult lead exposures in Wisconsin 1988-2005. WMJ 105(2):21-5.

Baghurst PA, McMichael AJ, Vimpani GV, Robertson EF, Clark PD, Wigg NR. 1987. Determinants of blood lead concentrations of pregnant women living in Port Pirie and surrounding areas. Med J Aust 146(2):69-73.

Baum CR, Shannon MW. 1997. The lead concentration of reconstituted infant formula. J Toxicol Clin Toxicol 35(4):371-5.

Benin AL, Sargent JD, Dalton M, Roda S. 1999. High concentrations of heavy metals in neighborhoods near ore smelters in northern Mexico. Environ Health Perspect 107(4):279-84.

Bolger PM, Carrington CD, Capar SG, Adams MA. 1991. Reductions in dietary lead exposure in the United States. Chem Speciat Bioavail 3:31-6.

Bolger PM, Yess NJ, Gunderson EL, Troxell TC, Carrington CD. 1996. Identification and reduction of sources of dietary lead in the United States. Food Addit Contam 13(1):53-60.

Brown MJ, Hu H, Gonzales-Cossio T, Peterson KE, Sanin LH, Kageyama ML, et al. 2000. Determinants of bone and blood lead concentrations in the early postpartum period. Occup Environ Med 57(8):535-41.

Burke M. 2004. Leaded gasoline phaseout becoming a reality. Environ Sci Technol 38(17):326A.

California Department of Health Services. 2003. State health department issues health warning on lead-contaminated chapulines (grasshoppers). Sacramento, CA: California Department of Health Services.

Carrington CD, Bolger PM, Scheuplein RJ. 1996. Risk analysis of dietary lead exposure. Food Addit Contam 13(1):61-76.

Centers for Disease Control and Prevention. 1993. Lead poisoning associated with use of traditional ethnic remedies—California, 1991-1992. MMWR Morb Mortal Wkly Rep 42(27):521-4.

Centers for Disease Control and Prevention. 1998. Lead poisoning associated with imported candy and powdered food coloring—California and Michigan. MMWR Morb Mortal Wkly Rep 47(48):1041-3.

Centers for Disease Control and Prevention 2004a. Lead poisoning associated with ayurvedic medications—Five States 2000-2003. MMWR Morb Mortal Wkly Rep 53(26):582-4.

Centers for Disease Control and Prevention. 2004b. Blood lead levels in residents of homes with elevated lead in tap water—District of Columbia, 2004. MMWR Morb Mortal Wkly Rep 53(12):268-70.

Centers for Disease Control and Prevention. 2005. Blood lead levels—United States, 1999-2002. MMWR Morb Mortal Wkly Rep 54(20):513-6.

Centers for Disease Control and Prevention. 2006. Adult blood lead epidemiology and surveillance—United States, 2003-2004. MMWR Morb Mortal Wkly Rep 55(32):876-9.

Centers for Disease Control and Prevention. 2007. Lead exposure among females of childbearing age—United States, 2004. MMWR Morb Mortal Wkly Rep 56(16):397-400.

Centers for Disease Control and Prevention. 2009. Children with elevated blood lead levels related to home renovation, repair, and painting activities —- New York State, 2006—2007. MMWR Morb Mortal Wkly Rep 58(03):55-8.

Cheng TJ, Wong RH, Lin YP, Hwang YH, Horng JJ, Wang JD. 1998. Chinese herbal medicine, sibship, and blood lead in children. Occup Environ Med 55(8):573-6.

Corbett RW, Ryan C, Weinrich SP. 2003. Pica in pregnancy: does it affect pregnancy outcomes? MCN Am J Matern Child Nurs 28(3):183-9; quiz 190-1.

Cortez-Lugo M, Tellez-Rojo MM, Gomez-Dantes H, Hernandez-Avila M. 2003. [Trends in atmospheric concentrations of lead in the metropolitan area of Mexico city, 1988-1998]. Salud Publica Mex 45(Suppl 2):S196-202.

Dykeman R, Aguilar-Madrid G, Smith T, Juárez-Pérez CA, Piacitelli GM, Hu H, et al. 2002. Lead exposure in Mexican radiator repair workers. Am J Ind Med 41(3):179-87.

Edwards CH, Johnson AA, Knight EM, Oyemade UJ, Cole OJ, Westney OE, et al. 1994. Pica in an urban environment. J Nutr 124(6 Suppl):954S-62S.

Eisenberg DM, Davis RB, Ettner SL, Appel S, Wilkey S, Van Rompay M, et al. 1998. Trends in alternative medicine use in the United States, 1990-1997: results of a follow-up national survey. JAMA 280(18):1569-75.

Eisenberg DM, Kessler RC, Foster C, Norlock FE, Calkins DR, Delbanco TL. 1993. Unconventional medicine in the United States. Prevalence, costs, and patterns of use. N Engl J Med 328(4):246-52.

Ernst E. 2002. Heavy metals in traditional Indian remedies. Eur J Clin Pharmacol 57(12):891-6.

Factor-Litvak P, Cushman LF, Kronenberg F, Wade C, Kalmuss D. 2001. Use of complementary and alternative medicine among women in New York City: a pilot study. J Altern Complement Med 7(6):659-66.

Feldman RG. 1978. .Urban lead mining: lead intoxication among deleaders. N Engl J Med 298:1143-5.

Fernandez GO, Martinez RR, Fortoul TI, Palazuelos E. 1997. High blood lead levels in ceramic folk art workers in Michoacan, Mexico. Arch Environ Health 52(1):51-5.

Finster ME, Gray KA, Binns HJ. 2004. Lead levels of edibles grown in contaminated residential soils: a field survey. Sci Total Environ 320(2-3):245-57.

Fischbein A, Anderson KE, Shigeru S, Lilis R, Kon S, Sarkoi L, Kappas A. 1981. Lead poisoning from do-it -yourself heat guns for removing lead paint: report of two cases. Environ Res 24:425-31.

Fletcher AM, Gelberg KH, Marshall EG. 1999. Reasons for testing and exposure sources among women of childbearing age with moderate blood lead levels. J Commun Health 24(3):215-27.

Garvey GJ, Hahn G, Lee RV, Harbison RD. 2001. Heavy metal hazards of Asian traditional remedies. Int J Environ Health Res 11(1):63-71.

Geissler PW, Shulman CE, Prince RJ, Mutemi W, Mnazi C, Friis H, et al. 1998. Geophagy, iron status and anaemia among pregnant women on the coast of Kenya. Trans R Soc Trop Med Hyg 92(5):549-53.

Graber N, Gabinskaya T, Forman J, Gertner M. 2006. Prenatal lead exposure in New York City immigrant communities [poster]. In: Pediatric Academic Societies (PAS) 2006 Annual Meeting, April 29-May 3, 2006, San Francisco.

Graziano JH, Popovac D, Factor-Litvak P, Shrout P, Kline J, Murphy MJ, et al. 1990. Determinants of elevated blood lead during pregnancy in a population surrounding a lead smelter in Kosovo, Yugoslavia. Environ Health Perspect 89:95-100.

Hackley B, Katz-Jacobson A. 2003. Lead poisoning in pregnancy: a case study with implications for midwives. J Midwifery Womens Health 48(1):30-8.

Hamilton S, Rothenberg SJ, Khan FA, Manalo M, Norris KC. 2001. Neonatal lead poisoning from maternal pica behavior during pregnancy. J Natl Med Assoc 93(9):317-9.

Handley MA, Hall C, Sanford E, Diaz E, Gonzalez-Mendez E, Drace K, et al. 2007. Globalization, binational communities, and imported food risks: results of an outbreak investigation of lead poisoning in Monterey County, California. Am J Public Health 97(5):900-6.

Hepner DL, Harnett MJ, Segal S, Camann W, Bader M, Tsen LC. 2002. Herbal medicinal products during pregnancy: are they safe? Br J Obstet Gynaecol 109(12):1425-6.

Hernandez Avila M, Romieu I, Rios C, Rivero A, Palazuelos E. 1991. Lead-glazed ceramics as major determinants of blood lead levels in Mexican women. Environ Health Perspect 94:117-20.

Hernandez-Avila M, Gonzalez-Cossio T, Palazuelos E, Romieu I, Aro A, Fishbein E, et al. 1996. Dietary and environmental determinants of blood and bone lead levels in lactating postpartum women living in Mexico City. Environ Health Perspect 104(10):1076-82.

Hibbert R, Bai Z, Navia J, Kammen DM, Zhang J. 1999. High lead exposures resulting from pottery production in a village in Michoacán State, Mexico. J Expos Anal Environ Epidemiol 9(4):343-51.

Hipkins KL, Materna BL, Payne SF, Kirsch LC. 2004. Family lead poisoning associated with occupational exposure. Clin Pediatr (Phila) 43(9):845-9.

Horner RD, Lackey CJ, Kolasa K, Warren K. 1991. Pica practices of pregnant women. J Am Diet Assoc 91(1):34-8.

Hunter J, de Kleine R. 1984. Geophagy in Central America. Geographic Rev 74:157-69.

Jacobs DE. 1998. Occupational exposures to lead-based paint in structural steel demolition and residential renovation work. Int J Environ Pollut 9(1):1-14.

Jacobs DE, Clickner RP, Zhou JY, Viet SM, Marker DA, Rogers JW, et al. 2002. The prevalence of lead-based paint hazards in U.S. housing. Environ Health Perspect 110(10):A599-606.

Jacobs DE, Mielke H, Pavur N. 2003. The high cost of improper removal of lead-based paint from housing: A case report. Environ Health Perspect 111:185-6.

Klitzman S, Sharma A, Nicaj L, Vitkevich R, Leighton J. 2002. Lead poisoning among pregnant women in New York City: risk factors and screening practices. J Urban Health 79(2):225-37.

Kosnett MJ. 2009. Health effects of low dose lead exposure in adults and children, and preventable risk posed by the consumption of game meat harvested with lead ammunition. In: Watson RT, Fuller M, Pokras M, Hunt WG, editors. Ingestion of lead from spent ammunition: implications for wildlife and humans. Boise, ID: The Peregrine Fund. DOI 10.4080/ilsa.2009.0103. Available at https://www.peregrinefund.org/lead_conference/PDF/0103 Kosnett.pdf [accessed 2010 May 6].

Lanphear BP, Matte TD, Rogers J, Clickner RP, Dietz B, Bornschein RL, et al. 1998. The contribution of lead-contaminated house dust and residential soil to children's blood lead levels. A pooled analysis of 12 epidemiologic studies. Environ Res 79(1):51-68.

Lee MG, Chun OK, Song WO. 2005. Determinants of the blood lead level of US women of reproductive age. J Am Coll Nutr 24(1):1-9.

Legge TM. 1901. Industrial lead poisoning. J Hyg 1:96-108.

Legge TM, Goadby KW. 1912. Lead poisoning and lead absorption. London: Edward Arnold. p. 129, 192. (Cited in Barltrop D. Transfer of lead to the human foetus. Mineral Metabol Pediatr 1969:135-51.)

Levesque B, Duchesne JF, Gariepy C, Rhainds M, Dumas P, Scheuhammer AM, et al. 2003. Monitoring of umbilical cord blood lead levels and sources assessment among the Inuit. Occup Environ Med 60(9):693-5.

Lopez LB, Ortega Soler CR, de Portela ML. 2004. [Pica during pregnancy: a frequently underestimated problem]. Arch Latinoam Nutr 54(1):17-24.

Lynch E, Braithwaite R. 2005. A review of the clinical and toxicological aspects of 'traditional' (herbal) medicines adulterated with heavy metals. Expert Opin Drug Saf 4(4):769-78.

Mahaffey KR. 1990. Environmental lead toxicity: nutrition as a component of intervention. Environ Health Perspect. Nov;89:75-8.

Manton WI, Angle CR, Stanek KL, Kuntzelman D, Reese YR, Kuehnemann TJ. 2003. Release of lead from bone in pregnancy and lactation. Environ Res 92(2):139-51.

Marino PE, Landrigan PJ, Graef J, Nussbaum A, Bayan G, Boch K, et al. 1990. A case report of lead paint poisoning during renovation of a Victorian farmhouse. Am J Public Health 80(10):1183-5.

Markowitz SB, Nunez CM, Klitzman S, Munshi AA, Kim WS, Eisinger J, et al. 1994. Lead poisoning due to hai ge fen. The porphyrin content of individual erythrocytes. JAMA 271(12):932-4.

Matte TD, Figueroa JP, Ostrowski S, Burr G, Jackson-Hunt L, Keenlyside RA, et al. 1989. Lead poisoning among household members exposed to lead-acid battery repair shops in Kingston, Jamaica. Int J Epidemiol 18(4): 874-81.

Matte TD, Proops D, Palazuelos E, Graef J, Hernandez Avila M. 1994. Acute high-dose lead exposure from beverage contaminated by traditional Mexican pottery. Lancet 344(8929):1064-5.

McKelvey W, Gwynn RC, Jeffery N, Kass D, Thorpe LE, Garg RK, et al. 2007. A biomonitoring study of lead, cadmium, and mercury in the blood of New York City adults. Environ Health Perspect 115(10):1435-41.

MedlinePlus [Internet]. 2009. Pica. Bethesda, MD: National Library of Medicine. Available from http://www.nlm.nih.gov/medlineplus/ency/article/001538.htm [accessed 2009 February 22].

Miranda ML, Kim D, Hull AP, Paul CJ, Galeano MA. 2007. Changes in blood lead levels associated with use of chloramines in water treatment systems. Environ Health Perspect 115(2):221-5. Epub 2006 Nov 7.

Moghraby SA, Abdullah MA, Karrar O, Akiel AS, Shawaf TA, Majid YA. 1989. Lead concentrations in maternal and cord blood in women users of surma eye cosmetics. Ann Trop Paediatr 9(1):49-53.

Mojdehi GM, Gurtner J. 1996. Childhood lead poisoning through kohl. Am J Public Health 86(4):587-8.

National Institute for Occupational Safety and Health. 1995. Report to Congress on workers' home contamination study conducted under The Workers' Family Protection Act (29 U.S.C. 671a). Atlanta: U.S. Dpeartment of Health and Human Services. DHHS (NIOSH) Publication No. 95-123. Available at http://www.cdc.gov/niosh/95-123.html [accessed 2010 May 6].

Nchito M, Geissler PW, Mubila L, Friis H, Olsen A. 2004. Effects of iron and multimicronutrient supplementation on geophagy: a two-by-two factorial study among Zambian schoolchildren in Lusaka. Trans R Soc Trop Med Hyg 98(4):218-27.

New York City Department of Health and Mental Hygiene. Annual Report 2006 for Preventing Lead Poisoning in New York City. New York, 2006.

Occupational Safety and Health Administration. 1984. Occupational exposure to lead; effective date of compliance plan requirements for certain industries; final rule (standard number 1910.1025). Fed Reg 49:23175.

Occupational Safety and Health Administration. 1993. Lead exposure in construction - interim rule (standard number 1926.62). Fed Reg 58:26590-649.

Parry C, Eaton J. 1991. Kohl: a lead-hazardous eye makeup from the Third World to the First World. Environ Health Perspect 94:121-3.

Partnership for Clean Fuels and Vehicles. 2007. The global campaign to eliminate leaded gasoline: progress as of January 2007. Nairobi, Kenya: Partnership for Clean Fuels and Vehicles.

Paul C. 1860. Etude sur l'intoxication lente par les préparations de plomb et son infuence sur le production de la conception [Studies on the chronic poisoning by lead compounds and its infuence on the fecundity). Arch Gén de Med 15:344-60.

Reissman DB, Matte TD, Gurnitz KL, Kaufmann RB, Leighton J. 2002. Is home renovation or repair a risk factor for exposure to lead among children residing in New York City? J Urban Health 79(4):L502-11.

Reynold S, Seem R, Fourtes L, Sprince N, Johnson J, Walkner L, Whitten P. 1999. Prevalence of elevated blood leads and exposure to lead in construction trades in Iowa and Illinois. Am J Ind Med 36:307-16.

Riess ML, Halm JK. 2007. Lead poisoning in an adult: lead mobilization by pregnancy? J Gen Intern Med 22(8):1212-5.

Romieu I, Palazuelos E, Hernandez-Avila M, Rios C, Munoz I, Jimenez C, et al. 1994. Sources of lead exposure in Mexico City. Environ Health Perspect 102(4):384-9.

Romieu I, Palazuelos E, Meneses F, Hernandez-Avila M. 1992. Vehicular traffic as a determinant of blood-lead levels in children: a pilot study in Mexico City. Arch Environ Health 47(4):246-9.

Ross EA, Szabo NJ, Tebbett IR. 2000. Lead content of calcium supplements. JAMA 284(11): 1425-1429.

Rothenberg SJ, Karchmer S, Schnaas L, Perroni E, Zea F, Fernandez Alba J. 1994. Changes in serial blood lead levels during pregnancy. Environ Health Perspect 102(10):876-80.

Saper RB, Kales SN, Paquin J, Burns MJ, Eisenberg DM, Davis RB, et al. 2004. Heavy metal content of ayurvedic herbal medicine products. JAMA 292(23):2868-73.

Saper RB, Phillips RS, Sehgal A, Khouri N, Davis RB, Paquin J, Thuppil V, Stefanos K. 2008. Lead, mercury, and arsenic in US- and Indian-manufactured ayurvedic medicines sold via the Internet. JAMA 300:915-23.

Scelfo GM, Flegal AR. 2000. Lead in calcium supplements. Environ Health Perspect 108(4):309-19.

Shannon M. 2003. Severe lead poisoning in pregnancy. Ambul Pediatr 3(1):37-9.

Simpson E, Mull JD, Longley E, East J. 2000. Pica during pregnancy in low-income women born in Mexico. West J Med 173(1):20-4; discussion 25.

Smulian JC, Motiwala S, Sigman RK. 1995. Pica in a rural obstetric population. South Med J 88(12):1236-40.

Sprinkle RV. 1995. Leaded eye cosmetics: a cultural cause of elevated lead levels in children. J Fam Pract 40(4):358-62.

Sule S, Madugu HN. 2001. Pica in pregnant women in Zaria, Nigeria. Niger J Med 10(1):25-7.

Tait PA, Vora A, James S, Fitzgerald DJ, Pester BA. 2002. Severe congenital lead poisoning in a preterm infant due to a herbal remedy. Med J Aust 177(4):193-5.

Tehranifar P, Leighton J, Auchincloss AH, Faciano A, Alper H, Paykin A, et al. 2008. Immigration and risk of childhood lead poisoning: findings from a case control study of New York City children. Am J Public Health 98(1): 92-7.

U.S. Department of Housing and Urban Development. 1995. Guidelines for the evaluation and control of lead-based paint hazards in housing. Chapter 4. Washington, DC: U.S. Department of Housing and Urban Development.

U.S. Environmental Protection Agency. 1973. Regulations of fuel and fuel additives. Fed Reg 38(6, Part III): 1257 (January 10, 1973).

U.S. Environmental Protection Agency. 1991. Maximum contaminant level goals and national primary drinking water regulations for lead and copper; final rule. Fed Reg 56(11):26460-4.

U.S. Environmental Protection Agency. 1996. Prohibition on gasoline containing lead or lead additives for highway use. Fed Reg 61(23):3834 (February 2, 1996).

U.S. Environmental Protection Agency. 2001. Lead; Identification of Dangerous Levels of Lead; Final Rule (40 CFR Part 745, 2001). Federal Register / Vol. 66, No. 4 / Friday, January 5, 2001.

U.S. Environmental Protection Agency. 2007a. National primary drinking water regulations for lead and copper: short-term regulatory revisions and clarifications; final rule. Fed Reg 72(195):57781-820.

U.S. Environmental Protection Agency. 1997b. Reducing lead hazards when remodeling your home. Washington, DC: U.S. Environmental Protection Agency.

U.S. Food and Drug Administration. 1993. FDA actions addressing lead in candy and candy wrappers. Fed Reg 58:33860.

U.S. Food and Drug Administration. 2001. FDA alerts public to possible health risk associated with certain tamarind candy lollipops from Mexico. Washington, DC: Center for Food Safety and Applied Nutrition.

U.S. Food and Drug Administration. 2006. Lead in candy likely to be consumed frequently by small children: recommended maximum level and enforcement policy. Washington, DC: Center for Food Safety and Applied Nutrition.

Vahter M, Counter SA, Laurell G, Buchanan LH, Ortega F, Schutz A, et al. 1997. Extensive lead exposure in children living in an area with production of lead-glazed tiles in the Ecuadorian Andes. Int Arch Occup Environ Health 70(4):282-6.

Walsh MP. 2007. The global experience with lead in gasoline and the lessons we should apply to the use of MMT. Am J Ind Med 50(11):853-60.

CHAPTER 5 – BLOOD LEAD TESTING IN PREGNANCY AND INFANCY

Binns HJ, Campbell C, Brown MJ. 2007. Interpreting and managing blood lead levels < 10 µg/dL in children and reducing childhood exposures to lead: recommendations of the CDC's Advisory Committee on Lead Poisoning Prevention. Pediatrics 120:e1285-98.

Centers for Disease Control and Prevention. 1991. Preventing lead poisoning in young children: a statement by the Centers for Disease Control. Atlanta, GA: U.S. Department of Health and Human Services.

Centers for Disease Control and Prevention. 2002. Managing elevated blood lead levels among young children: recommendations from the Advisory Committee on Childhood Lead Poisoning Prevention. Atlanta, GA: U.S. Department of Health and Human Services.

Centers for Disease Control and Prevention. 2005. Preventing lead poisoning in young children: a statement by the Centers for Disease Control. Atlanta, GA: U.S. Department of Health and Human Services.

Gulson BL, Mahaffey KR, Jameson CW, Mizon KJ, Korsch MJ, Cameron MA, et al. 1998. Mobilization of lead from the skeleton during the postnatal period is larger than during pregnancy. J Lab Clin Med 131(4):324-9.

Hu H. 1991. Knowledge of diagnosis and reproductive history among survivors of childhood plumbism. Am J Public Health. 81(8):1070-2.

Hu H, Hashimoto D, Besser M. 1996. Levels of lead in blood and bone of women giving birth in a Boston hospital. Arch Environ Health 51(1):52-8.

Hu H, Hernandez-Avila M. 2002. Invited commentary: lead, bones, women, and pregnancy—the poison within? Am J Epidemiol 156(12):1088-91.

Klitzman S, Sharma A, Nicaj L, Vitkevich R, Leighton J. 2002. Lead poisoning among pregnant women in New York City: risk factors and screening practices. J Urban Health 79(2):225-37.

Minnesota Department of Health. 2004. Blood lead screening risk questionnaire for pregnant women in Minnesota [updated December 2007]. Available at http://www.health.state.mn.us/divs/eh/lead/reports/pregnancy/pregnancy1page.pdf [accessed 2010 May 6].

New York City Department of Health and Mental Hygiene. 2006. Recommended lead risk assessment questions for pregnant women, guidelines for health care providers on the prevention, identification, and medical management of lead poisoning in pregnant women in New York City, June 30, 2006. Available at http://www.nyc.gov/html/doh/downloads/pdf/lead/lead-pregnant-letter.pdf [accessed 2009 July 8].

Osterloh JD, Kelly TJ. 1999. Study of the effect of lactational bone loss on blood lead concentrations in humans. Environ Health Perspect 107:187-194.

Parsons PJ, Chisolm JJ, Delves HT, Griffin R, Gunter EW, Slavin W, et al. 2001. Analytical procedures for the determination of lead in blood and urine, approved guideline. NCCLS document C40-A (ISBN 1-56238-437-6). Wayne, PA: NCCLS.

Pineau A, Fauconneau B, Rafael M, Viallefont A, Guillard O. 2002. Determination of lead in whole blood: comparison of the LeadCare blood lead testing system with Zeeman longitudinal electrothermal atomic absorption spectrometry. J Trace Elem Med Biol;16(2):113-7.

Rischitelli G, Nygren P, Bougatsos C, Freeman M, Helfand M. 2006. Screening for elevated lead levels in childhood and pregnancy: an updated summary of evidence for the U.S. Preventive Services Task Force. Pediatrics 118(6):e1867-95.

Rothenberg SJ, Khan F, Manalo M, Jiang J, Cuellar R, Reyes S, et al. 2000. Maternal bone lead contribution to blood lead during and after pregnancy. Environ Res 82(1):81-90.

Shannon M. 2003. Severe lead poisoning in pregnancy. Ambul Pediatr 3(1):37-9.

Shannon M, Rifai N. 1997. The accuracy of a portable instrument for analysis of blood lead in children. Ambulatory Child Health 3:249-54.

Stefanak MA, Bourguet CC, Benzies-Styka T. 1996. Use of the Centers for Disease Control and Prevention childhood lead poisoning risk questionnaire to predict blood lead elevations in pregnant women. Obstet Gynecol 87(2):209-212.

Tellez-Rojo MM, Hernandez-Avila M, Gonzalez-Cossio T, Romieu I, Aro A, Palazuelos E, et al. 2002. Impact of breastfeeding on the mobilization of lead from bone. Am J Epidemiol 155(5):420-8.

U.S. Preventive Services Task Force. 2006. Screening for elevated blood lead levels in children and pregnant women. Pediatrics 118:2514-8.

CHAPTER 6 –MANAGEMENT OF PREGNANT AND LACTATING WOMEN EXPOSED TO LEAD

American Academy of Pediatrics Committee on Environmental Health. 2005. Lead exposure in children: prevention, detection and management. Pediatrics 116:1036-46.

American College of Obstetrics and Gynecology. 2004. ACOG Practice Bulletin: nausea and vomiting of pregnancy. Obstet Gynecol 103(4):803-14.

Association of Occupational and Environmental Clinics. 2007. Medical management guidelines for lead-exposed adults. Washington, DC: Association of Occupational and Environmental Clinics. Available at http://www.aoec.org/documents/positions/MMG_FINAL.pdf [accessed 29 August 2008].

Anderson H, Islam K. 2006. Trends in occupational and adult lead exposures in Wisconsin 1988-2005. WMJ 105(2):21-5.

Binns HJ, Gray KA, Chen T, Finster ME, Peneff N, Schaefer P, et al. 2004. Evaluation of landscape coverings to reduce soil lead hazards in urban residential yards: the Safer Yards project. Environ Res 96(2):127-38.

Binns HJ, Campbell C, Brown MJ. 2007. Interpreting and managing blood lead levels of less than 10 [micro]g/dL in children and reducing childhood exposure to lead: recommendations of the Centers for Disease Control and Prevention Advisory Committee on Childhood Lead Poisoning Prevention. Pediatrics 120(5):e1285-98.

Bugle C, Rubin HB. 1993. Effects of a nutritional supplement on coprophagia: a study of three cases. Res Dev Disabil 14(6):445–56.

Centers for Disease Control and Prevention. 2002. Managing elevated blood lead levels among young children: recommendations from the Advisory Committee on Childhood Lead Poisoning Prevention. Atlanta, GA: U.S. Department of Health and Human Services.

Centers for Disease Control and Prevention. 2007. Lead exposure among females of childbearing age—United States, 2004. MMWR Morb Mortal Wkly Upd 56(6):397-400.

Corbett RW, Ryan C, Weinrich SP. 2003. Pica in pregnancy: does it affect pregnancy outcomes? MCN Am J Matern Child Nurs 28(3):183-9; quiz 190-1.

Dixon S, Wilson J, Clark C, Galke W, Succop P, Chen M. 2005. Effectiveness of lead-hazard control interventions on dust lead loadings: Findings from the evaluation of the HUD Lead-Based Paint Hazard Control Grant Program. Environ Res 98:303-14.

Dixon S, McLaine P, Kawecki C, Maxfield R, Duran S, Hynes P, et al. 2006. The effectiveness of low-cost soil treatments to reduce soil and dust lead hazards: the Boston lead safe yards low cost lead in soil treatment, demonstration and evaluation. Environ Res 102:113-24.

Edwards C, Johnson A, Knight E, Oyemade U, Cole O, Westney O, et al. 1994. Pica in an urban environment. J Nutr 124(6 Suppl):954S-62S. Fletcher, et al, 2007.

Fletcher AM, Gelberg KH, Marshall EG. 1999. Reasons for testing and exposure sources among women of childbearing age with moderate blood lead levels. J Commun Health 24(3):215-27.

Friedman JM. 2000. Teratology society: presentation to the FDA public meeting on safety issues associated with the use of dietary supplements during pregnancy. Teratology 62:134–7.

Geissler PW, Shulman CE, Prince RJ, Mutemi W, Mnazi C, Friis H, et al. 1998. Geophagy, iron status and anaemia among pregnant women on the coast of Kenya. Trans R Soc Trop Med Hyg 92(5):549-53.

Goh H, Iwat B, Kahng S. 1999. Multicomponent assessment of treatment of pica. J Appl Behav Anal 32(3): 297-316.

Institute of Medicine. 1990. Nutrition during pregnancy, part 2: nutrient supplements. Washington, DC: National Academy Press.

Kettaneh A, Eclache V, Fain O, Sontag C, Uzan M, Carbillon L, et al. 2005. Pica and food craving in patients with iron-deficiency anemia: a case-control study in France. Am J Med 118(2):185-8.

Kosnett M, Wedeen R, Rothenberg S, Hipkins K, Materna B, Schwartz B, et al. 2007. Recommendations for medical management of adult lead exposure. Environ Health Perspect 115(3):463.

Kosnett MJ. 2009. Health effects of low dose lead exposure in adults and children, and preventable risk posed by the consumption of game meat harvested with lead ammunition. In: Watson RT, Fuller M, Pokras M, Hunt WG, editors. Ingestion of lead from spent ammunition: implications for wildlife and humans. Boise, ID: The Peregrine Fund. DOI 10.4080/ilsa.2009.0103. Available at https://www.peregrinefund.org/lead_conference/ PDF/0103 Kosnett.pdf [accessed 2010 May 6].

Marcus DM, Snodgrass WR. 2005. Do no harm: avoidance of herbal medicines during pregnancy. Obstet Gynecol 105(5 Pt 1):1119-22. Comment in Obstet Gynecol 2005;106(2):409-10; author reply 410-1.

McAdam DB, Sherman JA, Sheldon JB, Napolitano DA. 2004. Behavioral interventions to reduce the pica of persons with developmental disabilities. Behav Modif 28(1):45-72.

Nchito M, Geissler P, Mubila L, Friis H, Olsen A. 2004. Effects of iron supplementation on geophagy: a two-by-two factorial study among Zambian schoolchildren in Lusaka. Trans Royal Soc Trop Med Hyg 98:218-27.

Occupational Safety and Health Administration. 1979. Medical surveillance guidelines. Washington, DC: Occupational Safety and Health Administration. Available at http://www.osha.gov/pls/oshaweb/owadisp.show_ document?p_table=STANDARDS&p_id=10033 [accessed 2010 May 6].

Pace G, Toyer E. 2000. The effects of a vitamin supplement on the pica of a child with severe mental retardation. J Appl Behav Anal 33(4):619-22.

Piazza C, Fisher W, Hanley G, LeBlanc L, Worsdell A, Lindauer S, et al. 1998. Treatment of pica through multiple analyses of its reinforcing functions. J Appl Behav Anal 31(2):165-89.

Rainville AJ. 1998. Pica practices of pregnant women are associated with lower maternal hemoglobin level at delivery. J Am Diet Assoc 98(3):293-6.

Smulian JC, Motiwala S, Sigman RK. 1995. Pica in a rural obstetric population. South Med J 88(12):1236-40.

U.S. Environmental Protection Agency. 1991. Maximum contaminant level goals and national primary drinking water regulations for lead and copper; final rule. Fed Reg 56(11):26460-4.

CHAPTER 7 – NUTRITION

Affenito SG, Thompson DR, Franko DL, Striegel-Moore RH, Daniels SR, Barton BA, et al. 2007. Longitudinal assessment of micronutrient intake among African-American and white girls: the National Heart, Lung, and Blood Institute growth and health study. J Am Diet Assoc 107:1113-23.

Ahamed M, Siddiqui MK. 2007. Environmental lead toxicity and nutritional factors. Clin Nutr 26:400-8.

American College of Obstetricians and Gynecologists. 2008. Anemia in pregnancy. Washington, DC: American College of Obstetricians and Gynecologists. ACOG Practice Bulletin 95.

Baghurst PA, McMichael AJ, Vimpani GV, Robertson EF, Clark PD, Wigg NR. 1987. Determinants of blood lead concentrations of pregnant women living in Port Pirie and surrounding areas. Med J Aust 146:69-73.

Ballew C, Bowman B. 2001. Recommending calcium to reduce lead toxicity in children: a critical review. Nutr Rev 59:71-9.

Barton JC, Conrad ME, Harrison L, Nuby S. 1978 J Lab Clin Med 91:366-76.

Beard JL. 2000. Effectiveness and strategies of iron supplementation during pregnancy. Am J Clin Nutr 7 (suppl):1288S-94S.

Black RE, Allan LH, Bhutta ZA, Caulfield LE. 2008. Maternal and child 1. Maternal and child undernutrition: global and regional exposures and health consequences. Lancet 371:243-60.

Bodnar ML, Scanlon KS, Freedman DS, Siega-Riz AM, Cogswell ME. 2001 High prevalence of postpartum anemia among low-income women in the United States. Am J Obstet Gynecol 185:438-43.

Bodnar LM, Catov JM, Roberts JM, Simhan HN. 2007a. Prepregnancy obesity predicts poor vitamin D status in mothers and their neonates. J Nutr 137:2437-42.

Bodnar LM, Simhan HN, Powers RW, Frank MP, Cooperstein E, Roberts JM. 2007b. High prevalence of vitamin D insufficiency in black and white pregnant women residing in the Northern United States and their neonates. J Nutr 137:447-52.

Bogden JD, Louria DB, Oleske JM. 2001. Regarding dietary calcium to reduce lead toxicity. Nutr Rev 59(9):307-8.

Bradman A, Eskenazi B, Sutton P, Athanasoulis M, Goldman LR. 2003. Iron deficiency associated with higher blood lead in children living in contaminated environments. Environ Health Perspect 109:1079-84.

Calvo M, Whiting SJ. 2006. Public health strategies to overcome barriers to optimal vitamin D status in populations with special needs. J Nutr 136:1135-9.

Cerklewski FL, Forbes RM. 1976. Influence of dietary selenium on lead toxicity in the rat. J Nutr 206:778-83.

Choi JW, Kim SK. 2003 Association between blood lead concentrations and body iron status in children. Arch Dis Child 88:791-2.

Cogswell NW, Kettel-Khan L, Ramakrishnan U. 2003. Iron supplement use among women in the United States: science, policy and practice. J Nutr 133:1974S-7S.

Dawson EB, Evans DR, Harris WA, Teter MC, McGanity WJ. 1999. The effect of ascorbic acid supplementation on the blood lead levels of smokers. J Am Coll Nutr 18:166-70.

Dunlop AL, Gardiner PM, Shellhaas CS, Menard MK, McDiarmid MA. The clinical content of preconception care: the use of medications and supplements amon women of reproductive age. Am J Obstet Gynecol. 2008 Dec;199(6 Suppl 2):S367-72.

Ervasti M, Kotisari S, Keinonen S, Punnonen K. 2007. Use of advanced red blood cell and reticulocyte indices improves the accuracy in diagnosing iron deficiency in pregnant women at term. Eur J Haematol 79:539-45.

Ervin RB, Wang CY, Wright JD, Kennedy-Stephenson J. 2004. Dietary intake of selected minerals for the United States population: 1999-2000. Adv Data 341:1-5.

Ettinger AS, Lamadrid-Figueroa H, Tellez-Rojo MM, Mercado-Garcia A, Peterson KE, Schwartz J, et al. 2009. Effect of calcium supplementation on blood lead levels in pregnancy: a randomized placebo-controlled trial. Environ Health Perspect 117(1):26-31.

Ettinger AS, Peterson K, Amasiriwardena C, Hu H, Hernandez-Avila M. 2004. Relation of dietary nutrient intake to lead in blood, bone and breast milk among lactating women at one-month postpartum. Epidemiology 15(4):S189.

Ettinger AS, Tellez-Rojo MM, Amarasiriwardena C, Peterson KE, Schwartz J, Aro A, et al. 2006. Influence of maternal bone lead burden and calcium intake on levels of lead in breast milk over the course of lactation. Am J Epidemiol 163:48-56.

Farias P, Borja-Aburto VH, Rios C, Hertz-Picciotto I, Rojas-Lopez M, Chavez-Ayala R. 1996. Blood lead levels in pregnant women of high and low socioeconomic status in Mexico City. Environ Health Perspect 104:1070-4.

Finch C. 1994. Regulators of iron balance in humans. Blood 84:1697-1702.

Frith-Terhune AL, Cogswell ME, Khan LK, Will JC, Ramakrishnan U. 2000. Iron deficiency anemia: higher prevalence in Mexican American than in non-Hispanic white females in the third National Health and Nutrition Examination Survey, 1988-1994. Am J Clin Nutr 72:963-8.

Fulgoni V 3rd, Nicholls J, Reed A, Buckley R, Kafer K, Huth P, et al. 2007. Dairy consumption and related nutrient intake of African-American adults and children in the United States: continuing survey of food intakes by individuals 1994-1996, 1998 and the National Health and Nutrition Examination Survey 1999-2000. J Am Diet Assoc 107:256-64.

Fullmer CS. 1995. Dietary calcium levels and treatment interval determine the effects of lead ingestion on plasma 1, 25-dihydroxyvitamin D concentration in chicks. J Nutr 125:1328-33.

Gao X, Wilde PE, Lichtenstein AH, Tucker KL. 2006. Meeting adequate intake for dietary calcium without dairy foods in adolescents aged 9 to 18 years (National Health and Nutrition Examination Survey 2001-2002). J Am Diet Assoc 106:1759-65.

Gardiner PM, Nelson L, Shellhaas CS, Dunlop AL, Long R, Andrist S, Jack BW. 2008. The clinical content of preconception care: nutrition and dietary supplements. Am J Obstet Gynecol 199(6 Suppl 2):S345-56.

Godwin HA. 2001. The biological chemistry of lead Curr Opin Chem Biol 5:223-7.

Graziano JH, Popovac D, Factor-Litvak P, Shrout P, Kline J, Murphy MJ, et al. 1990. Determinants of elevated blood lead during pregnancy in a population surrounding a lead smelter in Kosovo, Yugoslavia. Environ Health Perspect 89:95-100.

Gulson BL, Mahaffey KR, Jameson CW, Mizon KJ, Korsch MJ, Cameron MA, et al. 1998. Mobilization of lead from the skeleton during the postnatal period is larger than during pregnancy. J Lab Clin Med 131:324-9.

Gulson BL, Pounds JG, Mushak P, Thomas BJ, Gray B, Korsch MJ. 1999. Estimation of cumulative lead release (lead flux) from the maternal skeleton during pregnancy and lactation. J Lab Clin Med 134(6:6)31-640.

Gulson BL, Mizon KJ, Korsch MJ, Taylor AJ. 2006. Low blood lead levels do not appear to be further reduced by dietary supplements. Environ Health Perspect 114:1186-92.

Gulson BL, Mizon KJ, Palmer JM, Korsch MJ, Taylor AJ, Mahaffey KR. 2004. Blood lead changes during pregnancy and postpartum with calcium supplementation. Environ Health Perspect 112(15):1499-507.

Hamir AN, Sullivan ND, Handson PD. 1982. The effects of age and diet on the absorption of lead from the gastrointestinal tract of dogs. Aust Vet J 58:266-8.

Hammad TA, Sexton M, Langenberg P. 1996. Relationship between blood lead and dietary iron intake in preschool children. A cross-sectional study. Ann Epidemiol 6:30-3.

Harville EW, Schram M, Watt-Morse M, Chantaia K, Anderson JJ, Hertz-Picciotta I. 2004. Calcium intake during pregnancy among white and African-American pregnant women in the United States. J Am Coll Nutr 23:43-50.

Heaney RP, Davies KM, Chen TC, Holick MF, Barger-Lux MJ. 2003. Human serum 25-hydroxycholecalciferol response to extended oral dosing with cholecalciferol. Am J Clin Nutr 77:204-10.

Heard MJ, Chamberlain AC. 1982. Effect of minerals and food on uptake of lead from the gastrointestinal tract in humans. Hum Toxicol 1:411-8.

Hernandez-Avila M, Sanin LH, Romieu I, Palazuelos E, Tapia-Conyer R, Olaiz G, et al. 1997. Higher milk intake during pregnancy is associated with lower maternal and umbilical cord lead levels in postpartum women. Environ Res 74:116-21.

Hernandez-Avila M, Gonzalez-Cossio T, Hernandez-Avila JE, Romieu I, Peterson KE, Aro A, et al. 2003. Dietary calcium supplements to lower blood lead levels in lactating women. Placebo-controlled trial. Epidemiology 14:206-12.

Hertz-Picciotto I, Schramm M, Watt-Morse M, Chantala K, Anderson J, Osterloh J. 2000. Patterns and determinants of blood lead during pregnancy. Am J Epidemiol 152(9):829-37.

Hollis BW, Wagner CL. 2004. Assessment of dietary vitamin D requirements during pregnancy and lactation. Am J Clin Nutr 79:717-26.

Hollis BW. 2005. Circulating 25-hydroxyvitamin D levels indicative of vitamin D sufficiency: implications for establishing a new effective dietary intake recommendation for vitamin D. J Nutr 135:317-22.

Holick MF. 2003. Vitamin D: A millennium perspective. J Cell Biochem 88:296–307.

Holick MF. 2004. Sunlight and vitamin D for bone health and prevention of autoimmune diseases, cancers, and cardiovascular disease. Am J Clin Nutr 80:1678S-88S.

Holick MF. 2007. Vitamin D deficiency. N Engl J Med 357:266-81.

Horton R. 2008. Maternal and child undernutrition: an urgent opportunity. Lancet 371(9608):179.

Hotz C, Peerson JM, Brown KH. 2003. Suggested lower cutoffs of serum zinc concentrations for assessing zinc status: reanalysis of the second National Health and Nutrition Examination Survey data (1976-1980). Am J Clin Nutr 78:756-64.

Hsu PC, Guo YL. 2002. Antioxidant nutrients and lead toxicity. Toxicology 180:33-44.

Institute of Medicine. 1990. Nutrition during pregnancy. Committee on Nutritional Status During Pregnancy and Lactation, Food and Nutrition Board. Washington, DC: National Academy Press.

Institute of Medicine. 1997. Dietary reference intakes: calcium, phosphorus, magnesium, vitamin D, and fluoride. Food and Nutrition Board. Washington, DC: National Academy Press.

Institute of Medicine. 2001. Dietary reference intakes for vitamin A, vitamin K, arsenic, boron, chromium, copper, iodine, iron, manganese, molybdenum, nickel, silicon, vanadium, and zinc. Food and Nutrition Board. Washington, DC: National Academy Press.

Janakiraman V, Ettinger A, Mercado-Garcia A, Hu H, Hernandez-Avila M. 2003. Calcium supplements and bone resorption in pregnancy: a randomized crossover trial. Am J Prev Med 24:260-4.

Johnson MA. 2001. High calcium intake blunts pregnancy-induced increases in maternal blood lead. Nutr Rev 59(5):152-6.

Kim HS, Lee SS, Hwangbo Y, Ahn KD, Lee BK. 2003. Cross-sectional study of blood lead effects on iron status in Korean lead workers. Nutrition 19:571-6.

Kovacs CS, Kronenberg HM. 1997. Maternal-fetal calcium and bone metabolism during pregnancy, puerperium, and lactation. Endocr Rev 18(6):832-72.

Kraemer L, Zimmerman MB, editors. 2007. Nutritional anemia. Basel: Sight and Life Press.

Kwong WT, Friello P, Semba RD. 2004. Interactions between iron deficiency and lead poisoning: epidemiology and pathogenesis. Sci Total Environ 330(1-3):21-37.

Lacasana-Navarro M, Romieu I, Sanin-Aguirre LH, Palazuelos-Rendon E, Hernandez-Avila M. 1996. Calcium intake and blood lead in women in reproductive age. Rev Invest Clin 48:425-30.

Lee M-G, Chun OK, Song WO. 2005. Determinants of the blood lead level of US women of reproductive age. Am Coll Nutr 24:1-9.

Leong W-I, Bowlus CL, Talkvist J, Lonnerdal B. 2003. Iron supplementation during infancy – effects on expression of iron transporters, iron absorption, and iron utilization in rat pups. Am J Clin Nutr 78:1203-11.

Lonnerdal B. Dietary factors influencing zinc absorption. J Nutr. 2000 May;130(5S Suppl):1378S-83S.

Looker AC, Harris TB, Madans JH, Sempos CT. 1993. Dietary calcium and hip fracture risk: the NHANES I epidemiologic follow-up study. Ostoporos Int 3:177-84.

Looker AC, Dallman PR, Carroll MD, Gunter EW, Johnson CL. 1997. Prevalence of iron deficiency in the United States. JAMA 277:973-6.

Looker AC, Loyevsky M, Gordeuk VR. 1999. Increased serum transferring saturation is associated with lower serum transferring receptor concentration. Clin Chem 45:2191-9.

Looker AC, Pfeiffer CM, Lacher DA, Schleicher RL, Picciano MF, Yetley EA. 2008. Serum 25-hydroxyvitamin D status of the US population: 1988-1994 compared with 2000-2004. Am J Clin Nutr 88:1519-27.

Ma J, Johns RA, Stafford RS. 2007. Americans are not meeting current calcium recommendations. Am J Clin Nutr 85:1361-6.

Mahaffey KR. 1980. Nutrient-lead interactions. In: Singhal RL, Thomas JA, editors. Lead toxicity. Baltimore and Munich: Urban and Schwarzenberg. p. 425-60.

Mahaffey KR. 1983. Biotoxicity of lead: influence of various factors. Fed Proc 42(6):1730-4.

Mahaffey KR. 1985. Factors modifying susceptibility to lead toxicity. In: Mahaffey KR, editor. Dietary and environmental lead: human health effects. Amsterdam: Elsevier Scientific Press. p. 373-415.

Mahaffey KR, Goyer R, Haseman JK. 1973. Dose-response to lead ingestion in rats fed low dietary calcium. J Lab Clin Med 83:92-100.

Mahaffey KR, McKinney J, and Reigart JR. 1992. Lead and compounds. In: Lippmann, editor Critical review of environmental toxicants. First ed. New York: Van Nostrand Reinhold, New York. p. 360-91.

Mahaffey-Six K, Goyer RA. 1972. The influence of iron deficiency on tissue content and toxicity of ingested lead in the rat. J Lab Clin Med 79:128-36.

Manton WI, Angle CR, Stanek KL, Kuntzelman D, Reese YR, Kuehnemann TJ. 2003. Release of lead from bone in pregnancy and lactation. Environ Res 92:139-51.

Markowitz ME, Rosen JF, Bijur PE. 1990. Effects of iron deficiency on lead excretion in children with moderate lead intoxication. J Pediatr 116:360-4.

Moore C, Murphy MM, Keast DR, Holick MF. 2004. Vitamin D intake in the United States. J Am Diet Assoc 104:980-3.

Morgan EH, Oates PS. 2002 Mechanisms and regulation of intestinal iron absorption. Blood Cells Mol Dis 29:384-99.

National Institutes of Health. 1994. Optimal calcium intake. NIH Consens Statement 1994 June 6-8;12(4):1-31.

Osterloh JD, Kelly TJ. 1999. Study of the effect of lactational bone loss on blood lead concentrations in humans. Environ Health Perspect 107:187-94.

Pounds JG, Long GJ, Rosen JF. 1991. Cellular and molecular toxicity of lead in bone. Environ Health Perspect 91:17-32.

Prentice A. 2000a. Maternal calcium metabolism and bone mineral status. Am J Clin Nutr 71(suppl):1312S-6S.

Prentice A. 2000b. Calcium in pregnancy and lactation. Ann Rev Nutr 20:247-72.

Ros C, Mwanri L. 2003. Lead exposure, interactions and toxicity: food for thought. Asia Pac J Clin Nutr 12: 388-95.

Rosen JF, Chesney RW, Hamstra A, DeLuca HF, Mahaffey KR. 1980. Reduction in 1,25-dihydroxyvitamin D in children with increased lead absorption. N Engl J Med 302:1128-31.

Ross EA, Szabo NJ, Tebbett IR. 2000. Lead content of calcium supplements. JAMA 284(11):1425-9.

Sauk JJ, Somerman MJ. 1991. Physiology of bone: mineral compartment proteins as candidates for environmental perturbation by lead. Environ Health Perspect 91:9-16.

Schell LM, Denham M, Stark AD, Gomez M, Ravenscroft J, Parsons PJ, et al. 2003. Maternal blood lead concentration, diet during pregnancy, and anthropometry predict neonatal blood lead in a socioeconomically disadvantaged population. Environ Health Perspect 111:195-200.

Scelfo GM, Flegal AR. 2000. Lead in calcium supplements. Environ Health Perspect 108(4):309-13.

Simon JA, Hudes ES. 1999. Relationship of ascorbic acid to blood lead levels. JAMA 281:2289-93.

Smith CM, DeLuca HF, Tanaka Y, Mahaffey KR. 1981. Effect of lead ingestion on functions of vitamin D and its metabolites. J Nutr 111:1321-9.

Song WO, Chun OK, Kerver J, Cho S, Chung CE, Chung SJ. 2006. Ready-to-eat breakfast cereal consumption enhances milk and calcium intake in the US population. J Am Diet Assoc 106:1783-89.

Specker BL, Vieira NE, O'Brien KO, Ho ML, Heubi JE, Abrams SA, et al. 1994. Calcium kinetics in lactating women with high and low calcium intakes. Am J Clin Nutr 59:593-9.

Specker B. 2004. Vitamin D requirements during pregnancy. Am J Clin Nutr 80(suppl):1740S-7S.

Stowe HD, Vandevelde M. 1979. Lead-induced encephalopathy in dogs fed high fat, low calcium diets. J Neuropathol Exp Neurol 38:463-74.

Tellez-Rojo MM, Bellinger DC, Arroyo-Quiroz C, Lamadrid-Figueroa H, Mercado-Garcia A, Schnaas-Arrieta L, et al. 2006. Longitudinal associations between blood lead concentrations lower than 10 microg/dL and neurobehavioral development in environmentally exposed children in Mexico City. Pediatrics 118:e323-30.

Wagner CL, Greer FR, and the American Academy of Pediatrics Section on Breastfeeding and Committee on Nutrition. 2008. Prevention of rickets and vitamin D deficiency in infants, children, and adolescents. Pediatrics. 122;1142-52. Erratum appears in Pediatrics. 2009;123:197.

Wang Q, Luo W, Zheng W, Liu Y, Xu H, Zheng G, et al. 2007a. Iron supplementation prevents lead-induced disruption of the blood-brain barrier during rat development. Toxicol Appl Pharmacol 219:33-41.

Wang Q, Luo W, Zhang W, Dai Z, Chen Y, Chen J. 2007b. Iron supplementation protects against lead-induced apoptosis through MAPK pathway in weanling rat cortex. Neurotoxicol 28:850-9.

Wasserman G, Graziano JH, Factor-Litvak P, Popovac, D, Musabegovic MN, Vrenezi N, et al. 1992. Independent effects of lead exposure and iron deficiency anemia on developmental outcome at age 2 years. J. Pediatr 121:695-703.

Wasserman GA, Graziano JH, Factor-Litvak P, Popovac D, Morina N, Musabegovic A, et al. 1994. Consequences of lead exposure and iron supplementation on childhood development at age 4 years. Neurotoxicol Teratol 16:233-40.

Weinberg LG, Berner LA, Groves JE. 2004. Nutrient contributions of dairy foods in the United States. Continuing survey of food intakes by individuals, 1994-1995, 1998. J Am Diet Assoc 104:895-902.

West WL, Knight EM, Edwards CH, Manning M, Spurlock B, James H, et al. 1994. Maternal low level lead and pregnancy outcomes. J Nutr 124: 981S-6S.

Willoughby RA, Thirapatsakun T, McSherry BJ. 1972. Influence of rations low in calcium and phosphorus on blood and tissue lead concentrations in the horse. Am J Vet Res 33:1165-73.

Wright RO, Shannon MW, Wright RJ, Hu H. 1999. Association between iron deficiency and low-level lead poisoning in an urban primary care clinic. Am J Public Health 89:1049-53.

Wright RO, Tsaih SW, Schwartz J, Wright RJ, Hu H. 2003. Association between iron deficiency and blood lead level in a longitudinal analysis of children followed in an urban primary care clinic. J Pediatr 142(1):9-14.

CHAPTER 8 – CHELATION OF THE PREGNANT WOMAN, FETUS, AND NEWBORN INFANT

Abendroth K. 1971. [Excellent effect of sodium-citrate-EDTA-combination therapy in severe lead poisoning during pregnancy]. Dtsch Gesundheitsw 26(45):2130-1. [in German.]

Adamovich K. 1987. [Effect of exchange transfusion on blood lead levels in newborn infants] Kinderarztl Prax. 55(4):197-200. [in German.]

Angle CR, McIntire MS. 1964. Lead poisoning during pregnancy. Fetal tolerance of calcium disodium edetate. Am J Dis Child 108:436-9.

Aposhian HV. 1982. Biological chelation: 2,3-dimercapto-propanesulfonic acid and meso-dimercaptosuccinic acid. Adv Enzyme Regul 20:301-19.

Bearer CF, Linsalata N, Yomtovian R, Walsh M, Singer L. 2000. Blood transfusions: a hidden source of lead exposure. Lancet 62:332.

Bearer CF, O'Riordan MA, Powers R. 2003. Lead exposure from blood transfusion to premature infants. J Pediatr 137(4): 549-54.

Brown MJ, Willis T, Omalu B, Leiker R. 2006. Deaths resulting from hypocalcemia after administration of edetate disodium: 2003-2005. Pediatrics 118(2):e534-6.

Centers for Disease Control and Prevention. 1991. Preventing lead poisoning in young children: a statement by the Centers for Disease Control. Atlanta, GA: U.S. Department of Health and Human Services.

Chisolm JJ. 1968. The use of chelating agents in the treatment of acute and chronic lead intoxication in childhood. J Pediatr 73(1):1-38.

Ghafour SY, Khuffash FA, Ibrahim HS, Reavey PC. 1984. Congenital lead intoxication with seizures due to prenatal exposure. Clin Pediatr (Phila) 23(5):282-3.

Graziano JH, Lolacono NJ, Moulton T, Mitchell ME, Slavkovich V, Zarate C. 1991. Controlled study of meso-2, 3-dimercaptosuccinic acid for the management of childhood lead intoxication. J Pediatr 120(1):133-9.

Guzman DD, Velez LI, Shepherd JG, Goto CS. 2000. Calcium EDTA and DMSA chelation of a neonate with congenital lead intoxication. J Toxicol Clin Toxicol 38:548-549.

Hamilton S, Rothenberg SJ, Khan FA, Manalo M, Norris KC. 2001. Neonatal lead poisoning from maternal pica behavior during pregnancy. J Natl Med Assoc 93(9):317-9.

Horowitz BZ, Mirkin DB. 2001. Lead poisoning and chelation in a mother-neonate pair. J Toxicol Clin Toxicol 39(7):727-31.

Klitzman S, Sharma A, Nicaj L, Vitkevich R, Leighton J. 2002. Lead poisoning among pregnant women in New York City: risk factors and screening practices. J Urban Health 79(2):225-37.

Markowitz M. 2000. Lead poisoning. Pediatr Rev 21(10):327-35.

Mycyk MB, Leikin JB. 2004. Combined exchange transfusion and chelation therapy for neonatal lead poisoning. Ann Pharmacother 38(5):821-4.

National Research Council. 2000. Scientific frontiers in developmental toxicology and risk assessment. Washington, DC: National Academy Press.

Olmedo RE, Rella JG, Hoffman RS, Nelson LS. 1999. Lead poisoning in late pregnancy due to maternal pica. 1999 NACCT Abstracts. Clin Toxicol 37:626.

Piomelli S. 1996. Lead poisoning. In: Behrman RE, Kliegman RM, Arvin AM, editors. Nelson textbook of pediatrics. Philadelphia: WB Saunders. p. 2010–3.

Powell ST, Bolisetty S, Wheaton GR. 2006. Succimer therapy for congenital lead poisoning from maternal petrol sniffing. Med J Aust 184(2):84-5.

Rogan WJ, Dietrich KN, Ware JH, Dockery DW, Salganik M, Radcliffe J, et al. 2001. The effect of chelation therapy with succimer on neuropsychological development in children exposed to lead. N Engl J Med 344(19):1421-6.

Rothenberg SJ, Schnaas-Arrieta L, Ugartechea JC, Perroni-Hernandez E, Perez-Guerrero IA, Cansino-Prtiz S, et al. 1992. A documented case of perinatal lead poisoning. Am J Public Health 82(4):613-4.

Sensirivatana R, Supachadhiwong O, Phancharoen S, Mitrakul C. 1983. Neonatal lead poisoning. An unusual clinical manifestation. Clin Pediatr (Phila) 22(8):582-4.

Singh N, Donovan CM, Hanshaw JB. 1978. Neonatal lead intoxication in a prenatally exposed infant. J Pediatr 93(6):1019-21.

Stedman's. 2008. Stedman's medical dictionary. Baltimore, MD: Lippincott Williams and Wilkins.

Tait PA, Vora A, James S, Fitzgerald DJ, Pester BA. 2002. Severe congenital lead poisoning in a preterm infant due to a herbal remedy. Med J Aust 177(4):193-5.

Timpo AE, Amin JS, Casalino MB, Yuceoglu AM. 1979. Congenital lead intoxication. J Pediatr 94(5):765-7.

Walsh MJ, Pali M, Ferguson T. An unusual case of in-utero lead exposure J Toxicol Clin Toxicol 2000; 38:547-548.

CHAPTER 9 – BREASTFEEDING

Abadin HG, Hibbs BF, Pohl HR. 1997. Breast-feeding exposure of infants to cadmium, lead, and mercury: a public health viewpoint. Toxicol Ind Health 13(4):495-517.

Agency for Healthcare Research and Quality. 2007. Breastfeeding and maternal and infant health outcomes in developed countries. Rockville, MD: U.S. Department of Health and Human Services.

American Academy of Pediatrics. 2001. Transfer of drugs and other chemicals into human milk. Pediatrics 108(3):776-89.

American Academy of Pediatrics. 2005. Breastfeeding and the use of human milk. Pediatrics 115:496-506.

Arenz S, Ruckerl R, Koletzko B, von Kries R. 2004. Breast-feeding and childhood obesity—a systematic review. Int J Obes 28:1247-56.

Bachrach VR, Schwarz E, Bachrach LR. 2003. Breastfeeding and the risk of hospitalization for respiratory disease in infancy: a meta-analysis. Arch Pediatr Adolesc Med 157:237-43.

Baum CR, Shannon MW. 1997. The lead concentration of reconstituted infant formula. J Toxicol Clin Toxicol 35(4):371-5.

Bolger PM, Yess NJ, Gunderson EL, Troxell TC, Carrington CD. 1996. Identification and reduction of sources of dietary lead in the United States. Food Addit Contam 13(1):53-60.

Chien PF, Howie PW. 2001. Breast milk and the risk of opportunistic infection in infancy in industrialized and non-industrialized settings [review]. Adv Nutr Res 10:69-104.

Counter SA, Buchanan LH, Ortega F. 2004. Current pediatric and maternal lead levels in blood and breast milk in Andean inhabitants of a lead-glazing enclave. J Occup Environ Med 46(9):967-73.

Ettinger AS, Tellez-Rojo MM, Amarasiriwardena C, Gonzalez-Cossio T, Peterson KE, Aro A, et al. 2004a. Levels of lead in breast milk and their relation to maternal blood and bone lead levels at one month postpartum. Environ Health Perspect 112(8):926-31.

Ettinger AS, Tellez-Rojo MM, Amarasiriwardena C, Bellinger D, Peterson K, Schwartz J, et al. 2004b. Effect of breast milk lead on infant blood lead levels at 1 month of age. Environ Health Perspect 112(14):1381-5.

Ettinger AS, Tellez-Rojo MM, Amarasiriwardena C, Schwartz J, Peterson KE, Aro A, et al. 2006. Influence of maternal bone lead burden and calcium intake on levels of lead in breast milk over the course of lactation. Am J Epidemiol 163:48-56.

Gulson BL, Jameson CW, Mahaffey KR, Mizon KJ, Patison N, Law AJ, et al. 1998. Relationships of lead in breast milk to lead in blood, urine, and diet of the infant and mother. Environ Health Perspect 106(10):667-74.

Gulson BL, Mizon KJ, Palmer JM, Patison N, Law AJ, Korsch MJ, et al. 2001. Longitudinal study of daily intake and excretion of lead in newly born infants. Environ Res 85(3):232-45.

Gulson BL, Mizon KJ, Korsch MJ, Palmer JM, Donnelly JB. 2003. Mobilization of lead from human bone tissue during pregnancy and lactation—a summary of long-term research. Sci Total Environ 303(1-2):79-104.

Hernandez-Avila M, Smith D, Meneses F, Sanin LH, Hu H. 1998. The influence of bone and blood lead on plasma lead levels in environmentally exposed adults. Environ Health Perspect 106(8):473-7.

Ip S, Chung M, Raman G, Chew P, Magula N, DeVine D, et al. 2007. Breastfeeding and maternal and infant health outcomes in developed countries. Evidence report/technology assessment No. 153. AHRQ Publication No. 07-E007. Rockville, MD: Agency for Healthcare Research and Quality.

Kwan ML, Buffler PA, Abrams B, Kiley VA. 2004. Breastfeeding and the risk of childhood leukemia: a meta-analysis. Public Health Rep 119:521-35.

Lawrence RA. 1997. A review of the medical benefits and contraindications to breastfeeding in the United States. Maternal and child health technical information bulletin. Arlington, VA: National Center for Education in Maternal and Child Health.

Lawrence RA, Lawrence RM. 2005. Breastfeeding. A Guide for the Medical Profession. 6th ed. Philadelphia: Elsevier Mosby, Inc.

Li PJ, Sheng YZ, Wang QY, Gu LY, Wang YL. 2000. Transfer of lead via placenta and breast milk in human. Biomed Environ Sci 13(2):85-9.

Lonnerdal B. 1985. Dietary factors affecting trace element bioavailability from human milk, cow's milk and infant formulas. Prog Food Nutr Sci 9(1-2):35-62.

Manton WI, Angle CR, Stanek KL, Kuntzelman D, Reese YR, Kuehnemann TJ. 2003. Release of lead from bone in pregnancy and lactation. Environ Res 92(2):139-51.

Manton WI, Angle CR, Stanek KL, Reese YR, Kuehnemann TJ. 2000. Acquisition and retention of lead by young children. Environ Res 82(1):60-80.

Manton WI, Cook JD. 1984. High accuracy (stable isotope dilution) measurements of lead in serum and cerebrospinal fluid. Br J Ind Med 41(3):313-9.

Manton WI, Rothenberg SJ, Manalo M. 2001. The lead content of blood serum. Environ Res 86(3):263-73.

Namihira D, Saldivar L, Pustilnik N, Carreon GJ, Salinas ME. 1993. Lead in human blood and milk from nursing women living near a smelter in Mexico City. J Toxicol Environ Health 38(3):225-32.

O'Flaherty EJ. 1993. Physiologically based models for bone-seeking elements. IV. Kinetics of lead disposition in humans. Toxicol Appl Pharmacol 118(1):16-29.

O'Flaherty EJ. 1995. Physiologically based models for bone-seeking elements. V. Lead absorption and disposition in childhood. Toxicol Appl Pharmacol. 131(2):297-308.

Owen CG, Martin RM, Whincup PH, et al. Does breastfeeding influence risk of type 2 diabetes in later life? A quantitative analysis of published evidence. Am J Clin Nutr 2006;84(5):1043-54.

Rabinowitz M, Leviton A, Needleman H. 1985. Lead in milk and infant blood: a dose-response model. Arch Environ Health 40(5):283-6.

Rothenberg SJ, Karchmer S, Schnaas L, Perroni E, Zea F, Fernandez Alba J. 1994. Changes in serial blood lead levels during pregnancy. Environ Health Perspect 102(10):876-80.

Schutz A, Bergdahl IA, Ekholm A, Skerfving S. 1996. Measurement by ICP-MS of leadin plasma and whole blood of lead workers and controls. Occup Environ Med 53(11):736-40.

Shannon M. 1998. Lead poisoning from an unexpected source in a 4-month-old infant. Environ Health Perspect 106(6):313-6.

Shannon M, Graef JW. 1989. Lead intoxication from lead-contaminated water used to reconstitute infant formula. Clin Pediatr (Phila) 28(8):380-2.

Sowers MR, Scholl TO, Hall G, Jannausch ML, Kemp FW, Li X, et al. 2002. Lead in breast milk and maternal bone turnover. Am J Obstet Gynecol 187(3):770-6.

Tellez-Rojo MM, Hernandez-Avila M, Gonzalez-Cossio T, Romieu I, Aro A, Palazuelos E, et al. 2002. Impact of breastfeeding on the mobilization of lead from bone. Am J Epidemiol 155(5):420-8.

U.S. Department of Health and Human Services. 2000. HHS blueprint for action on breastfeeding. Washington, DC: U.S. Department of Health and Human Services.

U.S. Environmental Protection Agency. 1997. Chapter 14-breast milk intake. Exposure factors handbook, volume II, update. EPA/600/P-95/002Fa. Washington, DC: U.S. Environmental Protection Agency.

U.S. Food and Drug Administration. 2007. Total diet study statistics on element results. Revision 4.1, market baskets 1991-3 through 2005-4. College Park, MD: Center for Food Safety and Applied Nutrition.

World Health Organization Collaborative Study Team on the Role of Breastfeeding on the Prevention of Infant Mortality. 2000. Effect of breastfeeding on infant and child mortality due to infectious diseases in less developed countries: a pooled analysis. Lancet 355(9202):451-5.

APPENDICES

Institute of Medicine. 1997. Dietary reference intakes for calcium, phosphorus, magnesium, vitamin D and fluoride. Food and Nutrition Board. Washington, DC: National Academy Press.

Institute of Medicine. 1998. Dietary reference intakes for thiamin, riboflavin, niacin, vitamin B6, folate, vitamin B12, pantothenic acid, biotin, and choline. Food and Nutrition Board. Washington, DC: National Academy Press.

Institute of Medicine. 2000. Dietary reference intakes for vitamin a, vitamin k, arsenic, boron, chromium, copper, iodine, iron, manganese, molybdenum, nickel, silicon, vanadium, and zinc. Food and Nutrition Board. Washington, DC: National Academy Press.

Institute of Medicine. 2000. Dietary reference intakes: applications in dietary assessment. Food and Nutrition Board. Washington, DC: National Academy Press.

Institute of Medicine. 2001. Dietary reference intakes for vitamin c, vitamin e, selenium, and carotenoids. Food and Nutrition Board. Washington, DC: National Academy Press.

Institute of Medicine. 2003. Dietary reference intakes: applications in dietary planning. Food and Nutrition Board. Washington, DC: National Academy Press.

Institute of Medicine. 2004. Dietary reference intakes for water, potassium, sodium, chloride, and sulfate. Food and Nutrition Board. Washington, DC: National Academy Press.

Institute of Medicine. 2005. Dietary reference intakes for energy, carbohydrate, fiber, fat, fatty acids, cholesterol, protein, and amino acids (macronutrients). Food and Nutrition Board. Washington, DC: National Academy Press.

Institute of Medicine. 2006. Dietary reference intakes research synthesis: workshop summary. Food and Nutrition Board. Washington, DC: National Academy Press.

Parsons PJ, Chisolm JJ, Delves HT, Griffin R, Gunter EW, Slavin W, et al. 2001. Analytical procedures for the determination of lead in blood and urine, approved guideline. NCCLS document C40-A (ISBN 1-56238-437-6). Wayne, PA: NCCLS.

Appendices

Appendix I
Existing State Legislation Related to Lead and Pregnant Women

Existing State Legislation Related to Lead and Pregnant Women

SCREENING LAW(S):

New York Public Health Law §1370-a(2)
Summary: Requires dept to promulgate and enforce regulations for screening children and **pregnant women** for lead poisoning, and for follow-up treatment for those with positive results.

New York Public Health Law §1370-c
Summary: Authorizes dept to establish screening intervals and methods, which shall be followed by every physician or other provider of medical care to children or **pregnant women**.

Connecticut Gen. Stat. §19a-111
The commissioner shall establish, in conjunction with recognized professional medical groups, guidelines consistent with the CDC for assessment of the risk of lead poisoning, screening for lead poisoning and treatment and follow-up care of individuals including children with lead poisoning, women who are **pregnant** and women who are planning **pregnancy**.

RISK REDUCTION LAW(S):

Maryland Code §6-801- 6-852; Article 48A §734-737; Real Property § 8-208.2
Comply with specific Risk Reduction standards when notified of certain conditions such as chipping paint or the presence in the unit of a child or **pregnant woman** with an elevated blood lead level of 15 µg/dl or higher.

Minnesota Statute §144.9504
Lead risk assessment. (a) An assessing agency shall conduct a lead risk assessment of a residence according to the venous blood lead level and time frame set forth in clauses (1) to (4) for purposes of secondary prevention: within ten working days of a **pregnant female** in the residence being identified to the agency as having a venous blood lead level equal to or greater than ten micrograms of lead per deciliter of whole blood.
Subd. 5. Lead orders. (a) An assessing agency, after conducting a lead risk assessment, shall order a property owner to perform lead hazard reduction on all lead sources that exceed a standard adopted according to section 144.9508.

EDUCATION LAW(S):

Michigan Comp. Laws §333.5473a(2-3)
Summary: Requires department to establish and conduct educational programs to educate homeowners and remodelers of lead-safe practices and methods of lead-hazard reduction activities; (4): requires department to recommend appropriate maintenance practices for owners of residential property and day care facilities designed to prevent lead poisoning in children 6 years or younger and **pregnant women**.

PROPOSED LEGISLATION (NOT ENACTED):

California – Requires the Department to make available to all health care providers that administer **perinatal care** services informational materials on lead and require providers to make this information available to **pregnant women**.
New York – Bill aimed at eliminating lead hazards in housing which is or will be occupied by **pregnant women** or children 7 years of age or less.
Ohio - Requires the Director to produce an educational audio-video recording on lead poisoning prevention for at-risk **pregnant women**.

Appendix II
Charge Questions to the Lead and Pregnancy Work Group

Charge Questions to the Lead and Pregnancy Work Group

Subgroup 1. Prevalence, Risk and Screening
This group was asked to review literature including but not limited to:
- Distribution of BLLs and other measures of lead body burden in:
  – women of childbearing-age
  – pregnant women at various gestational ages
  – lactating women
  – newborns
- Risk factors/sources for elevated blood lead levels in pregnant and lactating women and the newborns
- Relationship between:
  – maternal blood/bone lead levels and newborn blood lead levels
  – pregnancy BLLs and postpartum BLLs?

Based on subgroup findings, address the following questions:
- When should pregnant women be screened for lead poisoning and when should screening occur? Are there questions that can predict which woman should be screened?
- What culturally sensitive interventions should be recommended to reduce exposure to potential sources?

Subgroup 2. Maternal, Pregnancy and Child Outcomes
This group was asked to review literature including but not limited to:
- Impact of elevated blood lead levels on:
  – fertility (spontaneous abortion, stillbirth)
  – maternal health (pregnancy induced hypertension)
  – pregnancy outcomes (preterm delivery, gestational age, birth weight, birth length, head circumference)
  – neurodevelopment outcomes due to prenatal exposure
  – behavioral outcomes due to prenatal exposure

Based on subgroup findings, address the following questions:
- When blood lead levels are elevated, what guidance should medical providers be providing to:
  – women of child-bearing age regarding delaying of pregnancy?
  – pregnant women about potential outcomes?

Subgroup 3. Management, Treatment and Other Interventions
This group was asked to review literature including but not limited to:
- Breast milk exposure including:
  – Amount transmitted to baby
  – Benefits vs. hazards of breast feeding when blood lead levels are elevated
- Effectiveness of nutritional supplementation during pregnancy and lactation
- Indications/Contraindications/Adverse effects of chelation on:
  – pregnant woman, fetus, and newborns

Based on subgroup findings, address the following questions:
- What is the follow-up testing schedule at various blood lead levels for pregnant and lactating women and for the newborns?
- At what blood lead level, if any, should women be advised against breastfeeding?
- What nutrition counseling or nutritional supplements should be recommended?
- What chelating agents should be employed?
- What interventions should be provided by public health agencies at various blood lead levels?

Appendix III
Commonly Ingested Substances in Pregnancy-related Pica, Reasons for Use, and Country/Race-Ethnicity or Origin

Commonly-ingested Substances in Pregnancy-related Pica, Reasons for Use, and Country/Race-Ethnicity of Origin

Substance/Name	Reason Used (If known or reported)	Country	Race/Ethnicity or Regional Affiliation
Bean Stones		**Mexico**	
Clay		**Asia** India	Hindu
Clay		**Caribbean** Trinidad Jamaica	Hindu
Clay		**Africa**: Uganda, Kenya, Zambia Ghana South Africa	
Clay		**Middle East** Saudi Arabia	
Clay (Cipula, Kipula, Akipula, Askipula)		**Central America** Belize	
Clay, Clay Pottery (Tierra Santa, Benditos)		**Mexico**	
Clay		**North America** US	African-Americans (South, particularly rural areas) Immigrants
Corn Starch	Nausea/GI upset	US	African-Americans (South)
Dirt or soil		**Mexico**	
Ice/Refrigerator Frost	Relieve thirst, cool down	**North America** US Mexico	African-Americans (South)
Milk of Magnesia (Solid)		**Mexico**	

Appendix IV
List of Occupations and Hobbies That Involve Lead Exposure

List of Occupations and Hobbies that Involve Lead Exposure

Lead Related Occupations and Industries

Ammunition/explosives production
Automotive repair shops
Battery manufacturing and recycling
Brass, bronze, copper or lead foundries
Bridge, tunnel and elevated highway/subway construction
Cable/wire stripping, splicing or production
Ceramic manufacturing
Firing range work
Glass recycling, stained glass and glass manufacturing
Home renovation/restoration
Lead Abatement
Lead production or smelting
Machining or grinding lead alloys
Manufacturing and installation of plumbing components
Manufacturing of industrial machinery and equipment
Metal scrap yards and other recycling operations
Motor vehicle parts and accessories
Occupations using firearms
Plastics manufacturing
Pottery making
Production and use of chemical preparations
Rubber manufacturing
Sandblasting, sanding, scraping, burning or disturbing lead paint
Use of lead based paints
Welding or torch-cutting painted metal

Hobbies and Activities That May Cause Lead Exposure

Making stained glass and painting on stained glass
Copper Enameling
Bronze Casting
Making pottery and ceramic ware with lead glazes and paints
Casting ammunition, fishing weights or lead figurines
Collecting, painting or playing games with lead figurines
Jewelry making with lead solder
Electronics with lead solder
Furniture refinishing
Glassblowing with leaded glass
Print making and other fine arts
Liquor distillation
Hunting and target shooting
Remodeling/renovating homes built before 1978

Appendix V
Alternative Cosmetics, Food Additives, and Medicines That Contain Lead

Alternative Cosmetics, Food Additives, and Medicines that Contain Lead

Exposure Source	Description/Exposure Pathway
Albayalde or *albayaidle*	Used by mainly by Mexicans and Central Americans to treat vomiting, colic, apathy and lethargy.
Al Kohl (Middle East, India, Pakistan, some parts of Africa)	A gray or black eye cosmetic applied to the conjunctival margins of the eyes for medicinal and cosmetic reasons. Can contain up to 83% lead. It is believed to strengthen and protect the eyes against disease and may be used as an umbilical stump remedy. Also known as simply as **kohl**.
Al Murrah	Used as a remedy for colic, stomach aches and diarrhea in Saudi Arabia.
Anzroot	A remedy from the Middle East used to treat gastroenteritis.
Azarcon	Also known as **alarcon**, **coral**, **luiga**, **maria luisa**, or **rueda**. Bright orange powder used to treat "empacho" (an illness believed to be caused by something stuck in the gastrointestinal tract, resulting in diarrhea and vomiting). Azarcon is 95% lead.
Ayurvedic medicine (Tibet)	Traditional medicines that may contain lead. Some examples include: **guglu, sundari kalp, jambrulin**
Ba-Baw-San or *Ba-Bow-Sen* (China)	Herbal medicine used to detoxify "fetal poisoning" and treat colic pain or to pacify young children.
Bali goli	A round, flat black bean which is dissolved in "gripe water" and used within Asian Indian cultures for stomach ache.
Bint Al Zahab (Iran)	Rock ground into a powder and mixed with honey and butter given to newborn babies for colic and early passage of meconium after birth.
Bint Dahab (Saudi Arabia; means "daughter of gold")	A yellow lead oxide used by local jewelers and as a home remedy for diarrhea, colic, constipation and general neonatal uses.
Bokhoor (Kuwait)	A traditional practice of burning wood and lead sulfide to produce pleasant fumes to calm infants.
Cebagin	Used in the Middle East as a teething powder.
Chuifong tokuwan	A pill imported from Hong Kong used to treat a wide variety of ailments.
Cordyceps	Used in China as a treatment for hypertension, diabetes and bleeding.
Deshi Dewa	A fertility pill used in Asia and India.
Farouk	A teething powder from Saudi Arabia.
Ghasard	Brown powder used in Asian Indian cultures as a tonic to aid in digestion.
Greta (Mexico)	Yellow powder used to treat "empacho" (see **azarcon**); can be obtained through pottery suppliers, as it is also used as a glaze for low-fired ceramics. Greta is 97% lead.
Hai Ge Fen (Concha cyclinae sinensis)	A Chinese herbal remedy derived from crushed clam shells.
Henna	Used as a hair dye and for temporary tattoos in the Middle East and India - may contain lead.

Jin Bu Huan (China)	An herbal medicine used to relieve pain.
Kandu	A red powder from Asia and India used to treat stomach ache.
Koo Sar	Red pills from China used to treat menstrual cramps.
Kushta	Used for diseases of the heart, brain, liver, and stomach and as an aphrodisiac and tonic in India and Pakistan.
Litargirio	A yellow or peach-colored powder used as a deodorant, a foot fungicide and a treatment for burns and wound healing particularly by people from the Dominican Republic.
Lozeena	An orange powder used to color rice and meat that contains 7.8%-8.9% lead.
Pay-loo-ah (Vietnam)	A red powder given to children to cure fever or rash.
Po Ying Tan (China)	An herbal medicine used to treat minor ailments in children.
Santrinj (Saudi Arabia)	An amorphous red powder containing 98% lead oxide used principally as a primer for paint for metallic surfaces, but also as a home remedy for "gum boils" and "teething."
Surma (India)	Black powder used as an eye cosmetic and as teething powder or umbilical stump remedy.
Tibetan herbal vitamin	Used to strengthen the brain.
Traditional Saudi medicine	Orange powder prescribed by a traditional medicine practitioner for teething; also has an antidiarrheal effect.

Appendix VI
Recommendations for Medical Management of Adult Lead Exposure

Recommendations for Medical Management of Adult Lead Exposure

Michael J. Kosnett,[1] Richard P. Wedeen,[2] Stephen J. Rothenberg,[3,4] Karen L. Hipkins,[5] Barbara L. Materna,[6] Brian S. Schwartz,[7,8] Howard Hu,[9] and Alan Woolf[10]

[1]Division of Clinical Pharmacology and Toxicology, Department of Medicine, University of Colorado Health Sciences Center, Denver, Colorado, USA; [2]Department of Veterans Affairs, New Jersey Health Care System, East Orange, New Jersey, USA; [3]CINVESTAV-IPN (Centro de Investigaciones y de Estudios Avanzados-Instituto Politécnico Nacional), Merida, Yucatan, Mexico; [4]National Institute of Public Health, Cuernavaca, Morelos, Mexico; [5]Public Health Institute, Occupational Lead Poisoning Prevention Program, Richmond, California, USA; [6]California Department of Health Services, Occupational Health Branch, Richmond, California, USA; [7]Departments of Environmental Health Sciences and Epidemiology, Johns Hopkins Bloomberg School of Public Health, Baltimore, Maryland, USA; [8]Department of Medicine, Johns Hopkins School of Medicine, Baltimore, Maryland, USA; [9]Department of Environmental Health Sciences, University of Michigan School of Public Health, Ann Arbor, Michigan, USA; [10]Program in Environmental Health, Division of General Pediatrics, Children's Hospital, Boston, Massachusetts, USA

Research conducted in recent years has increased public health concern about the toxicity of lead at low dose and has supported a reappraisal of the levels of lead exposure that may be safely tolerated in the workplace. In this article, which appears as part of a mini-monograph on adult lead exposure, we summarize a body of published literature that establishes the potential for hypertension, effects on renal function, cognitive dysfunction, and adverse female reproductive outcome in adults with whole-blood lead concentrations < 40 µg/dL. Based on this literature, and our collective experience in evaluating lead-exposed adults, we recommend that individuals be removed from occupational lead exposure if a single blood lead concentration exceeds 30 µg/dL or if two successive blood lead concentrations measured over a 4-week interval are ≥ 20 µg/dL. Removal of individuals from lead exposure should be considered to avoid long-term risk to health if exposure control measures over an extended period do not decrease blood lead concentrations to < 10 µg/dL or if selected medical conditions exist that would increase the risk of continued exposure. Recommended medical surveillance for all lead-exposed workers should include quarterly blood lead measurements for individuals with blood lead concentrations between 10 and 19 µg/dL, and semiannual blood lead measurements when sustained blood lead concentrations are < 10 µg/dL. It is advisable for pregnant women to avoid occupational or avocational lead exposure that would result in blood lead concentrations > 5 µg/dL. Chelation may have an adjunctive role in the medical management of highly exposed adults with symptomatic lead intoxication but is not recommended for asymptomatic individuals with low blood lead concentrations. Key words: adult lead exposure, blood lead, chelation, medical management, medical surveillance, pregnancy. Environ Health Perspect 115:463–471 (2007). doi:10.1289/ehp.9784 available via http://dx.doi.org/ [Online 22 December 2006]

As a likely consequence of its capacity to interfere with biochemical events present in cells throughout the body, inorganic lead exerts a wide spectrum of multisystemic adverse effects. These health impacts range from subtle, subclinical changes in function to symptomatic, life-threatening intoxication. In recent years, research conducted on lead-exposed adults has increased public health concern over the toxicity of lead at low dose. These findings support a reappraisal of the levels of lead exposure, sustained for either short or extended periods of time, that may be safely tolerated in the workplace. In this article we offer health-based recommendations on the management of lead-exposed adults aimed at primary and secondary prevention of lead-associated health problems. As noted in the introduction to this mini-monograph (Schwartz and Hu 2007) the authors of this article are an independent subgroup of an expert panel (8 of 13 members) originally convened by the Association of Occupational and Environmental Clinics (www.aoec.org) to address these management issues. In deriving the recommendations in this article, we took note of a body of literature that establishes the potential for adverse health effects at blood lead concentrations or exposure levels permissible under current workplace regulations established in the 1970s by the U.S. Occupational Safety and Health Administration (OSHA). These regulations generally require removal from lead exposure when whole-blood lead concentrations exceed 50 or 60 µg/dL. These values are considerably above blood lead concentrations of the general population of the United States, which had a geometric mean of 12.8 µg/dL in the late 1970s (National Center for Health Statistics 1984), and a recent value of 1.45 µg/dL [U.S. Centers for Disease Control and Prevention (CDC) 2005].

In setting forth our perspective on the recommended medical management of adult lead exposure, the narrative of this article focuses on four categories of health effects—hypertension, decrement in renal function, cognitive dysfunction, and adverse reproductive outcome—that have been the subject of much recent research. The discussion of these end points highlights those studies, that by virtue of their design and scope, were particularly influential in establishing the authors' concerns regarding the potential for adverse health effects at low to moderate levels of lead exposure in adults. Collectively, these effects support the preventive medical management strategies that are recommended in the tables. A review of the extensive literature on the health effects of lead is beyond the scope of this article, but the reader is referred to reviews on the cardiovascular and cognitive impacts of lead on adults that appear elsewhere in this mini-monograph (Navas-Acien et al. 2007; Shih et al. 2007), as well as a review on recent lead literature prepared by the U.S. Environmental Protection Agency (EPA) for its Air Quality Criteria for Lead (U.S. EPA 2006).

Table 1 is a summary of the adverse health risks associated with different blood lead concentrations and presents corresponding medical management recommendations that range from discussion of risks and

This article is part of the mini-monograph "Lead Exposure and Health Effects in Adults: Evidence, Management, and Implications for Policy."

Address correspondence to M. Kosnett, 1630 Welton St., Ste. 300, Denver, CO 80202 USA. Telephone: (303) 571-5778. Fax: (303) 571-5820. E-mail: Michael.Kosnett@uchsc.edu

The findings and conclusions in this article are those of the authors and do not necessarily represent the views of CDHS. All other authors declare no competing financial interest.

The participation of H.H. was supported in part by National Institute of Environmental Health Sciences grants R01 ES05257, R01 ES10798, and R01 ES07821, and Center grant ES0002.

MJK is an independent consultant who has provided paid consultation to community groups, industrial corporations, and governmental agencies regarding the health effects of occupational and environmental exposure to lead. He received no funding from any party for his contributions to this manuscript. B.L.M. and K.L.H. are affiliated with the Occupational Health Branch, California Department of Health Services (CDHS).

Received 3 October 2006; accepted 21 December 2006.

reduction of lead exposure at low levels to removal from lead exposure accompanied by probable chelation therapy at the highest levels. The designation of risks as either "short-term" or "long-term," depending on whether the risks are associated with exposure lasting less than or more than 1 year, reflects a qualitative understanding of the duration of lead exposure that may be required to elicit certain adverse health effects of lead. For some of the long-term risks, such as hypertension, research employing noninvasive K-shell X-ray fluorescence measurement of lead in bone, a biomarker of long-term cumulative exposure, suggests that several years of sustained elevations in blood lead may be necessary for a significant risk to emerge. The use of 1 year as a cut-point in the table is not intended to represent a sharp division, in terms of cumulative dose, between what might constitute a short-term versus a long-term risk nor does it imply that a significant long-term risk begins to exist as soon as 1 year is surpassed. Blood lead, a measure of the amount of lead circulating in the tissues, reflects both recent exogenous exposure as well as endogenous redistribution of lead stored in bone.

The categorization of risks in Table 1 by discrete intervals of blood lead concentration is a qualitative assessment. In clinical practice, substantial interindividual variability in the susceptibility to symptomatic adverse effects of lead is commonly observed. Factors that might influence the risk of lead toxicity in adults include preexisting disease affecting relevant target organs (e.g., hypertension, renal disease, or neurologic dysfunction), nutritional deficiencies that modify the absorption or distribution of lead (e.g., low dietary calcium or iron deficiency), advanced age, and genetic susceptibility. Although recent studies suggest that polymorphisms in specific genes may modify the toxicokinetics and renal effects of lead (Theppeang et al. 2004; Weaver et al. 2006; Wu et al. 2003), research findings at present are insufficient to conclusively identify genotypes that confer increased risk.

Table 1. Health-based management recommendations for lead-exposed adults.

Blood lead level (µg/dL)	Short-term risks (lead exposure < 1 year)	Long-term risks (lead exposure ≥ 1 year)	Management
< 5	None documented	None documented	None indicated
5–9	Possible spontaneous abortion Possible postnatal developmental delay	Possible spontaneous abortion Possible postnatal developmental delay Possible hypertension and kidney dysfunction	Discuss health risks Reduce lead exposure for women who are or may become pregnant
10–19	Possible spontaneous abortion Possible postnatal developmental delay Reduced birth weight	Possible spontaneous abortion Reduced birth weight Possible postnatal developmental delay Hypertension and kidney dysfunction Possible subclinical neurocognitive deficits	As above for BLL 5–9 µg/dL, plus: Decrease lead exposure Increase biological monitoring Consider removal from lead exposure to avoid long-term risks if exposure control over an extended period does not decrease BLL < 10 µg/dL, or if medical condition present that increases risk with continued exposure[a]
20–29	Possible spontaneous abortion Possible postnatal developmental delay Reduced birth weight	Possible spontaneous abortion Possible postnatal developmental delay Reduced birth weight Hypertension and kidney dysfunction Possible subclinical neurocognitive deficits	Remove from lead exposure if repeat BLL measured in 4 weeks remains ≥ 20 µg/dL
30–39	Spontaneous abortion Possible postnatal developmental delay Reduced birth weight	Spontaneous abortion Reduced birth weight Possible postnatal developmental delay Hypertension and kidney dysfunction Possible neurocognitive deficits Possible nonspecific symptoms[b]	Remove from lead exposure
40–79	Spontaneous abortion Reduced birth weight Possible postnatal developmental delay Nonspecific symptoms[b] Neurocognitive deficits Sperm abnormalities	Spontaneous abortion Reduced birth weight Possible postnatal developmental delay Nonspecific symptoms[b] Hypertension Kidney dysfunction/nephropathy Subclinical peripheral neuropathy Neurocognitive deficits Sperm abnormalities Anemia Colic Possible gout	Remove from lead exposure Refer for prompt medical evaluation Consider chelation therapy for BLL > 50 µg/dL with significant symptoms or signs of lead toxicity
≥ 80	Spontaneous abortion Reduced birth weight Possible postnatal developmental delay Nonspecific symptoms[b] Neurocognitive deficits Encephalopathy Sperm abnormalities Anemia Colic	Spontaneous abortion Reduced birth weight Possible postnatal developmental delay Nonspecific symptoms[b] Hypertension Nephropathy Peripheral neuropathy Neurocognitive deficits Sperm abnormalities Anemia Colic Gout	Remove from lead exposure Refer for immediate/urgent medical evaluation Probable chelation therapy

BLL, blood lead level.
[a]Medical conditions that may increase the risk of continued exposure include chronic renal dysfunction (serum creatinine > 1.5 mg/dL for men and > 1.3 mg/dL for women, or proteinuria), hypertension, neurologic disorders, and cognitive dysfunction. [b]Nonspecific symptoms may include headache, fatigue, sleep disturbance, anorexia, constipation, arthralgia, myalgia, and decreased libido.

Health Effects at Low Dose

Hypertension. Animal investigations support a pressor effect of lead at low dose (Fine et al. 1988; Gonick et al. 1997; Vaziri 2002). Epidemiologic investigations conducted in large general population samples (e.g., Harlan 1988; Nash et al. 2003; Pocock et al. 1988; Schwartz 1988) suggest lead may elevate blood pressure in adults at blood lead concentrations < 20 µg/dL. In some human studies of the link between blood lead and blood pressure, the relationship appeared to be influenced by subjects' sex or race (e.g., Den Hond et al. 2002; Staessen et al. 1996; Vupputuri et al. 2003). Three meta-analyses of studies examining the relationship between blood lead and blood pressure found relatively consistent effects of blood lead on blood pressure. The studies showed statistically significant coefficients for a 2-fold increase in blood lead of 1.0 mmHg (Nawrot et al. 2002; Staessen et al. 1994) or 1.25 mmHg (Schwartz 1995) for systolic blood pressure, and 0.6 mmHg for diastolic blood pressure (Nawrot et al. 2002; Staessen et al. 1994). The study populations analyzed in these meta-analyses included many with blood lead concentrations < 20 µg/dL.

Further support for the impact of low-level lead exposure on blood pressure has emerged from studies employing K-shell X-ray fluorescence measurement of lead in bone, a biomarker of long-term cumulative lead exposure. In two major studies drawn from samples of the general population, bone lead concentration was a significant predictor of the risk of hypertension (Hu et al. 1996; Korrick et al. 1999). Findings from the study by Hu et al. (1996) illustrate the associated risk. In that general population sample of middle-aged to elderly men (n = 590), the average blood lead concentration was 6.3 µg/dL. On the basis of the subjects' ages (mean 67 ± 7.2 years), it may be expected that they lived most of their adult lives at a time when the blood lead concentration of the general population ranged from 10 to 25 µg/dL (Hofreuter et al. 1961; Mahaffey et al. 1982; Minot 1938). Comparing the lowest with the highest quintile of bone lead among that cohort, a tibia bone lead increment of 29 µg/g was associated with a 1.5 odds ratio (OR) for hypertension [95% confidence interval (CI), 1.1–1.8]. Given the slope of 0.05 that has described the linear relationship between tibia bone lead concentration and cumulative blood lead index in subjects with chronic lead exposure in many studies (Hu et al. 2007), this increment in bone lead is roughly equivalent to a cumulative blood lead index of 580 µg/dL · years (i.e., 29 ÷ 0.05 = 580). Considered in the context of a 40-year working lifetime, the risk of lead-associated hypertension may be significantly reduced by preventive measures that lower chronic workplace blood lead concentrations from the 20s and 30s µg/dL range to < 10 µg/dL. For example, a change in average workplace blood lead concentration from 25 to 10 µg/dL over a 40-year working lifetime would reduce a worker's cumulative blood lead index by 600 µg/dL · years, slightly more than the 580 µg/dL · years cited above.

Hypertension is a significant risk factor for cardiovascular and cerebrovascular mortality. As reviewed in an accompanying article in this mini-monograph (Navas-Acien et al. 2007), studies conducted in general population cohorts have consistently observed a positive association between lead exposure and cardiovascular disease. Because of their size and design, studies derived from the National Health and Nutrition Evaluation Surveys (NHANES) are particularly notable. A 16-year longitudinal analysis of the general population cohort studied between 1976 and 1980 as part of NHANES II found that blood lead concentrations of 20–29 µg/dL at baseline were associated with 39% increased mortality from circulatory system disease compared with subjects with blood lead < 10 µg/dL [relative risk (RR) 1.39; 95% CI, 1.01–1.91] (Lustberg and Silbergeld 2002). Two studies recently examined the longitudinal relationship between blood lead concentration and cardiovascular mortality among participants in NHANES III. In a 12-year longitudinal study of participants in NHANES III, ≥ 40 years of age (n = 9,757), the subgroup with blood lead concentration ≥ 10 µg/dL (median, 11.8) had a relative risk of cardiovascular mortality of 1.59 (95% CI, 1.28–1.98) compared with subjects with blood lead < 5 µg/dL (Schober et al. 2006). In a 12-year longitudinal analysis of subjects ≥ 17 years of age (n = 13,946), the relative risk for cardiovascular mortality was 1.53 (95% CI, 1.21–1.94), comparing a blood lead of 4.92 µg/dL (80th percentile of the distribution) with a blood lead of 1.46 µg/dL (20th percentile of the distribution) (Menke et al. 2006).

Renal effects. Renal injury that appears after acute high-dose lead exposure may include reversible deficits in proximal tubular reabsorption and prerenal azotemia induced by renal vasoconstriction and/or volume depletion (Coyle et al. 200; Wedeen et al. 1979). In a minority of exposed individuals, years of chronic, high-dose lead exposure may result in chronic lead nephropathy, a slowly progressive interstitial fibrosis characterized by scant proteinuria (Lilis et al. 1968). Epidemiologic investigations of renal function in workers with lower levels of chronic lead exposure have yielded variable findings. For example, in a cohort of approximately 800 current and former lead workers with mean blood lead of 32 ± 15 µg/dL, there was no significant linear relationship between blood lead concentration and two measures of renal function, serum creatinine and creatinine clearance (Weaver et al. 2003). There was an interaction between age and tibia lead concentration, a biomarker of cumulative lead exposure, on these same biomarkers, resulting in a trend toward worse renal function with increasing bone lead in the oldest tercile of workers (> 46 years of age) but improved renal function with increasing bone lead in the youngest workers (≤ 36 years of age). The authors suggested that lead-induced hyperfiltration, a finding noted in other studies, might presage the eventual development of lead-induced renal insufficiency. Both blood lead and tibia lead were correlated with increased urinary N-acetyl-β-D-glucosaminidase (NAG), a biomarker of early biological effect on the renal tubule, but in an analysis of a smaller subset of the lead workers (n = 190) that controlled for the relatively low levels of urinary cadmium (1.1 ± 0.78 µg/g creatinine), only the relationship with tibia lead and NAG remained significant (Weaver et al. 2003). Among a cohort of 70 active lead workers with a median blood lead concentration of 32 µg/dL (range, 5–47), there were modest correlations between blood lead and urinary β-2-microglobulin (r = 0.27; p = 0.02), and between cumulative blood lead index and NAG (r = 0.25; p = 0.04) (Gerhardsson et al. 1992).

Several studies conducted in general population samples have reported an association between blood lead concentration and common biomarkers of renal function (serum creatinine and creatinine clearance). In a cross-sectional investigation of a subcohort of middle-aged to elderly men enrolled in the Normative Aging Study (n = 744), there was a negative correlation between blood lead (mean, 8.1 ± 3.9 µg/dL; range, < 4.0–26.0 µg/dL) and measured creatinine clearance, after natural log transformation of both variables and adjustment for other covariates (Payton et al. 1994). Among an adult population that included subjects with environmental cadmium exposure [n = 965 men (geometric mean blood lead, 11.4 µg/dL; range, 2.3–72.5 µg/dL); n = 1,016 women (geometric mean blood lead, 7.5 µg/dL; range, 1.7–60.3 µg/dL)], log-transformed blood lead concentration was inversely correlated with measured creatinine clearance (Staessen et al. 1992). In a population-based study of Swedish women 50–59 years of age (n = 820), low levels of blood lead (mean 2.2 µg/dL; 5th–95th percentiles, 1.1–4.6 µg/dL) were inversely correlated with creatinine clearance and glomerular filtration rate, after adjusting for age, body mass index, urinary or blood cadmium, hypertension, diabetes, and regular use of nonsteroidal anti-inflammatory drug (NSAID) medication (Akesson et al. 2005).

Individuals with other risk factors for renal disease, notably hypertension and diabetes, may be more susceptible to an adverse impact of low-level lead exposure on renal function. Among adults participating in NHANES III (n = 15,211), blood lead was a risk factor for elevated serum creatinine (defined as ≥ 99th percentile of the analyte's race and sex specific distributions, generally > 1.2–1.5 mg/dL) and "chronic kidney disease" (defined as an estimated glomerular filtration rate < 60 mL/min) only among subjects with hypertension (n = 4813) (Muntner et al. 2003). Compared with hypertensives in the lowest quartile of blood lead (range, 0.7–2.4 µg/dL), hypertensive subjects in the next highest quartile of blood lead (range, 2.5–3.8 µg/dL) had a covariate adjusted OR for elevated serum creatinine of 1.47 (95% CI, 1.03–2.10) and for chronic kidney disease of 1.44 (95% CI, 1.00–2.09). At the next highest quartile of blood lead (range, 3.9–5.9 µg/dL), the covariate-adjusted OR for elevated serum creatinine was 1.80 (95% CI, 1.34–2.42), and for chronic kidney disease it was 1.85 (95% CI, 1.32–2.59). In a subcohort of middle-aged to elderly men participating in the Normative Aging Study (n = 427, blood lead 4.5 ± 2.5 µg/dL), multiple regression analysis revealed that log-transformed blood lead was positively correlated with serum creatinine in hypertensive but not normotensive subjects (Tsaih et al. 2004). In a longitudinal study of this cohort over a mean of 6 years, an interaction between lead and diabetes yielded a positive association between baseline blood lead concentration and change in serum creatinine that was strongest in diabetic subjects (Tsaih et al. 2004). An interaction with diabetes was also present in the association of tibial lead concentration with longitudinal change in serum creatinine (Tsaih et al. 2004). Although these general population studies are consistent with an adverse effect of lead exposure on renal function at notably low levels, the extent to which diminished renal function may itself result in increased body lead burden has not been fully elucidated.

Cognitive dysfunction. A few studies examining relatively small numbers of workers (n ≤ 100) with blood lead concentrations ranging approximately 20–40 µg/dL have associated lead exposure with subclinical decrements in selective domains of neurocognitive function (Barth et al. 2002; Hänninen et al. 1998; Mantere et al. 1984; Stollery 1996). Among a large cohort of current and former inorganic lead workers studied in Korea, a cross-sectional analysis (n = 803 workers) (Schwartz et al. 2001) and a 3-year longitudinal analysis (n = 576 workers)

(Schwartz et al. 2005) found that blood lead concentrations across the approximate range of 20–50 µg/dL were associated with subclinical neurocognitive deficits. Among a small population of former lead workers (n = 48) and age-matched controls with similar blood lead concentrations (approximately 5 µg/dL in both groups; range, 1.6–14.5 µg/dL; mean age, 39.8 years), increases in current blood lead concentration within the entire study population were correlated with poorer performance on several tests of neurocognitive function but on only one measure was cumulative lead exposure (measured in the workers) associated with poorer performance (Winker et al. 2005).

In the population-based sample of adults 20–59 years of age participating in the NHANES III study (n = 4937), there was no relationship between blood lead concentration (geometric mean, 2.51 µg/dL) and covariate-adjusted performance on neurocognitive function (Krieg et al. 2005). However, significant associations have emerged in some studies of older adults with slightly higher blood lead concentrations. In a rural subset of elderly women (mean age, 71.1 ± 4.7 years; n = 325) with background, community lead exposure (geometric mean blood lead concentration, 4.8 µg/dL; range, 1–21 µg/dL), certain measures of neuropsychologic function (Trailmaking part B and Digit Symbol test) were performed more poorly by women in the upper 15th percentile of blood lead (blood lead ≥ 8 µg/dL, n = 38; Muldoon et al. 1996). However, in the slightly younger subset of elderly women who resided in an urban area (mean age, 69.4 ± 3.8 years; n = 205), no relationship between blood lead (geometric mean, 5.4 µg/dL) and neuropsychologic performance was discernible (Muldoon et al. 1996). In a general population sample of middle-aged to elderly men (n = 141; mean age, 66.8 ± 6.8 years) with a mean blood lead concentration of 5.5 ± 3.5 µg/dL examined as part of the Normative Aging Study, increased blood lead concentration was associated with poorer performance on neuropsychologic assessment of memory, verbal ability, and mental processing speed (Payton et al. 1998). In a larger subset of men (n = 736; mean age, 68.2 ± 6.9 years) from the Normative Aging Study assessed with the Mini-Mental Status Examination (MMSE), the OR for having a test score associated with an increased risk of dementia was 3.4 (95% CI, 1.6–7.2) comparing the mean blood lead of the highest quartile (mean, 8.9 µg/dL) to that of the lowest quartile (mean, 2.5 µg/dL) (Wright et al. 2003). There was a positive interaction between age and blood lead, which is consistent with a lead-associated acceleration in age-related neurodegeneration.

As reviewed in an accompanying article in this mini-monograph (Shih et al. 2007), there is evidence that at low levels of lead exposure, biomarkers of cumulative lead exposure, such as lead in bone, may be associated with an adverse impact on neurocognitive function that is not reflected by measurement of lead in blood. Among subjects from the Normative Aging Study (n = 466; mean age, 67.4 ± 6.6 years) examined for longitudinal change in MMSE score over an average of 3.5 ± 1.1 years, higher patella bone lead concentrations, a biomarker of cumulative lead exposure, predicted a steeper decline in performance (Weisskopf et al. 2004). By comparison, baseline blood lead concentration (median, 4 µg/dL; interquartile range = 3, 5) did not predict change in MMSE score. In a longitudinal analysis of performance on a battery of cognitive tests in a subset of the Normative Aging Study, bone lead measurements were predictive of worsening performance over time on tests of visuospatial/visuomotor ability (Weisskopf et al. 2007). In a cross-sectional analysis of 985 community dwelling residents 50–70 years of age, increasing tibia bone lead concentrations were significantly associated with decrements in cognitive function, whereas an impact of blood lead (mean, 3.46 ± 2.23 µg/dL) was not apparent (Shih et al. 2006).

Reproductive outcome in women. Adverse effects on reproductive outcome constitute a special risk of lead exposure to women of reproductive age. A nested case–control study examined the association of blood lead concentration with spontaneous abortion in a cohort of 668 pregnant women seeking prenatal care in Mexico City (Borja-Aburto et al. 1999). After matching for maternal age, education, gestational age at study entry, and other covariates, the OR for spontaneous abortion before 21 weeks gestation was 1.13 (95% CI, 1.01–1.30) for every 1 µg/dL increase in blood lead across the blood lead range of 1.4–29 µg/dL. Compared with the reference category of < 5 µg/dL of blood lead, women whose blood lead levels were 5–9, 10–14, and > 15 µg/dL had ORs for spontaneous abortion of 2.3, 5.4, and 12.2, respectively (test for trend, p = 0.03). Although several earlier studies failed to detect this substantial impact, they may have been subject to methodologic limitations not present in the Mexico City investigation (Hertz-Picciotto 2000).

Several studies have found that lead exposure during pregnancy affects child physical development measured during the neonatal period and early childhood. In an extensively studied cohort of 272 full-term, parturient women from Mexico City with environmental lead exposure common to the region (mean maternal blood lead, 8.9 ± 4.1 µg/dL; mean tibia bone lead, 9.8 ± 8.9 µg/g; range, 12–38 µg/g), every increase of 10 µg/g in maternal tibia lead was associated with a 73-g (95% CI, 25–121) decrease in birth weight (Gonzalez-Cossio et al. 1997). The impact of tibia bone lead on birth weight was nonlinear and was most pronounced in mothers with the highest quartile of bone lead (> 15–38 µg/g) where the decrement relative to the lowest quartile was estimated to be 156 g. Primarily in the same cohort, a maternal patella lead concentration > 24.7 µg/g was associated with an OR of 2.35 (95% CI, 1.26–4.40) for a neonate with one category smaller head circumference at birth, assessed as a five-category–ordered variable (Hernandez-Avila et al. 2002). In a different Mexico City cohort, each doubling of maternal blood lead at 36 weeks of pregnancy (geometric mean, 8.1 µg/dL; 25th–75th percentile, 5–12 µg/dL) was associated with a decrease of 0.37 cm (95% CI, 0.57–0.17) in the head circumference of a 6-month-old infant (Rothenberg et al. 1999b).

Prenatal lead exposure assessed by umbilical cord blood lead concentration has been inconsistently associated with an adverse effect on neurobehavioral development in childhood. However, recent studies suggest that mobilization of maternal bone lead during pregnancy may contribute to fetal lead exposure in ways that may be incompletely reflected by the single measurement of umbilical cord whole-blood lead (Chuang et al. 2001; Tellez-Rojo et al. 2004). In a prospective study conducted in Mexico City of 197 mother–infant pairs, a statistically significant adverse effect of umbilical cord blood lead (mean, 6.7 ± 3.4 µg/dL; range, 1.2–21.6 µg/dL) was also accompanied by an independent adverse effect of maternal bone lead burden on the 24-month Mental Development Index (MDI) of the Bayley Scales of Infant Development, which decreased 1.6 points (95% CI, 0.2–3.0) for every 10-µg/g increase in maternal patellar lead (mean, 17.9 ± 15.2 µg/g; range, < 1–76.6 µg/g) (Gomaa et al. 2002).

A prospective study that measured maternal plasma lead and maternal whole-blood lead during pregnancy found that maternal plasma lead during the first trimester was the stronger predictor of infant mental development at 24 months of age (Hu et al. 2006). In this cohort, first trimester maternal plasma lead was 0.016 ± 0.014 µg/dL and first trimester maternal whole-blood lead was 7.07 ± 5.10 µg/dL (n = 119). Adjusting for covariates that included maternal age, maternal IQ, child sex, childhood weight and height for age, and childhood whole-blood lead at 24 months, an increase of one SD in $\log_e$ (natural log)–transformed plasma lead in the first trimester was associated with a 3.5-point decrease in score on the 24-month

MDI of the Bayley Scales of Infant Development. The corresponding impact of one SD increase in $\log_e$ maternal whole blood during the first trimester was a 2.4-point decrease in the 24-month MDI. The logarithmic relationship between maternal plasma and blood lead concentrations and infant MDI indicated that the strongest effects occurred among mothers with the lowest plasma and blood lead concentrations.

Two long-term prospective studies that conducted multiple measurements of maternal blood lead during pregnancy and childhood have identified an adverse impact of low-level prenatal lead exposure on postnatal neurobehavioral development extending beyond infancy. Applying a repeated measures linear regression technique to analysis of age-appropriate IQ test data obtained in 390 children 3–7 years of age, the Yugoslavia Prospective Lead Study found independent adverse effects of both prenatal and postnatal blood lead. After controlling for the pattern of change in postnatal blood lead and other covariates, IQ decreased 1.8 points (95% CI, 1.0–2.6) for every doubling of prenatal blood lead, which was assessed as the average of maternal blood lead at midpregnancy and delivery (mean, 10.2 ± 14.4 µg/dL; n = 390) (Wasserman et al. 2000). The Mexico City Prospective Lead Study used generalized linear mixed models with random intercept and slope to assess the impact on IQ measured at 6–10 years of age of blood lead measurements systematically obtained during weeks 12, 20, 24, and 36 of pregnancy, at delivery, and at multiple points throughout childhood (Schnaas et al. 2006). Geometric mean blood lead during pregnancy was 8.0 µg/dL (range, 1–33 µg/dL; n = 150); from 1 through 5 years it was 9.8 µg/dL (2.8–36.4 µg/dL), and from 6 through 10 years it was 6.2 µg/dL (range, 2.2–18.6 µg/dL). IQ at 6 to 10 years of age, assessed by the Wechsler Intelligence Scale for Children—Revised, decreased significantly only with increasing natural-log third-trimester blood lead, controlling for other blood lead measurements and covariates. Every doubling of third trimester blood lead (geometric mean of maternal blood lead at weeks 28 and 36 = 7.8 µg/dL, 5th–95th percentile: range, 2.5–24.6 µg/dL) was associated with an IQ decrement of 2.7 points (95% CI, 0.9–4.4). Notably, the nonlinear (i.e., log-linear) relationships detected in the Yugoslavia and Mexico City studies indicate that across a maternal blood lead range of 1–30 µg/dL, an increase in blood lead from 1 to 10 µg/dL will account for more than half the IQ decrement.

Two independent cohorts have provided evidence that maternal lead burden during pregnancy may be associated with increased risk of pregnancy hypertension and/or elevated blood pressure during pregnancy. In a

retrospective study of 3,210 women during labor and delivery, increasing umbilical cord blood lead levels (mean, 6.9 ± 3.3 µg/dL; range, 0–35 µg/dL) were associated with increased systolic blood pressure during labor (1.0 mmHg for every doubling of blood lead) and increased odds of hypertension (not further defined) recorded any time during pregnancy (OR = 1.3; 95% CI, 1.1–1.5) for every doubling of blood lead (Rabinowitz et al. 1987). A prospective study of third trimester blood lead (geometric mean, 2.3 ± 1.4 µg/dL; range, 0.5–36.5 µg/dL) in 1,188 predominantly Latina immigrants showed that, in the immigrants, every doubling in blood lead was associated with increased third-trimester systolic blood pressure (1.2 mmHg; 95% CI, 0.5–1.9) and diastolic blood pressure (1.0 mmHg; 95% CI, 0.4–1.5) (Rothenberg et al. 1999a). A study of a subset of the same cohort (n = 637) without regard to immigration status found that every 10-µg/g increase in calcaneus (heel) bone lead increased the OR of third trimester pregnancy hypertension (systolic > 90 and/or diastolic > 140 mmHg) by 1.86 (95% CI, 1.04–3.32) (Rothenberg et al. 2002).

Medical Surveillance for Lead-Exposed Workers

The OSHA workplace standard for lead exposure in general industry (adopted in 1978) and a corresponding standard for lead exposure in construction trades (adopted in 1993) set forth medical surveillance requirements that include baseline and periodic medical examinations and laboratory testing. Details of the two standards, which establish distinct criteria for the implementation of surveillance, can be found on the OSHA website (OSHA 2002). Because of the concern regarding adverse health effects of lead associated with the lower levels of exposure discussed in this article, we recommend a revised schedule of medical surveillance activities (Table 2). Unlike the OSHA medical surveillance requirements, which apply only to workers exposed to airborne lead levels ≥ 30 µg/m[3] as an 8-hr time-weighted average, the recommendations in Table 2 are intended to apply to all lead-exposed workers who have the potential to be exposed by lead ingestion, even in the absence of documented elevations in air lead levels (Sen et al. 2002). As shown in Table 2, the level of a worker's current blood lead measurement, as well as possible changes in lead-related exposure, influences the recommended time interval for subsequent blood lead measurements. Blood lead measurements should be obtained from a clinical laboratory that has been designated by OSHA as meeting the specific proficiency requirements of the OSHA lead standards. OSHA maintains a list of these laboratories on its website (OSHA 2005). Venous blood should be used for biological monitoring of adult lead exposures, except where prohibited by medical or other reasons. Routine measurement of zinc protoporphyrin, a requirement of the OSHA lead standards, is not recommended in Table 2 because it is an insensitive biomarker of lead exposures in individuals with blood lead concentrations < 25 µg/dL (Parsons et al. 1991).

The content of the baseline or preplacement history and physical examination for lead-exposed workers should continue to follow the comprehensive scope set forth in the OSHA lead standard for general industry. Measurement of serum creatinine will identify individuals with chronic renal dysfunction who may be subject to increased health risks from lead exposure. With the potential exception of an annual blood pressure measurement and a brief questionnaire regarding the presence of medical conditions (such as renal insufficiency) that might increase the risk of adverse health effects of lead exposure, medical evaluations for lead-exposed workers should be unnecessary as long as blood lead concentrations are maintained < 20 µg/dL. Annual education of lead workers regarding the nature and control of lead hazards, and ongoing access to health counseling regarding lead-related health risks are recommended as preventive measures.

Lead Exposure during Pregnancy and Lactation

As summarized earlier in this article, the recent findings concerning lead-related adverse reproductive outcomes render it advisable for pregnant women to avoid occupational or avocational lead exposure that would result in blood lead concentrations > 5 µg/dL. Calcium supplementation during pregnancy may be especially important for women with past exposure to lead. Calcium decreases bone resorption during pregnancy (Janakiraman et al. 2003) and may minimize release of lead from bone stores and subsequent fetal lead exposure (Gomaa et al. 2002).

Maternal body lead burden and external lead exposure influence the lead concentration of breast milk (Ettinger et al. 2006; Gulson et al. 1998). The few studies that used ultraclean techniques and mass spectrometry analyses report human breast milk concentrations ranging from 0.6 to 3% of maternal blood lead (Ettinger et al. 2004b; Gulson et al. 1998; Manton et al. 2000; Sowers et al. 2002). Using 1% as a guide, it can be estimated that nursing mothers with a blood lead concentration < 20 µg/dL will have breast milk with a concentration < 2 µg/L, a value that approximates the amount of lead in infant formula (Gulson et al. 2001). A recent randomized clinical

trial among Mexican women with mean blood lead concentrations of approximately 9 µg/dL found that calcium supplementation during lactation may reduce the lead concentration of breast milk by 5–10% (Ettinger et al. 2006). Breast feeding should be encouraged for almost all women (Ettinger et al. 2004a; Sanin et al. 2001; Sinks and Jackson 1999), with decisions concerning women with very high lead exposure addressed on an individual basis.

Medical Treatment of Elevated Blood Lead Concentration and Overt Lead Intoxication

Removal from all sources of hazardous lead exposure, whether occupational or nonoccupational, constitutes the first and most fundamental step in the treatment of an individual with an elevated blood lead concentration. A careful history that inquires about a broad spectrum of potential lead sources is recommended (Occupational Lead Poisoning Prevention Program 2006). Removal from occupational lead exposure will usually require transfer of the individual out of any environment or task that might be expected to raise the blood lead concentration of a person not using personal protective equipment above background levels (i.e., 5 µg/dL). If there has been a history of an affected individual bringing lead-contaminated shoes, work clothes, or equipment home from the workplace, evaluation of vehicles and the home environment for significant levels of lead-containing dust might be considered (Piacitelli et al. 1995). Although such "take-home" exposure might contribute to further lead exposure of the worker, it ordinarily poses more of a potential risk to young children and pregnant or nursing women who share the worker's home environment (Hipkins et al. 2004; Roscoe et al. 1999).

Medical treatment of individuals with overt lead intoxication involves decontamination, supportive care, and judicious use of chelating agents. Comprehensive discussion of such treatment is beyond the scope of this article but has been reviewed in recent medical toxicology texts (Kosnett 2001, 2005). A variety of chelating agents has been demonstrated to decrease blood lead concentrations and increase urinary lead excretion. A recent double-blind randomized clinical trial of oral chelation in young children with blood lead concentrations ranging from 22 to 44 µg/dL found that the drug succimer lowered blood concentrations transiently but did not improve cognitive function (Dietrich et al. 2004; Rogan et al. 2001). Although anecdotal evidence suggests that chelation has been associated with improvement in symptoms and decreased mortality in patients with lead encephalopathy, controlled clinical trials demonstrating efficacy are lacking. Treatment recommendations are therefore mostly empiric, and decisions regarding the initiation of chelation therapy for lead intoxication have occasionally engendered controversy.

In our experience, adults with blood lead concentrations ≥ 100 µg/dL almost always warrant chelation, as levels of this magnitude are often associated with significant symptoms and may be associated with an incipient risk of encephalopathy or seizures. Occasionally, patients with very high blood lead concentrations may have no overt symptoms. Patients with blood lead concentrations of 80–99 µg/dL, with or without symptoms, can be considered for chelation treatment, as may some symptomatic individuals with blood lead concentrations of 50–79 µg/dL. These demarcations are imprecise, however, and decisions on chelation should be made on a case-by-case basis after consultation with an

Table 2. Health-based medical surveillance recommendations for lead-exposed workers.

Category of exposure	Recommendations
All lead-exposed workers[a]	Baseline or preplacement medical history and physical examination, baseline BLL, serum creatinine
BLL (µg/dL)	
	See Table 1 for pregnancy concerns
10–19	As above for BLL < 10 µg/dL, plus:
	BLL every 3 months
	Evaluate exposure, engineering controls, and work practices
	Consider removal (see Table 1)
	Revert to BLL every 6 months after 3 BLLs < 10 µg/dL
	monitor as above

BLL, blood lead level.
[a]Lead-exposed means handling or disturbing materials with a significant lead content in a manner that could reasonably be expected to cause potentially harmful exposure through inhalation or ingestion.

experienced specialist in occupational medicine or medical toxicology.

Hair lead analysis or measurement of urine lead concentration seldom provide exposure information of clinical value beyond that provided by the history and the measurement of blood lead concentration. Chelation initiated exclusively on the basis of hair or urine lead levels or chelation of asymptomatic individuals with low blood lead concentrations is not recommended.

Adults with overt lead intoxication will generally experience improvement in symptoms after removal from lead exposure and decline in blood lead concentration. This clinical observation on improvement in overt symptoms finds some support from the relatively limited number of studies that have examined the impact of naturally declining blood lead concentrations on cognitive function in occupationally exposed subjects (Chuang et al. 2005; Lindgren et al. 2003; Winker et al. 2006). Improvement or resolution of neurocognitive or neurobehavioral symptoms may sometimes lag the decline in blood lead concentration, possibly because of the relatively slower removal of lead from the central nervous system (Cremin et al. 1999; Goldstein et al. 1974). The pace of improvement can be highly variable, and may range from weeks to a year or more depending on the magnitude of intoxication. Anecdotal experience and analogy to other forms of brain injury suggest a potential role for rehabilitative services (e.g., physical therapy, cognitive rehabilitation) in enhancing the prospect for recovery, and in demonstrating the capacity for safe return to work. Short-term improvement in neurocognitive function associated with a decline in blood lead concentration does not obviate concern that long-term cumulative lead exposure may nonetheless have a deleterious effect on cognitive reserve, and may accelerate age-related decline in cognitive function (Schwartz et al. 2005; Weisskopf et al. 2004).

Additional Management Considerations

With appropriate engineering controls, safe work practices, and personal protective equipment, workers without a previous history of substantial lead exposure should be able to work with lead in a manner that minimizes the potential for hazardous levels of exposure. For such workers, elevations in blood lead concentration that result from unforeseen transient increases in exposure will often decline promptly once the exposure is controlled. However, in a worker with a long history of high exposure, redistribution of lead from a large internal skeletal burden may result in a prolonged elevation of blood lead concentration despite marked reductions in external lead dose.

The recommendations for management of adult lead exposure contained in this article are derived from consideration of risks to health, and have not been the subject of a cost-benefit analysis examining economic feasibility or social impacts. Nonmedical, socioeconomic factors will likely influence how workers, employers, and clinicians respond to the recommendations. In particular, the blood lead concentrations for which some major interventions, such as removal from lead exposure, are recommended are considerably lower than those explicitly specified in the current OSHA lead standards (OSHA 2002). The OSHA standards do require an employer to implement reductions in exposure recommended by a physician who determines an employee has a "detected medical condition" that places him or her at increased risk of "material impairment to health." This nonspecific provision could form the basis for implementation of protective workplace action at the lower blood concentrations recommended by the authors. Nonetheless, clinicians should inform patients that such recommendations may be contested by an employer or an insurer, and could potentially jeopardize their job benefits or work

status. Prudent case management that considers the worker's perspective on their unique health risks and employment situation will usually be advisable.

Interpretative Guidance for Clinical Laboratory Report Forms

Clinical laboratories routinely offer brief interpretative guidance on the forms that report the result of blood lead concentrations. There is considerable variability among laboratories regarding the content of such guidance, and laboratories exercise their own discretion regarding the source and detail of the information they provide. Unlike the management guidance chart for childhood blood lead concentrations published by the CDC (2002), which is often reproduced by clinical laboratories, no corresponding CDC guidance exists for blood lead concentrations measured in adults. Notwithstanding the limitations inherent in an abbreviated tabular format, Table 3 represents a guidance chart for adult blood lead measurements that is proposed for use by clinical laboratories.

REFERENCES

Akesson A, Lundh T, Vahter M, Bjellerup, Lidfeltdt J, Nerbrand C, et al. 2005. Tubular and glomerular kidney effects in Swedish women with low environmental cadmium exposure. Environ Health Perspect 113:1627–1631.

Barth A, Schaffer AW, Osterode W, Winker R, Konnaris C, Valic E, et al. 2002. Reduced cognitive abilities in lead-exposed men. Int Arch Occup Environ Health 75:394–398.

Borja-Aburto VH, Hertz-Picciotto I, Lopez MR, Farias P, Rios C, Blanco J. 1999. Blood lead levels measured prospectively and risk of spontaneous abortion. Am J Epidemiol 150: 590–597.

CDC. 2002. Managing Elevated BLLs Among Young Children. Atlanta:Centers for Disease Control and Prevention, National Center for Environmental Health.

CDC. 2005. Third National Report on Human Exposure to Environmental Chemicals. NCEH Publ no 05-0570. Atlanta:Centers for Disease Control and Prevention.

Chuang HY, Chao KY, Tsai SY. 2005. Reversible neurobehavioral performance with reductions in blood lead levels—a prospective study on lead workers. Neurotox Teratol 27:497–504.

Chuang HY, Schwartz J, Gonzales-Cossio T, Lugo MC, Palazuelos E, Aro A, et al. 2001. Interrelations of lead levels in bone, venous blood, and umbilical cord blood with exogenous lead exposure through maternal plasma lead in peripartum women. Environ Health Perspect 109:527–532.

Coyle P, Kosnett MJ, Hipkins KL. 2005. Severe lead poisoning in the plastics industry: a report of three cases. Am J Ind Med 47:172–175.

Cremin JD, Luck ML, Laughlin NK, Smith DR. 1999. Efficacy of succimer chelation for reducing brain lead in a primate model of human lead exposure. Toxicol Appl Pharmacol 161:283–293.

Den Hond E, Nawrot T, Staessen JA. 2002. The relationship between blood pressure and blood lead in NHANES III. National Health and Nutritional Examination Survey. J Hum Hypertens 16:563–568.

Dietrich KN, Ware JH, Salganik M, Radcliff J, Rogan WJ, Rhoads GG, et al. 2004. Effect of chelation therapy on the neuropsychological and behavioral development of lead-exposed children after school entry. Pediatrics 114:19–26.

Ettinger AS, Tellez-Rojo MM, Amarasiriwardena C, Peterson KE, Schwartz J, Aro A, et al. 2006. Influence of maternal bone lead burden and calcium intake on levels of lead in breast milk over the course of lactation. Am J Epidemiol 163:48–56.

Table 3. Recommended interpretive guidance for clinical laboratories reporting adult blood lead concentrations.

Blood lead level (µg/dL)	Management recommendations and requirements[a] for adults
< 5	No action needed
5–9	Discuss health risks Reduce exposure for pregnancy
10–19	Discuss health risks. Decrease exposure. Monitor BLL Remove from exposure for pregnancy, certain medical conditions, long-term risks
20–29	Remove from exposure if repeat BLL in 4 weeks remains ≥ 20 µg/dL
30–79	Remove from exposure. Prompt medical evaluation and consultation advised for BLL > 40 µg/dL OSHA requirements may apply Chelation not indicated unless BLL > 50 µg/dL with significant symptoms

BLL, blood lead level. Primary management of lead poisoning is source identification and removal from exposure. A single BLL does not reflect cumulative body burden or predict long-term effects.
[a]Refer to OSHA general industry and construction lead standards for occupational exposure.

4

Ettinger AS, Tellez-Rojo MM, Amarasiriwardena C, Bellinger D, Peterson J, Schwartz J, Hu H, Hernandez-Avila M. 2004a. Effect of breast milk lead on infant blood lead levels at 1 month of age. Environ Health Perspect 112:1381–1385.

Ettinger AS, Tellez-Rojo MM, Amarasiriwardena C, Gonzalez-Cossio T, Peterson KE, Aro A, et al. 2004b. Levels of lead in breast milk and their relation to maternal blood and bone lead levels at one-month postpartum. Environ Health Perspect 112:926–931.

Fine BP, Vetrano T, Skurnick J, Ty A. 1988. Blood pressure elevation in young dogs during low-level lead poisoning. Toxicol Appl Pharmacol 93:388–393.

Gerhardsson L, Chettle DR, Englyst V, Nordberg GF, Nyhlin H, Scott MC, et al. 1992. Kidney effects in long-term exposed lead smelter workers. Br J Ind Med 49:186–192.

Goldstein GW, Asbury AK, Diamond I. 1974. Pathogenesis of lead encephalopathy. Uptake of lead and reaction of brain capillaries. Arch Neurol 31:382–389.

Gonzalez-Cossio T, Peterson KE, Sanín L, Fishbein SE, Palazuelos E, Aro A, et al. 1997. Decrease in birth weight in relation to maternal bone lead burden. Pediatrics 100:856–862.

Gomaa A, Hu H, Bellinger D, Schwartz J, Tsaih S, Gonzalez-Cossio T, et al. 2002. Maternal bone lead as an independent risk factor for fetal neurotoxicity: a prospective study. Pediatrics 110:110–118.

Gonick HC, Ding Y, Bondy SC, Ni Z, Vaziri ND. 1997. Lead-induced hypertension: interplay of nitric oxide and reactive oxygen species. Hypertension 30:1487–1492.

Gulson BL, Jameson CW, Mahaffey KR, Mizon KJ, Patison N, Law A, et al. 1998. Relationship of lead in breast milk to lead in blood, urine, and diet of the infant and mother. Environ Health Perspect 106:667–674.

Gulson BL, Mizon KJ, Korsch MJ, Mahaffey KR, Taylor AJ. 2001. Dietary intakes of selected elements from longitudinal 6-day duplicate diets for pregnant and nonpregnant subjects and elemental concentrations of breast milk and infant formula. Environ Res 87:160–174.

Hänninen H, Aitio A, Kovala T, Luukkonen R, Matikainen E, Mannelin T, et al. 1998. Occupational exposure to lead and neuropsychological dysfunction. Occup Environ Med 55:202–209.

Harlan WR. 1988. The relationship of blood lead levels to blood pressure in the U.S. population. Environ Health Perspect 78:9–13.

Hernandez-Avila M, Peterson KE, Gonzalez-Cossio T, Sanin LH, Aro A, Schnaas L, et al. 2002. Effect of maternal bone lead on length and head circumference at birth. Arch Environ Health 57:482–488.

Hertz-Picciotto I. 2000. The evidence that lead increases the risk for spontaneous abortion. Am J Ind Med 38:300–309.

Hipkins KL, Materna BL, Payne S, Kirsch L. 2004. Family lead poisoning due to occupation. Clin Pediatr 43:845–849.

Hofreuter DH, Catcott EJ, Keenan RG, Xintaras C. 1961. The public health significance of atmospheric lead. Arch Environ Health 3:568–574.

Hu H, Aro A, Payton M, Korrick S, Sparrow D, Weiss ST, et al. 1996. The relationship of bone and blood lead to hypertension. JAMA 275:1171–1176.

Hu H, Shih R, Rothenberg S, Schwartz BS. 2007. The epidemiology of lead toxicity in adults: measuring dose and consideration of other methodologic issues. Environ Health Perspect 115:455–462.

Hu H, Téllez-Rojo MM, Bellinger D, Smith D, Ettinger AS, Lamadrid-Figueroa H, et al. 2006. Fetal lead exposure at each stage of pregnancy as a predictor of infant mental development. Environ Health Perspect doi:10.1289/ehp.9067 available via http://dx.doi.org/ [Online 19 July 2006].

Janakiraman V, Hu H, Mercado-Garcia A, Hernandez-Avila M. 2003. A randomized crossover trial of nocturnal calcium supplements to suppress bone resorption during pregnancy. Am J Prev Med 24:260–264.

Korrick SA, Hunter DJ, Rotnitzky A, Hu H, Speizer FE. 1999. Lead and hypertension in a sample of middle-aged women. Am J Public Health 89:330–335.

Kosnett MJ. 2001. Lead. In: Clinical Toxicology (Ford M, Delaney KA, Ling L, Erickson T, eds). St. Louis:WB Saunders, 723–736.

Kosnett MJ. 2005. Lead. In: Critical Care Toxicology (Brent J, Wallace KL, Burkhart KK, Phillips SD, Donovan JW, eds). Philadelphia:Elsevier Mosby, 821–836.

Krieg EF, Chislip DW, Crespo CJ, Brightwell WS, Ehrenberg RL, Otto D. 2005. The relationship between blood lead levels and neurobehavioral test performance in NHANES III and

related occupational studies. Public Health Rep 120:240–251.

Lilis R, Gavrilescu N, Nestorescu B, Dumitriu C, Roventa A. 1968. Nephropathy in chronic lead poisoning. Br J Ind Med 25:196–202.

Lindgren KN, Ford DP, Bleeker ML. 2003. Pattern of blood lead levels over working lifetime and neuropsychological performance. Arch Environ Health 58:373–379.

Lustberg M, Silbergeld E. 2002. Blood lead levels and mortality. Arch Intern Med 162:2443–2449.

Mahaffey KR, Annest JL, Roberts J, Murphy RS. 1982. National estimates of blood lead levels: United States, 1976–1980. N Engl J Med 307:573–579.

Mantere P, Hänninen H, Hernberg S, Luukkonen R. 1984. A prospective follow-up study on psychological effects in workers exposed to low-levels of lead. Scand J Work Environ Health 10:43–50.

Manton WI, Angle CR, Stanek KL, Reese YR, Kuehnemann TJ. 2000. Acquisition and retention of lead by young children. Environ Res 82:60–80.

Menke A, Muntner P, Batuman V, Silbergeld EK, Guallar E. 2006. Blood lead below 0.48 μmol/L (10 μg/dL) and mortality among US adults. Circulation 114:1388–1394.

Minot AS. 1938. The physiological effects of small amounts of lead: an evaluation of the lead hazard of the average individual. Physiol Rev 18:554–577.

Muldoon SB, Cauley JA, Kuller LH, Morrow L, Needleman HL, Scott J, et al. 1996. Effects of blood lead levels on cognitive function of older women. Neuroepidemiology 15:62–72.

Muntner P, Vupputuri S, Coresh J, Batuman V. 2003. Blood lead and chronic kidney disease in the general United States population: results from NHANES III. Kidney Int 63:104–150.

Nash D, Magder L, Lustberg M, Sherwin R, Rubin R, Kaufmann R, et al. 2003. Blood lead, blood pressure, and hypertension in perimenopausal and postmenopausal women. JAMA 289:1523–1531.

National Center for Health Statistics. 1984. Blood lead levels for persons ages 6 months to 74 years. United States, 1976-1980. Vital and Health Statistics. Ser 11, no 233. Publ no (PHS) 84-1683. Washington, DC:National Center for Health Statistics.

Nawrot TS, Thijs L, Den Hond EM, Roels HA, Staessen JA. 2002. An epidemiological re-appraisal of the association between blood pressure and blood lead: a meta-analysis. J Hum Hypertens 16:123–131.

Navas-Acien A, Guallar E, Silbergeld EK, Rothenberg SJ. 2007. Lead exposure and cardiovascular disease—a systematic review. Environ Health Perspect 115:472–482.

Occupational Lead Poisoning Prevention Program. 2006. Common Jobs, Hobbies & Other Sources of Lead. Richmond, CA:California Department of Health Services, Occupational Health Branch. Available: http://www.dhs.ca.gov/ohb/olppp/leadsources.pdf [accessed 14 December 2006]

OSHA (U.S. Occupational Safety and Health Administration). 2002. Safety and Health Topics: Lead. Compliance. Available: http://www.osha.gov/SLTC/lead/compliance.html [accessed 14 December 2006].

OSHA (U.S. Occupational Safety and Health Administration). 2005. Blood Lead Laboratories Program Description and Background. Available: http://www.osha.gov/SLTC/bloodlead/program.html [accessed 14 December 2006].

Parsons PJ, Reilly AA, Hussain A. 1991. Observational study of erythrocyte portoporphyrin screening test for detecting low lead exposure in children; impact of lowering the blood lead action threshold. Clin Chem 37:216–225.

Payton M, Hu H, Sparrow D, Weiss ST. 1994. Low-level lead exposure and renal function in the Normative Aging Study. Am J Epidemiol 140:821–829.

Payton M, Riggs KM, Spiro A, Weiss ST, Hu H. 1998. Relations of bone and blood lead to cognitive function: the VA Normative Aging Study. Neurotoxicol Teratol 20:19–27.

Piacitelli GM, Whelan EA, Ewers LM, Sieber WK. 1995. Lead contamination in automobiles of lead-exposed bridge-workers. Appl Occup Environ Hyg 10:849–855.

Pocock SJ, Shaper AG, Ashby D, Delves HT, Clayton BE. 1988. The relationship between blood lead, blood pressure, stroke, and heart attacks in middle-aged British men. Environ Health Perspect 78:23–30.

Rabinowitz MB, Bellinger D, Leviton A, Needleman H, Schoenbaum S. 1987. Pregnancy hypertension, blood pressure during labor, and blood lead levels. Hypertension 10:447–451.

Rogan WJ, Dietrich KN, Ware JH, Docery DW, Salganik M,

Radcliffe J, et al. 2001. The effects of chelation therapy with succimer on neuropsychological development in children exposed to lead. N Engl J Med 344:1421–1426.

Roscoe RJ, Gittleman JL, Deddens JA, Petersen MR, Halperin WE. 1999. Blood lead levels among children of lead-exposed workers: a meta-analysis. Am J Ind Med 36:475–481.

Rothenberg SJ, Kondrashov V, Manalo M, Jiang J, Cuellar R, Garcia M, et al. 2002. Increases of hypertension and blood pressure during pregnancy with increased bone lead. Am J Epidemiol 156:1079–1087.

Rothenberg SJ, Manalo M, Jiang J, Cuellar R, Reyes S, Sanchez M, et al. 1999a. Blood lead levels and blood pressure during pregnancy in South Central Los Angeles. Arch Environ Health 54:382–389.

Rothenberg SJ, Schnaas L, Perroni E, Hernandez RN, Martinez S, Hernandez C. 1999b. Pre- and postnatal lead effect on head circumference: a case for critical periods. Neurotoxicol Teratol 21:1–11.

Sanín LH, González-Cossín T, Romieu I, Perterson KE, Ruíz S, Palazuelos E, Hernández-Avila M. Hu H. 2001. Effect of maternal lead burden on infant weight and weight gain at one month of age among breastfed infants. Pediatrics 107:1016–1023.

Schnaas L, Rothenberg SJ, Flores MF, Martinez S, Hernandez C, Osorio E, et al. 2006. Reduced intellectual development in children with prenatal lead exposure. Environ Health Perspect 111:791–797.

Schober SE, Miral B, Graudbard BI, Brody DJ, Flegal KM. 2006. Blood lead levels and death from all causes, cardiovascular disease, and cancer: results from the NHANES III mortality study. Environ Health Perspect 114:1538–1541.

Schwartz BS, Hu H. 2007. Adult lead exposure: time for change. Environ Health Perspect 115:451–454.

Schwartz BS, Lee BK, Lee GS, Stewart WF, Lee SS, Hwang KY, et al. 2001. Association of blood lead, dimercaptosuccinic acid-chelatable lead, and tibia lead with neurobehavioral test scores in South Korean lead workers. Am J Epidemiol 153:453–464.

Schwartz BS, Lee BK, Bandeen-Roche K, Stewart W, Bolla K, Links J, et al. 2005. Lead dose is associated with longitudinal decline in neurobehavioral test scores in South Korean lead workers. Epidemiology 16:106–113.

Schwartz J. 1988. The relationship between blood lead and blood pressure in NHANES II survey. Environ Health Perspect 78:15–22.

Schwartz J. 1995. Lead, blood pressure, and cardiovascular disease in men. Arch Environ Health 50:31–37.

Sen D, Wolfson H, Dilworth M. 2002. Lead exposure in scaffolders during refurbishment construction activity—an observational study. Occup Med 52:49–54.

Shih RA, Glass TA, Bandeen-Roche K, Carlson MC, Bolla KI, Todd AC, Schwartz BS. 2006. Environmental lead exposure and cognitive function in community-dwelling older adults. Neurology 14:1556–1562.

Shih RA, Hu H, Weisskopf MG, Schwartz BS. 2007. Cumulative lead dose and cognitive function in adults: a review of studies that measured both blood lead and bone lead. Environ Health Perspect 115:483–492.

Sinks T, Jackson RJ. 1999. International study finds breast milk free of significant lead contamination. Environ Health Perspect 107:A58–A59.

Sowers MR, Scholl TO, Hall G, Jannausch ML, Kemp FW, Li X, et al. 2002. Lead in breast milk and maternal bone turnover. Am J Obstet Gynecol 187:770–776.

Staeesen JA, Bulpitt CJ, Fagard R, Lauwerys RR, Roels H, Thijs L, Amery A. 1994. Hypertension caused by low-level lead exposure: myth or fact? J Cardiovasc Risk 1:87–97.

Staessen JA, Lauwerys RR, Buchet JP, Bulpitt CJ, Rondia D, Vanrenterghem Y, et al. 1992. Impairment of renal function with increasing blood lead concentrations in the general population. The Cadmibel Study Group. N Engl J Med 327: 151–156.

Staessen JA, Roels H, Fagard R. 1996. Lead exposure and conventional and ambulatory blood pressure: a prospective population study. PheeCad Investigators. JAMA 275: 1563–1570.

Stollery BT. 1996. Reaction time changes in workers exposed to lead. Neurotoxicol Teratol 18:477–483.

Tellez-Rojo MM, Hernandez-Avila M, Lamadrid-Figueroa H, Smith D, Hernandez-Cadena L, Mercado A, et al. 2004. Impact of bone lead and bone resorption on plasma and whole blood lead levels during pregnancy. Am J Epidemiol 160:668–678.

Theppeang K, Schwartz BS, Lee BK, Lustberg ME, Silbergeld EK, Kelsey KT, et al. 2004. Associations of patella lead with polymorphisms in the vitamin D receptor, delta-aminolevulinic acid dehydratase and endothelial nitric oxide synthase genes. J Occup Environ Med 46:528–537.

Tsaih SW, Korrick S, Schwartz J, Amarasiriwardena C, Aro A, Sparrow D, et al. 2004. Lead, diabetes, hypertension, and renal function: Normative Aging Study. Environ Health Perspect 112:1178–1182.

U.S. EPA. 2006. Air Quality Criteria for Lead (Final). Washington, DC:U.S. Environmental Protection Agency, National Center for Environmental Assessment. Available: http://cfpub.epa. gov/ncea/cfm/recordisplay.cfm?deid=158823 [accessed 14 December 2006].

Vaziri ND. 2002. Pathogenesis of lead-induced hypertension: role of oxidative stress. J Hypertens 20(suppl 3):S15–S20.

Vupputuri S, He J, Munter P, Bazzano L, Whelton PK, Batuman V. 2003. Blood lead level is associated with elevated blood pressure in blacks. Hypertension 41:463–468.

Wasserman GA, Liu X, Popovac D, Factor-Litvak P, Kline J, Waternaux C, et al. 2000. The Yugoslavia prospective lead study: contributions of prenatal and postnatal lead exposure to early intelligence. Neurotoxicol Teratol 22:811–818.

Weaver VM, Lee B-K, Ahn K-D, Lee G-S, Todd AC, Stewart WF, et al. 2003. Associations of lead biomarkers with renal function in Korean lead workers. Occup Environ Med 60:551–562.

Weaver VM, Lee BK, Todd AC, Ahn KD, Shi W, Jaar BG, et al. 2006. Effect modification by δ-aminolevulinic acid dehydratase, vitamin D receptor, and nitric oxide sythase gene polymorphisms on associations between patella lead and renal function in lead workers. Environ Res 102:61–69.

Wedeen RP, Mallik DK, Batuman V. 1979. Detection and treatment of occupational lead nephropathy. Arch Intern Med 139:53–57.

Weisskopf MG, Proctor SP, Wright RO, Schwartz J, Spiro A, Sparrow D, Nie H, Hu H. 2007. Cumulative lead exposure and cognitive performance among elderly men. Epidemiology 18: 59–66.

Weisskopf MG, Wright RO, Schwartz J, Spiro III A, Sparrow D, Aro A, et al. 2004. Cumulative lead exposure and prospective change in cognition among elderly men: the VA Normative Aging Study. Am J Epidemiol 160:1184–1193.

Winker R, Barth A, Ponocny-Seliger E, Pilger A, Osterode W, Rudiger HW. 2005. No cognitive deficits in men formerly exposed to lead. Wein Klin Wochenschr 117:755–760.

Winker R, Ponocny-Seliger E, Rudiger HW, Barth A. 2006. Lead exposure levels and duration of exposure absence predict neurobehavioral performance. Int Arch Occup Environ Health 79:123–127.

Wright RO, Tsaih SW, Schwartz J, Spiro A, McDonald K, Weiss ST, et al. 2003. Lead exposure biomarkers and mini-mental status exam scores in older men. Epidemiology 14:713–718.

Wu MT, Kelsey K, Schwartz J, Sparrow D, Weiss S, Hu H. 2003. A δ-aminolevulinic acid dehydratase (ALAD) polymorphism may modify the relationship of low level lead exposure to uricemia and renal function: the Normative Aging Study. Environ Health Perspect 111:335–341.

Appendix VII
Medical Management Guidelines for Lead-Exposed Adults
Association of Occupational and Environmental Clinics

Medical Management Guidelines for Lead-Exposed Adults
Revised 04/24/2007

Summary:

Overexposure to inorganic lead continues to be an important problem worldwide. The reduction of lead in the U.S. environment, largely accomplished through effective EPA regulatory efforts, has resulted in lowering the overall geometric mean whole blood lead level (BLL) for the general population in the United States from approximately 13 µg/dL (0.63 µmol/L) in the 1970s to less than 2 µg/dL (0.10 µmol/L) (CDC 2005; NCHS 1984). Lead exposure remains a significant public health and medical concern for thousands of children and adults exposed primarily through remaining lead-based paint in older housing stock as well as to workplace exposures, although other sources occur. For children and adults, the role of environmental investigation, identification and reduction or elimination of sources of exposure remains of primary importance. While the clinical care of lead-exposed children has been well established in the pediatric and public health communities, similar clinical recommendations for adults have not been widely available.

The purpose of this document is to provide useful advice to clinicians caring for adult patients who have been exposed to lead, whether at work, at home, through hobbies, in the community, through consumer products, retained bullets, or other sources. This document is derived, in part, from the input of an expert panel convened by the Association of Occupational and Environmental Clinics (AOEC). However, three clinical scholars then considered the medical evidence submitted by the expert panel and incorporated many of the conclusions reached by this panel. This paper, therefore, reflects a general consensus of the clinical views of AOEC members, not necessarily the expert panel, particularly in areas where the expert panel had been unable to come to consensus. The following points are emphasized:

1) Medical care serves as an adjunct to public health and industrial hygiene exposure control. Clinicians who evaluate patients with potential lead exposure should have appropriate referral mechanisms in place for prevention of further exposure to lead. Although one goal of health care is to remove the patient from exposure, the social consequences of potential disruption of housing or of income may be important and must be considered by the clinician.

2) Current occupational standards are not sufficiently protective and should be strengthened. Although the federal Occupational Safety and Health Administration's (OSHA) lead standards have provided guidance that has been beneficial for lead-exposed workers, these regulations have not been substantially changed since the late 1970s and thus are primarily based on health effects studies that are well over three decades old. There is an urgent need to revise them.

3) The clinical guidelines presented here are appropriate for adults, recognizing that younger adults, particularly those in workplace settings, may share developmental risks that place them closer to pediatric populations, and that maternal exposure, whether in the workplace or in the general environment, places the developing fetus at risk for exposure.

4) Clinicians should feel free to contact any of the member AOEC clinics for additional telephone advice, and are encouraged to refer patients when appropriate.

Background

Lead is used in over 100 industries. Job activities known to involve the use or disturbance of lead include: handling of lead-containing powders, liquids, or pastes; production of dust or fumes by melting, burning, cutting, drilling, machining, sanding, scraping, grinding, polishing, etching, blasting, torching, or welding lead-containing solids; and dry sweeping of lead-containing dust and debris. Adults also encounter lead in environmental settings and through activities such as home remodeling, particularly in homes built before 1978 that contain lead-based paint, lead-contaminated consumer products, traditional remedies, moonshine whiskey, hobbies, such as melting lead sinkers or use of target ranges, from retained bullets, and through other sources.

Lead is not an essential element and serves no useful purpose in the body. A substantial body of recent research demonstrates that multiple health effects can occur at levels once considered safe. The routes of exposure for inorganic lead are inhalation and ingestion. Once absorbed, lead is found in all tissues, but eventually 90% or more of the body burden is accumulated (or redistributed) into bone with a biological half-life of years to decades. Lead is excreted primarily in the urine. Lead does not remain in the bone permanently but is slowly released back into the blood.

The "dose" or quantity of lead that a person receives will be determined by the concentration of lead in the air and/or the amount ingested as well as the duration of such exposure. The BLL remains the predominant biological marker used in clinical assessment, workplace monitoring, public health surveillance, and regulatory decisions regarding removal from exposure under the OSHA lead standards.

Research tools capable of measuring cumulative lead exposure, such as the use of in-vivo K-shell X-ray fluorescence (K-XRF) instruments for the rapid, non-invasive measurement of lead in bone, have expanded recent understanding of long-term consequences from lead exposure on a population basis. These studies have demonstrated adverse effects of lead exposure across populations, including on neurologic, reproductive and renal function and on blood pressure, that occur at extremely low levels of exposure and appear not to have a threshold. However, because inter-individual differences are greater than population differences at lower lead levels, these effects are less important for clinical evaluation than they are for public health policy. The preponderance of the evidence for adverse effects at levels of exposure far below those currently permitted by OSHA speaks forcefully for an immediate reduction in permissible exposure levels in the workplace and for enhanced public health attention to those sources, including among self employed individuals, not currently subject to OSHA regulation.

Because lead interferes with biochemical processes occurring in cells throughout the body, adverse effects occur in multiple organ systems. The non-uniformity of symptoms that appear in exposed individuals, as well as a growing body of epidemiologic studies, suggest that wide variation exists in individual susceptibility to lead poisoning. Early overt symptoms in adults are often subtle and nonspecific, involving the nervous, gastrointestinal, or musculoskeletal systems. High levels of exposure can result in delirium, seizures, stupor, coma, or lead colic. Other overt signs and symptoms include hypertension, peripheral neuropathy, ataxia, tremor, gout, nephropathy, and anemia. In general, symptoms increase with increasing BLLs.

In addition to exposure that occurs from external sources, carefully performed lead isotope studies demonstrated that pregnancy and lactation are both associated with large increases in the release of lead from the maternal skeleton (Gulson et al. 2003). High levels of lead in women's bones at the time of childbirth corresponded to lower birth weight (Gonzalez-Cossio et al. 1997), lower weight gain from birth to one month of age (Sanin et al. 2001), and reduced head circumference and birth length (Hernandez-Avila et al. 2002).

In males, abnormal sperm morphology and decreased sperm count have been observed at BLLs of approximately 40 µg/dL (1.93 µmol/L) or less (Telisman et al. 2000). In the absence of effects on sperm count or concentration, the impact of paternal lead exposure on reproductive outcome is uncertain.

Recent research has examined several genetic polymorphisms that may influence lead uptake, distribution, and target organ toxicity. However, at this point in time, research findings are insufficient to conclusively identify subpopulations that may have increased susceptibility to lead toxicity based on specific genotypes. Other factors that might modify the risk of lead toxicity include pre-existing disease affecting relevant target organs (such as diabetic nephropathy or borderline hypertension), nutritional deficiencies (particularly of dietary cations such as iron and calcium), ethnicity, and aging.

CLINICAL ASSESSMENT OF LEAD EXPOSURE

Taking a detailed medical and occupational/environmental history is a fundamental step in the assessment of a person with lead exposure. It is important to ask about exposure to lead in current and previous jobs (Table 1), protections used, biological and air monitoring data, hygiene practices, knowledge and training, hobbies, traditional medications, moonshine use and other non-occupational sources (Table 2). A medical and reproductive history is essential in identifying individuals at increased risk of adverse health effects from lead exposure. Table 3 summarizes symptoms and target organ toxicity of lead at progressive BLLs. Physical exam findings in lead poisoning are frequently lacking. Gingival lead lines and wrist or foot drop are rarely seen.

Blood Lead Level and Zinc Protoporphyrin

The BLL is the most convenient and readily interpretable of the available lead biomarkers. It is mainly an estimate of recent external exposure to lead, but it is also in equilibrium with bone lead stores. The BLL alone is not a reliable indicator of prior or cumulative dose or total body burden; nor can a single BLL be used to confirm or deny the presence of chronic health effects thought due to lead exposure. The "normal" or "reference range" BLL is less than 5 µg/dL (0.24 µmol/L) for more than 90% (CDC 2005) of the adult population. When interpreting the BLL, key questions are whether the exposure has been 1) of short-term or long-term duration; 2) recent or in the remote past; and 3) of high or low intensity.

Erythrocyte protoporphyrin IX (EP), which can be measured as free EP (FEP) or zinc protoporphyrin (ZPP), is a measurement of biological effect and is an indirect reflection of lead exposure. Lead affects the heme synthesis pathway. Increases in EP or ZPP are not detectable until BLLs reach 20 to 25 µg/dL, (0.97-1.21 µmol/L) followed by an exponential rise relative to increasing BLLs. An increase in EP or ZPP usually lags behind an increase in BLL by two to six weeks.

Periodic testing of BLL and ZPP, called biological monitoring, is required by the OSHA lead standards for workers exposed to significant levels of airborne lead.

Other Laboratory Tests

Depending on the magnitude of lead exposure, a complete blood count, serum creatinine, blood urea nitrogen, and complete urinalysis may be indicated. Evaluation of reproductive status may be pertinent for some lead-exposed adults.

It is important to check BLLs of family members, particularly children, of lead-exposed individuals. Lead workers may unwittingly expose their families to lead dust brought home on clothes, shoes and in cars.

Except for rare circumstances, there is little or no value in measuring lead in urine or hair. Because of the pharmacokinetics of lead clearance, urine lead changes more rapidly and may vary independently of BLL. Urine lead is less validated than BLL as a biomarker of external exposure, or as a predictor of health effects. Lead in hair may be a reflection of external contamination rather than internal lead dose; laboratory analysis is not standardized.

EXPOSURE INVESTIGATION

The occupational and environmental exposure history is the first step in identifying the source of the lead exposure. Both because the cornerstone of intervention is source removal or reduction and because others may be at risk from exposure, the first step is to identify the source. A list of US Environmental Protection Agency accredited laboratories is available at http://www.epa.gov/lead/nllaplist.pdf. Assistance, especially for non-occupational problems such as herbal remedies, candy, moonshine etc. is available from the local and/or state health departments at http://www.apha.org/public_health/state.htm.

The clinician, with the patient's permission, should also contact the employer for further exposure information, such as air level monitoring, biologic monitoring and Material Safety Data Sheets (MSDSs). Work related exposure measurements should be readily available to the clinician. The federal OSHA standards are available at http://www.osha.gov/SLTC/lead/standards.html. Small businesses can obtain information at http://www.osha.gov/dcsp/smallbusiness/index.html

HEATH-BASED MEDICAL MANAGEMENT

The single most important aspect of treating lead poisoning is removal from exposure, yet there may be important socioeconomic constraints for a given individual that limit this approach. For this reason, the panel and the AOEC petition OSHA to update the requirements of the current lead standards and urge clinicians to engage public health and industrial hygiene professionals whenever lead exposure is suspected.

Documented health risks and medical management recommendations are summarized in Table 4. The table presents recommendations for a broad range of BLLs. Although the BLL range is categorized in discrete steps, the outcomes will not neatly conform to these arbitrary divisions, and expectation of health effects in the BLL categories will also be influenced by cumulation of dose. For example, clinical peripheral neuropathy can be present at the high end of the BLL 40 to 79 µg/dL (1.93-3.81 µmol/L) range, while it would not be expected to occur from lead exposure at the low end of the same range. The table is intended to assist clinicians in discussing the short-term and long-term health risks of lead exposure with their patients.

There are other instances where removal from lead exposure is warranted that are consistent with the OSHA lead standards. In addition to specific "trigger" BLLs for medical removal protection (MRP), under the OSHA lead standards (e.g. BLL 50 µg/dL (2.41 µmol/L) or greater) the physician can remove an individual from lead work due to a medical condition which places the employee "at increased risk of material impairment to health from exposure to lead", chronic renal dysfunction (serum creatinine > 1.5 mg/dL (133 µmol/L) for men, > 1.3 mg/dL (115 µmol/L) for women, or proteinuria), hypertension, neurological disorders, cognitive dysfunction, and pregnancy.

Central nervous system effects may have a delayed onset and may sometimes persist well after the BLL has dropped below the BLLs at which the OSHA lead standards permit return to work. These persistent effects could negatively impact work performance and safety in certain jobs. Anecdotal evidence, and analogy to other neurotoxic injury, suggests that individuals who develop overt neurological signs and symptoms from lead exposure above that permissible under current OSHA regulations may benefit from rehabilitative measures (e.g., physical therapy, cognitive rehabilitation) that have been used effectively in patients with other brain injuries, such as traumatic brain injury or stroke. Participation in a rehabilitation program may enhance the prospect for recovery, and may demonstrate the worker's capacity to safely return to work. [1]

Medical Surveillance

Medical surveillance is an essential part of an employer's lead safety program and includes biological monitoring with periodic BLL testing, medical evaluation, and treatment if needed, and intervention to prevent or control identified exposure. The BLL is the best available measure of total exposure from both inhalation and ingestion. Biological monitoring provides feedback to the employer and worker about the efficacy of workplace controls, helps avoid surprises, and saves costs such as medical removal.

Currently, under the OSHA standards, a worker must be included in a lead medical surveillance program if his/her airborne lead exposure is 30 $\mu g/m^3$ (eight-hour time-weighted average) or higher for more than 30 days per year. The panel believes that the trigger for medical surveillance should not rely solely on air monitoring results; instead, workers should be included in a medical surveillance program whenever they are handling or disturbing materials with a significant lead content in a manner that could reasonably be expected to cause potentially harmful exposure through inhalation or ingestion.

A medical surveillance program with increased frequency of BLL testing and early intervention for all lead-exposed workers is recommended to reduce health risks. The panel does not recommend routine ZPP testing as an early biomarker of lead toxicity; however, ZPP measurement is required by OSHA for certain levels of lead exposure. New employees and those newly assigned to lead work should have a preplacement lead medical examination and BLL test, followed by periodic BLL testing, blood pressure measurement, and health status review. Monthly BLL testing is recommended for the first three months of employment for an initial assessment of the adequacy of exposure control measures. Subsequently, testing frequency can be reduced to every six months as long as BLLs remain below 10 µg/dL (0.48 µmol/L). Any increase in BLL of 5 µg/dL (0.24 µmol/L) or greater should be addressed by re-examining control measures in place to see where improvements should be made and by increasing BLL monitoring if needed. If the task assignment changes to work with significantly higher exposures, the initial BLL testing schedule of monthly tests for the first three months at this task should be repeated.

The above schedule for BLL testing may be inadequate for certain situations where the exposures are very high and/or highly variable. In these situations, the BLL testing schedule should be tailored to address the special risks of different types of work and exposures. For example, a construction worker may have very high, intermittent exposures in contrast to someone working in a battery plant or other general industry setting with significant exposures but less day-to-day variability. Employees assigned to tasks where exposures are extremely high (e.g., abrasive blasting) should be tested more frequently than as recommended above,

---

i.e., at least monthly. In general, it is a good idea to do BLL testing at peak exposures to assess controls and, specifically for the construction trades, to test pre-, mid-, and post-job.

Because of the significant reduction of lead in the general environment, new workers enter lead jobs with very low BLLs while others who have worked with lead often have much higher BLLs and body burdens. With increased biological monitoring frequency to ensure that low BLLs are maintained, it is possible that some workers with lead-related health risks may be able to work safely in a lead-exposed environment. All lead-exposed workers should receive education about the health effects of lead and prevention information from the clinician and the employer, and they should be provided necessary protections including protective clothing, clean eating areas, and hygiene measures such as wash-up facilities and/or showers to prevent both ingestion of lead and take-home exposures.

Chelation Therapy

Primary management for adult lead poisoning is identification of the lead source and cessation of exposure. In adults, chelation therapy generally should be reserved for individuals with high BLLs and/or significant symptoms or signs of toxicity. There is no evidence-based guidance in this regard because of lack of appropriate studies.

Based upon the clinical experience and judgment of panel members, the following general recommendations concerning chelation are offered: chelation therapy is *recommended* for adults with BLLs 100 µg/dL (4.83 µmol/L) or greater, can be *strongly considered* for BLLs 80 to 99 µg/dL (3.86-4.78 µmol/L), and *possibly considered* for BLLs between 50 and 79 µg/dL (2.41-3.81 µmol/L) in the presence of lead-related symptoms. BLLs greater than 100 µg/dL (4.83 µmol/L) almost always warrant chelation as they are usually associated with significant symptoms and may be associated with an incipient risk of encephalopathy or seizures. These are general recommendations and clinicians may vary appropriately from these recommendations depending upon circumstances. Adults with a very high BLL (e.g., 90 µg/dL (4.34 µmol/L)) may remain asymptomatic. Oral chelation has largely supplanted parenteral agents. Chelation therapy relies on enhancing renal excretion, and remobilization of lead from other body stores may occur. Guidance on administration of chelating agents is available in several publications (e.g. Kosnett 2004). Clinicians unfamiliar with chelation protocols are encouraged to contact AOEC clinics (http://www.aoec.org/directory.htm or 1-888-347-2632) or with other physicians experienced in treating adults with lead poisoning for additional advice prior to instituting treatment.

On a population basis it is important to reduce fetal exposure to lead, and maternal lead levels less than 5 µg/dL are optimal. However, laboratory measures are not absolutely precise, and clinical judgment is needed in every patient encounter. Chelation should be used during pregnancy ONLY to protect the life and health of the mother and ONLY if the potential benefit to the mother justifies the potential risk to the fetus. This decision will need to be made on a case by case basis by the attending physician. Because of the increase in lead mobilized from maternal bone during pregnancy, clinicians should be aware that maternal blood lead levels may exhibit an upward trend in the second and third trimesters even in the absence of further exposure. Women with a history of long-term lead exposure or prior elevated BLL's should be monitored regularly during pregnancy for BLL elevation. If the occupational history or clinical evaluation suggests elevated bone lead stores, clinicians may wish to counsel patients on delaying conception until the risk of mobilization of lead from bone depots has been reduced.

Prophylactic chelation therapy of lead-exposed workers, to prevent elevated BLLs or to routinely lower BLLs to pre-designated concentrations believed to be "safe," is prohibited by OSHA. Non-traditional uses of chelation therapy are not advised. There is no established basis to initiate chelation based on results of hair analysis or, in most cases, urine lead levels nor for chelation of asymptomatic individuals with low blood lead concentrations. Chelation should be used during pregnancy only if the potential benefit justifies the potential risk to the fetus. Breast feeding during chelation therapy is not recommended. The effect of chelating agents on the fetus and newborn is unknown.

Pregnancy and Breast Feeding Concerns

Prevention of fetal and postnatal lead exposure of breastfed infants requires identification and control of sources of environmental and occupational lead exposures (both endogenous and exogenous) for pregnant and lactating women. The CDC has established 10 µg/dL (0.48 µmol/L) as a BLL of concern in children (CDC 2002).

Because fetal blood contains approximately 80% of the blood lead concentration of the mother, and because of the risk of spontaneous abortion, the panel's recommendation is that the mother's BLL should be kept below 5 µg/dL (0.24 µmol/L) from the time of conception through pregnancy. For women with a history of lead exposure, calcium supplementation during pregnancy may be especially important and may thus minimize release of lead from bone stores and subsequent fetal lead exposure.

In a recent prospective study, umbilical cord BLL and maternal bone lead measured shortly postpartum were independent risk factors for impaired mental development of the infants assessed at 24 months of age, even after controlling for contemporaneous BLL (Gomaa et al. 2002). Long-term prospective studies suggest that the adverse neurodevelopmental effects of prenatal lead exposure may not persist into adolescence if early postnatal exposure falls to background levels (Bellinger et al. 1990, 1992; Tong et al. 1996). However, maternal BLL measured during pregnancy has been associated with alterations in brainstem auditory response at in the offspring at age five (Rothenberg et al. 2000), and in retinal response at age 10 (Rothenberg et al. 2002b).

Lead does not concentrate in breast milk because it does not bind to nor dissolve in fat; thus, levels of lead are generally higher in a mother's blood than in her milk. Lead in human breast milk appears to be well-absorbed by breast fed infants. Nevertheless, breast feeding should be encouraged in most situations since the benefits generally outweigh the negatives. Decisions relating to lactating women with evidence of very high lead exposure should be made on an individual basis.

If elevated maternal blood lead is suspected or demonstrated, the source(s) of lead exposure in the mother's diet, home, and work environment should be identified and mitigated. Also, the clinician should monitor infant BLLs during the early weeks of breast feeding. Only upon detection and elimination of all other suspected lead sources without corresponding reduction of infant BLL should cessation of breast feeding be advised.

Retained Bullet

Gunshot injuries to the head, face, and neck may be associated with swallowed bullets, fragments, or pellets, which result in a rapid increase in blood lead in the first days following injury. After detection of bullet fragments in the gut with X-rays, efforts to promote gastrointestinal decontamination may result in a gradual reduction of blood lead over the following weeks. Retained bullets or fragments, particularly those in joint spaces, are risk factors for elevated BLL after injury. Decisions to remove bullet fragments imbedded in tissue should be made in consultation between the treating physician and the surgeon. Individuals with retained bullets should receive baseline and periodic blood lead testing to monitor their lead status. Follow-up blood lead levels may not be needed if the bullets are in muscle tissue and physicians are sure the lead fragments have not migrated from muscle into tissues more likely to allow lead uptake.

CONCLUSIONS

AOEC offers these Guidelines as a resource for health care providers, public health professionals, employers, and others to utilize in providing medical management of lead-exposed adults. In this document, the panel has summarized the current scientific evidence concerning the non-carcinogenic adverse health effects in adults from exposure to inorganic lead.

The toxic effects of lead can occur without overt symptoms. A substantial body of recent research demonstrates a high probability that lead exposure at levels previously thought to be of little concern can result in an increased risk of adverse chronic health effects if the exposure is maintained for many years, thereby resulting in a progressively larger cumulative dose. Such effects may include elevations in blood pressure and increased risk of hypertension, kidney disease, cognitive dysfunction and/or accelerated declines in cognitive function, and reproductive risks.

Prevention of lead exposure should remain the primary goal of health care providers, public health professionals, and employers. Biological monitoring, mainly by periodic measurement of blood lead levels (BLLs) for adults engaged in activity with potential exposure to lead, should be conducted routinely to assess the efficacy of primary prevention and to guide the clinician in determining whether exposure has become excessive. Clinicians are encouraged to advise patients of the risks associated with any elevation of lead level and to advocate strongly for environmental controls that would maintain BLLs below 10 µg/dL (0.48 µmol/L) wherever feasible.

TABLE 1

Jobs and Industries with Potential Lead Exposure

General Industry	
Lead production or smelting	Battery manufacturing or recycling
Brass, bronze, copper, or lead foundries	Automotive radiator repair
Ammunition/explosives production	Lead soldering
Scrap metal handling	Ceramic manufacturing
Firing ranges	Cable/wire stripping, splicing or production
Machining or grinding lead alloys	Rubber manufacturing
Manufacture of radiation shielding	Plastics manufacturing
Repair/replacement of refractory material in furnaces	Leaded glass manufacturing
	Paint/pigment manufacturing
Ship building/repairing/breaking	
Mining	

Construction	
Renovation, repair or demolition of structures with lead paint	Use or disturbance of lead solder, sheeting, flashing, or old electrical conduit
Welding or torch-cutting painted metal	Plumbing, particularly in older buildings
Sandblasting, sanding, scraping, burning, or disturbing lead paint	

TABLE 2

Non-occupational and Environmental Sources of Lead Exposure

Remodeling or painting pre-1978 housing	Lead solder in stained-glass artwork
Peeling paint	Lead-soldered cans
Ethnic medicines or folk remedies (e.g., azarcon, greta, pay-loo-ah, kandu, some Ayurvedics)	Lead-contaminated candies
	Backyard scrap metal recycling
Pica (ingestion of lead-containing nonfood items, e.g., soil or ceramics, plaster, or paint chips)	Moonshine (liquor from a homemade still)
	Antique pewter plates, mugs, utensils, toys
Retained lead bullet or fragments	Imported brass or bronze kettles, cookware
Melting lead for fishing weights, bullets, or toys	Lead-glazed tableware or cooking vessels
Imported vinyl miniblinds	Leaded crystal tableware
Recreational target shooting	Mine tailings
Lead-contaminated drinking water supply	Beauty products such as kohl eye make-up, certain hair dyes
Using lead glazes for ceramics	
Painting/stripping cars, boats, bicycles	

TABLE 3

Health Effects to Lead Exposed Adults by Blood Lead Level

Blood Lead Level (µg/dL) (µmol/L)				
5-9(0.24-0.43)	**10-19**(0.48-0.92)	**20-39**(0.97-1.88)	**40-79**(1.93-3.81)	**≥ 80**(≥ 3.86)

› Possible adverse population effects suggested by epidemiological studies	› Possible spontaneous abortion
	
	› Reduced newborn birth weight
	
	› Possible blood pressure changes
	
	› Possible renal dysfunction
		› Spontaneous abortion
		
		› Reduced newborn birth weight
		
		› Possible blood pressure changes
		
		› Possible renal dysfunction
		
		› Possible non-specific symptoms
		  -Headache
		  -Fatigue
		  -Sleep disturbance
		  -Anorexia
		  -Constipation
		  -Diarrhea
		  -Arthralgia
		  -Myalgia
		  -Decreased Libido
		  -Mood Swings, personality changes
		
		› Possible CNS effects
		  -Memory and attention deficits
			› Spontaneous abortion
			
			› Reduced newborn birth weight
			
			› Non-specific symptoms
			
			› CNS effects
			
			› Sperm effects
			  -lowered counts
			  -abnormal sperm
			
			› Subclinical peripheral neuropathy
			
			› Possible hypertension
			
			› Possible anemia
			
			› Possible renal damage
			
			› Possible gout
				› Spontaneous abortion
				
				› Reduced newborn birth weight
				
				› Non-specific symptoms
				
				› CNS effects
				
				› Sperm effects
				
				› Peripheral Neuropathy
				
				› Hypertension
				
				› Anemia
				
				› Abdominal Colic
				
				› Nephropathy
				
				› Gout

TABLE 4

Health Based Management Guidelines

Blood Lead Level (µg/dL) (µmol/L)			
5-9(0.24-0.43)	**10-29**(0.48-1.40)	**30-79****(1.45-3.81)****	**≥ 80**(≥ 3.86)

‣ Lead education
  -Occupational
  -Environmental
  -Reproductive
 	
‣ Follow-up blood
  lead levels (BLLs)
	‣ Consider clinical
	  assessment
	  -History:
	    occupational
	    environmental
	    medical
	  -Exam, labs
	  -Identify risk factors
	  -Family BLLs
	
	‣ Exposure investigation
	  -MSDSs
	  -Air testing
	  -Workplace
	    communication
	
	‣ Consider consultations
	  -Occupational Medicine
	  -Industrial Hygienist
	  -Public Health
	    department
	
	‣ Lead hazard reduction
	
	‣ Consider removal from
	  lead exposure if
	  warranted
	
	‣ Lead education
	
	‣ Follow-up BLLs
	  (See Medical
	  Surveillance
	  recommendations)
		‣ Lead education
		
		‣ Clinical assessment
		  -History
		  -Exam, labs (BUN, Cr,
		    CBC)
		  -Identify risk factors
		  -Family BLLs
		
		‣ Exposure Assessment
		
		‣ Consultations as
		  appropriate
		
		‣ Lead Hazard
		  Reduction
		
		‣ Removal from lead
		  exposure**
		
		‣ Possible chelation for
		  BLL>50 with signs or
		  symptoms of toxicity
		
		‣ Medical Surveillance
		  -Follow-up BLLs
		  -Follow-up clinical
		    assessments
		
		**Note this is the
		recommendation by
		AOEC. Consult the
		OSHA Standard for the
		levels currently defined in
		regulation which provides
		workers' protections.*
			‣ Immediate removal
			  from lead exposure
			
			‣ Refer for immediate/
			  urgent medical
			  evaluation and
			  consideration
			  of chelation therapy
			
			‣ Clinical assessment
			
			‣ Lead education
			
			‣ Exposure investigation
			
			‣ Consultations
			
			‣ Lead hazard reduction
			
			‣ Medical surveillance

ACKNOWLEDGEMENTS

These guidelines were adopted in May 2007 following approval by a three fourths majority of the AOEC member clinics. This version of the guidelines supercedes the prior version approved in December 2005.

AOEC wishes to acknowledge the authors of the final document: Rosemary Sokas, MD, MOH, Kathleen Fagan, MD, MPH, and Alan Ducatman, MD, MS.

While this paper does not necessarily reflect the views of the expert panel convened by AOEC in March 2003, AOEC also wishes to acknowledge their efforts. The final documents of the panel prepared for AOEC provided a significant contribution for this work.

Richard Wedeen, MD-CHAIR, Rose Goldman, MD, MPH, Dana Headapohl, MD, MPH, Karen Hipkins, RN, NP-C, MPH, Howard Hu, MD, MPH, ScD, Michael Kosnett, MD, MPH, Barbara Materna, PhD, CIH, Pamela Reich, BS, Stephen Rothenberg, PhD, Brian Schwartz, MD, MS, Eugene Shippen, MD, Laura Welch, MD, Alan Woolf, MD, MPH.

Affiliations and nominating organizations for the panelists and primary authors may be obtained from the AOEC office at 202-347-4976 or by e-mail from kkirkland@aoec.org

REFERENCES (*alphabetical order*)

Bellinger D, Leviton A, Sloman J. 1990. Antecedents and correlates of improved cognitive performance in children exposed *in utero* to low levels of lead. Environ Health Perspect 89:5-11.

CDC.2002. Managing Elevated BLLs Among Young Children. Atlanta, GA:Centers for Disease Control and Prevention, National Center for Environmental Health.

CDC.2005. Third National Report on Human Exposoure to Environmental Chemicals. NCEH Pub. No. 05-05-7, Lead CAS No. 7439-92-1. Atlanta: CDC. Available at: http://www.cdc.gov/exposurereport/3rd/pdf/thirdreport.pdf

González-Cossío T, Peterson KE, Sanín L, Fishbein SE, Palazuelos E, Aro A, Hernández-Avila M, Hu H. 1997. Decrease in birth weight in relation to maternal bone lead burden. Pediatrics 100:856-862.

Gulson BL, Mizon KJ, Korsch MJ, Palmer JM, Donnelly JB. 2003. Mobilization of lead from human bone tissue during pregnancy and lactation—a summary of long-term research. Sci Total Environ 303:79-104.

Hernandez-Avila M, Peterson KE, Gonzalez-Cossio T, Sanin LH, Aro A, Schnaas L, Hu H. 2002. Effect of maternal bone lead on length and head circumference at birth. Arch Environ Health 57: 482-488.

Kosnett MJ. 2004. Lead. In: Poisoning and Drug Overdose (Olson KR, ed.). New York:Lange Medical Publishing/McGraw Hill, 238–242.

NCHS. 1984. Blood lead levels for persons ages 6 months to 74 years. United States, 1976-1980. Vital and Health Statistics. Series 11, No. 233. Pub. No. (PHS) 84-1683. Washington, DC:National Center for Health Statistics.

Rothenberg SJ, Poblano A, Schnaas L. 2000. Brainstem auditory evoked response at five years and prenatal lead exposure. Neurotoxicol Teratol 22:503-510.

Rothenberg SJ, Schnaas L, Salgado-Valladares M, Casanueva E, Geller AM, Hudnell HK, Fox DA. 2002b. Increased ERG a-wave and b-wave amplitudes in 7-10 year old children resulting from prenatal lead exposure. J Investigative Ophthamology and Visual Science 43: 2036-2044.

Sanin LH, González-Cossín T, Romieu I, Perterson KE, Ruíz S, Palazuelos E, Hernández-Avila M. Hu H. 2001. Effect of maternal lead burden on infant weight and weight gain at one month of age among breastfed infants. Pediatrics 107:1016-1023.

Telisman S, Cvitkovic P, Jurasovic J, Pizent A, Gavella M, Rocic B. 2000. Semen quality and reproductive endocrine function in relation to biomarkers of lead, cadmium, zinc, and copper in men. Environ Health Perspect 108:45-53.

Tong S, Baghurst P, McMichael A, Sawyer M, Mudge J. 1996. Lifetime exposure to environmental lead and children's intelligence at 11-13 years: the Port Pirie cohort study. Br Med J 312:1569-1575.

Appendix VIII
Pregnancy Risk Assessment Form
New York City Department of Health and Mental Hygiene

EDC:_____   ID:_____

PREGNANCY RISK ASSESSMENT FORM

Instructions: Fill out the information on the first page using the Activity Report. The information on this page will be double-checked beginning on Page 2.

Case Name:_____
                Last   **Middle**   **First**

Expected Date of Confinement (EDC): _____/_____/_____
                                  Month   **Day**   **Year**

BLL at case assignment (µg/dL): _____   **Test date:** _____/_____/_____

Report date: _____/_____/_____   **DOB:** _____/_____/_____
              Month   **Day**   **Year**   **Month** **Day** **Year**

Address

Street:		Apt#:
City/Borough:	State:	Zip:

Home telephone number	(_____) _____ - _____	
Work telephone number	(_____) _____ - _____	☐ Not provided
Cell telephone number	(_____) _____ - _____	☐ Not provided

Prior LPPP Pregnant Woman Case: ☐ No   ☐ Yes

Prior or Current LeadQuest Child Case: ☐ No   ☐ Yes>> LI #_____
(18 years or younger)

Interview Language Information
Instructions: <u>In the office,</u> the primary language of the pregnant woman should be determined. If necessary, an interpreter from the family, the LPPP office, or telephone interpreting services can be used to assist in gathering information.

Please check off the language used by the pregnant woman during the interview and whether an <u>interpreter</u> was used:

Interview language:

☐ English   ☐ Spanish   ☐ Russian   ☐ Bengali   ☐ Hindi   ☐ Haitian-Creole   ☐ Urdu
☐ Other:_____

Interpreter Used:

☐ No   ☐ Yes
If yes>> **Type of interpreter used:**
☐ Family member   ☐ Friend   ☐ Telephone interpreting services
☐ LPPP staff   ☐ Other:_____

Staff member conducting interview:_____   1

Interview Date: _____/_____/_____   Time Started: _____

A. CONTACT INFORMATION
I would like to make sure the information we have in our records is correct.

1. What is the exact spelling of <u>your</u> name?
Instructions: Ask for the spelling of the name.

☐ Confirmed	Last Name	
☐ Confirmed	First Name	
☐ Confirmed	Middle Name	☐ NA

2. What is your date of birth?   _____/_____/_____
                              Month   Day   Year

3. Please confirm the address where you currently live.
Instructions: Confirm the address from Page 1. Check off the confirmed box if information is correct. Otherwise write in correct information.

☐ Confirmed	Street:		Apt#:
☐ Confirmed	City/Borough:	State:	Zip:

3a. How long have you been living at this address?

_____ year(s) _____ month(s) _____ day(s)

4. Please tell me your <u>current</u> home telephone number.
Instructions: Confirm the home phone number from Page 1. Check off the confirmed box if information is correct. Otherwise write in correct information.

☐ Confirmed   Home telephone number: (_____) _____- _____

4a. If you work, please tell me your work number:	(_____) _____ - _____ ☐ NA		
4b. If you have a cell phone, please tell me your cell number:	(_____) _____ - _____ ☐ NA		
4c. Which phone number is the best to reach you?	☐ Home	☐ Cell	☐ Work
4d. Which days of the week are the easiest to reach you? ☐ Mon ☐ Tues ☐ Wed ☐ Thurs ☐ Fri	☐ Sat	☐ Sun	☐ Any day
4e. When is the best time to reach you? _____	☐ a.m.	☐ p.m.	☐ Any time

B. HOUSEHOLD INFORMATION

Now I'd like to find out about the other people in your household because they may have been exposed to lead.

5. How many children under age 18 live with you? _____
Instructions: If no child(ren), go to Section C.

Please give me the name and date of birth of the child(ren). Let's start with the youngest child.
Instructions: Write in information. If more than 3 children, write on back of form.

	#1	#2	#3
Full Name *(ask for spelling)*	Last:_____ First:_____	Last:_____ First:_____	Last:_____ First:_____
Date of Birth	_____ / _____ / _____ Mo Day Year	_____ / _____ / _____ Mo Day Year	_____ / _____ / _____ Mo Day Year
Relationship to You	Daughter / Son Other:_____	Daughter / Son Other:_____	Daughter / Son Other:_____
BLL (µg/dL)	_____	_____	_____
Date of BLL	_____ / _____ / _____ Mo Day Year	_____ / _____ / _____ Mo Day Year	_____ / _____ / _____ Mo Day Year

Instructions: Provide education about blood lead testing for children.

C. MEDICAL INFORMATION

I need to write down contact information for your doctor and health insurance. If you have a card, letter or bill from the doctor or health insurance, I can copy down the information.
Instructions: Ask to see card and write down information. If no information shown, ask for spelling of name and address.

6. What is the contact information for your doctor?

Clinic Name:	
Doctor's Last Name:	First:
Street:	City/Borough:
State:	Zip:
Telephone number: (_____) _____ - _____	☐ Documents shown ☐ No documents shown

7. Do you currently have any type of health insurance such as PCAP or Medicaid?

☐ No >> *go to Q. 8*   ☐ Yes >>   ☐ Don't know >> *go to Q. 8*

7a. *If yes>> Instructions: Ask to see insurance card and write down information. If no card provided, ask for any information available.*

Plan Name	
ID #	
Additional Information	☐ Card shown ☐ No card shown

8. When was your <u>first</u> doctor or prenatal care visit during this pregnancy?	_____/_____/_____ Month Day Year	☐ Don't know
8a. When is your <u>next</u> doctor or prenatal care appointment?	_____/_____/_____ Month Day Year	☐ Not scheduled/ Don't have one
8b. How far along are you in your pregnancy right now?	_____(weeks)	☐ Don't know
8c. What is your expected due date?	_____/_____/_____ Month Day Year	☐ Don't know

8d. Are you currently taking a prenatal vitamin with calcium?

☐ No   ☐ Yes

9. At which hospital do you plan to have your baby?

Hospital Name:	
City/Borough:	State:
Comment:	☐ Don't know

10. In the past, were you ever told you had a high blood lead level or were you diagnosed with lead poisoning?

☐ No >> *go to Section D*	☐ Yes >>	☐ Don't know >> *go to Section D*

If yes >>

10a. What was the blood lead level?	_____µg/dL	☐ Don't know
10b. When was the blood test taken?	_____/_____/_____ Mo Day Year	☐ Don't know
10c. In what city and state was the blood test performed?	City:_____ State:_____ Country:_____	
10d. Were you pregnant at that time?	☐ No ☐ Yes	

D. DEMOGRAPHIC INFORMATION

Now, I'd like to learn more about your background.

11. What is the highest grade or year of school you have completed?
Instructions: Read out the categories. Do not read out Declined to answer.

☐ Never attended school or only attended kindergarten ☐ Some elementary or primary school ☐ Completed elementary or primary school ☐ Some high school ☐ Completed high school/ high school graduate ☐ Some college or technical school ☐ College graduate
☐ Declined to answer

12. Which of the following groups best describes your race or ethnicity? I'm going to first read out all the categories. You can tell me more than one category.
Instructions: Read out all categories first. Check as many as reported.

☐ African American or Black ☐ American Indian or Alaska Native ☐ Asian ☐ Hispanic or Latino ☐ Native Hawaiian or Other Pacific Islander ☐ White or Caucasian
Instructions: Do not read aloud. ☐ Other group not listed, *Instructions: If mentioned, write in response.* _____ ☐ Declined to answer

E. COUNTRY OF BIRTH/ FOREIGN TRAVEL

Now I have a few questions about where you were born and any trips you may have taken outside of the US. This information can help us identify possible ways you may have been exposed to lead. I am not interested in your immigration status.

13. In what country were __you__ born?	☐ U.S. >> *go to Q.14* ☐ Mexico ☐ Bangladesh ☐ Ecuador ☐ India ☐ Pakistan ☐ Other country: _____ ☐ Declined to answer

*Instructions: If woman was born in **Bangladesh, Ecuador, India, Mexico,** or **Pakistan** show list at the end of the form (Appendix A).*

13a. Where in *[Bangladesh, Ecuador, India, Mexico, or Pakistan]* **were you born?**

Bangladesh:_____

Ecuador:_____

India:_____

Mexico:_____

Pakistan:_____

☐ Don't know >> *go to Q. 13b*

Instructions: For ALL women born __outside of the US.__

13b. How long did you live there?	_____ day(s) _____ month(s) _____ year(s)
13c. When (what month and year) did you come to the US?	Month: _____ Year: _____

Instructions: For all women, including US-born women.
For foreign-born women – read first part of sentence. For US-born, start from 2nd line:

14. __Since leaving__ *[birth country]*,
Have you ever spent any time outside of the US? This includes any traveling, visiting family or friends, or living in another country.

☐ No >> *go to Section F*   ☐ Yes >>

14a. *If yes >> Instructions: Write down all information about time spent outside of US. Ask for all visits. If more than 3 times, write below.*

	#1	#2	#3
Country			
When did you stay there? (start w/ most recent)	_____/_____ Mo/Year	_____/_____ Mo/Year	_____/_____ Mo/Year
How long did you stay?	☐ Less than 1 month ☐ More than 1 month ☐ Don't know	☐ Less than 1 month ☐ More than 1 month ☐ Don't know	☐ Less than 1 month ☐ More than 1 month ☐ Don't know
How often do you travel there?	☐ 1x a year ☐ every 2 years ☐ every 5 years	☐ 1x a year ☐ every 2 years ☐ every 5 year	☐ 1x a year ☐ every 2 years ☐ every 5 years
Comments			

F. IMPORTED REMEDIES, FOODS, SPICES, COSMETICS AND POTTERY

Now I am going to ask you about some product(s) you may have used or come in contact with, such as medications and health remedies, foods and spices. Some of these products may be made in other countries and may contain lead. They could be products or items:

- sent by friends and family
- brought back from trips you may have taken
- bought in local stores
- or given to you by friends or family

I want to find out if you used any of these products during the past 12 months.

Instructions: Ask woman to show you products in the kitchen and medicine cabinets. Take note of any product(s) that may contain lead. If Yes to Questions 15 – 18, ask to see product(s). See sampling guidelines. Complete Non-Dust Chain of Custody Form.

15. [Imported Medicines] Have you used any imported...

Product	No	Yes >>	Sample Taken (Yes/No)	Comments/Observations
Medicines? (e.g. Products to help become pregnant or remedies for stomach problems)			Yes / No	
Ayurvedics? (e.g. Remedies based on traditional Indian medical system)			Yes / No	
Vitamins?			Yes / No	
Powder or pills?			Yes / No	
Herbs?			Yes / No	
Teas?			Yes / No	
Any other imported remedies?:_____			Yes / No	

16. [Imported Cosmetics] Have you used any imported…

Product	No	Yes >>	Sample Taken (Yes/No)	Comments/Observations
Cosmetics? (e.g. Eye makeup, hair dye)			Yes / No	
Deodorant?			Yes / No	
Any other imported cosmetics?:_____			Yes / No	

17. [Imported Food] Have you eaten any imported…

Product	No	Yes >>	Sample Taken (Yes/No)	Comments/Observations
Spices? (e.g. Orange or red spices)			Yes / No	
Foods?			Yes / No	
Snacks or candies? (e.g. Candy spiced with chili or sold in clay pots)			Yes / No	
Any other imported food?:_____			Yes / No	

18. [Imported Pottery] Have you been served food in or eaten from imported, antique or painted…

Product	No	Yes >>	Sample Taken (Yes/No)	Comments/Observations
Clay pots?			Yes / No	
Ceramic dishes, bowls, pitchers, or cups?			Yes / No	
Any other imported containers?:_____			Yes / No	

G. NON-FOOD ITEMS

Now I'd like to ask you about your eating habits during your pregnancy. Women often crave or have an urge to eat many different things when pregnant. Some women eat new foods when they are pregnant; some eat things that are recommended during pregnancy by family and friends; and some women also eat things that are **not** considered food.

19. At any time during your pregnancy, have you eaten, chewed on or mouthed anything that is not food? Some examples are paint chips, soil, clay, crushed pottery or other items.

☐ No >> *go to Section H*   ☐ Yes >>

19a. *If yes >> Instructions: Write in information in table.*

	#1	#2	#3
Item Name/Description			
Where did you get it?			
For how long have you been eating it?	_____ wks/mo/yrs	_____ wks/mo/yrs	_____ wks/mo/yrs
How often do/did you eat, on average? (daily, weekly, monthly)			
How much do you eat, on average?			
Why did you eat it?			
Sample Taken	No / Yes	No / Yes	No / Yes
Comments/Observations			

Instructions: See sampling guidelines and complete Non-Dust Chain of Custody Form.

H. OCCUPATION AND HOBBIES

Now I'd like to ask you about the jobs, hobbies or activities of people in the household.

20. Are you currently working?

☐ Yes >>	**20a. Please describe the work you do.**	
☐ No >>	**20b. Have you worked in the past?** ☐ No ☐ Yes >> **20c. Please describe your past work:** _____	

21. Have you or anyone in your household done any of the following jobs, hobbies or activities?

Job/hobby/activity	No Yes	Relationship to PW	Time Period/ How long? (mo/yrs)	Comment Section/ Current Status
Bridge painting or repair work	☐ No ☐ Yes	☐ Self ☐ Other: _____	_____ month(s) _____ year(s)	
Commercial building renovation or demolition	☐ No ☐ Yes	☐ Self ☐ Other: _____	_____ month(s) _____ year(s)	
Home renovation, repair or repainting	☐ No ☐ Yes	☐ Self ☐ Other: _____	_____ month(s) _____ year(s)	
Torch cutting or burning steel, welding	☐ No ☐ Yes	☐ Self ☐ Other: _____	_____ month(s) _____ year(s)	
Cable splicing, soldering, electronics repair	☐ No ☐ Yes	☐ Self ☐ Other: _____	_____ month(s) _____ year(s)	
Metal or car battery recycling; working in a scrap yard; radiator repair	☐ No ☐ Yes	☐ Self ☐ Other: _____	_____ month(s) _____ year(s)	
Working in a firing range; target shooting	☐ No ☐ Yes	☐ Self ☐ Other: _____	_____ month(s) _____ year(s)	
Jobs/Crafts like furniture refinishing, jewelry making, stained glass, pottery, ceramics, glass blowing; making fishing weights, bullets, or lead figures	☐ No ☐ Yes	☐ Self ☐ Other: _____	_____ month(s) _____ year(s)	
Other: _____	☐ No ☐ Yes	☐ Self ☐ Other: _____	_____ month(s) _____ year(s)	

I. PAINT HAZARDS

22. In the past 12 months, has there been water damage, deteriorated plaster or paint <u>in this home</u>?

☐ No >> *go to Q.23* ☐ Yes >> ☐ Don't know >> *go to Q.23*

22a. *If yes* >> **Can you please show me and describe the damage?**

Location/Room	
Describe Damage	
When did this occur? (mo/yr)	____/____ Mo/Year
Current Status	

23. In the past 12 months, has there been any renovation or repair work at your current address, at an address where you lived previously or another address where you have spent time?

☐ No >> *go to Q.24* ☐ Yes >> ☐ Don't know >> *go to Q.24*

23a. *If yes>>* **Please tell me what type of work and when the work was done.**

	#1	#2
Location/Room		
Work Description		
Address		
When was the work done? (mo/yr)	____/____ Mo/Year	____/____ Mo/Year
Current Status		

24. Do you plan to stay at this current address after your baby is born?

☐ No ☐ Yes ☐ Don't know

J. ALTERNATE CONTACT

Finally, I would like to ask for a contact person in case we cannot reach you.

25. Is there <u>another person, like a family member or friend, who lives at a different address</u>, whom we could contact?

☐ No >> *go to Q. 26*   ☐ Yes >>

25a. What is this person's relationship to you?

☐ Husband	☐ Boyfriend	☐ Mother	☐ Father	☐ Brother	☐ Sister	☐ Aunt
☐ Uncle	☐ Grandmother	☐ Grandfather	☐ Other: _____			

25b. Please tell me his/her name and telephone number?

Alternate contact's last name	
Alternate contact's first name	
Home number	(_____) _____ - _____ ☐ Not provided
Work number	(_____) _____ - _____ ☐ Not provided
Cell number	(_____) _____ - _____ ☐ Not provided

Instructions: Inform woman that she should notify alternate contact that we may contact him/her but only if we cannot get in touch with her.

26. Is there anything else you would like to tell me?
Instructions: Ask if there are any questions.

☐ No	☐ Yes >>_____ _____ _____

Time Ended: _____

Visual Inspection

Now I need to look around your home for possible sources of lead exposure. I may need to take some samples. The results of the tests will be provided to you as soon as they are available.

Instructions: Conduct visual inspection.

SUMMARY
Instructions: Check all those that apply. Then, ask if there are any questions.

Potential Lead Exposure

Yes   **No**

☐   ☐   Emigrated from or traveled to a foreign country with significant lead contamination

☐   ☐   Used imported health remedies, food or spices

☐   ☐   Used imported pottery or cosmetics

☐   ☐   Ate, chewed or mouthed non-food items

☐   ☐   Participated in an activity that may involve lead exposure

☐   ☐   Present during repair work that disturbed paint

Samples

Yes   **No**

☐   ☐   Imported health remedy/food/spice sample taken

☐   ☐   Imported pottery or cosmetic sample taken

☐   ☐   Nonfood sample(s) taken

Missing Information

Yes   **No**

☐   ☐   Doctor's contact information needed

☐   ☐   Health insurance information needed

Counseling and Education

Follow up with your doctor

- How often you will need a blood lead test is based on the results of your previous blood tests as well as your risk for further exposure.
- Discuss breastfeeding with your doctor. Breastfeeding is generally considered safe in most cases.

Eat a healthy diet during pregnancy

- It is important to eat foods with enough calcium, iron and vitamin C.
- Talk to your doctor to make sure you are getting enough of these nutrients. Your doctor may suggest changes to your diet or may prescribe a supplement to help you get enough of these nutrients.

Reduce your exposure to lead

- Avoid using medicines, spices, foods or cosmetics from other countries. They are more likely to contain lead than products made in the United States.
- Avoid using clay pots and dishes from other countries to cook, store or serve food. Do not use pottery that is chipped or cracked.
- Never eat non-food items such as clay, soil, pottery or paint chips.
- Stay away from any repair work being done in your home.
- Avoid jobs and hobbies that may involve contact with lead.

Get other household members tested for lead

- This is especially important for children younger than 6 years of age, children with developmental problems and pregnant women.
- Older children and adults should be tested if they may have had contact with lead.

For more information about lead poisoning

- Speak with your doctor.
- You can contact me at 212-676-6379.
- Call 311 and ask for the BAN-LEAD information line.
- Go to www.nyc.gov/lead.

Ask if there are any questions.

APPENDIX A: Question 13a.

Instructions: Please show this list to the woman and ask her to tell you/point to the area where she was born. Then return to Q.13a on page 6 and write in name of area. If the area is not on the list, please write in the area and ask for the spelling.

Mexico

☐ Aguascalientes	☐ Guerrero	☐ Quintana Roo
☐ Baja California	☐ Hidalgo	☐ San Luis Potosí
☐ Baja California Sur	☐ Jalisco	☐ Sinaloa
☐ Campeche	☐ México	☐ Sonora
☐ Chiapas	☐ Michoacán (de Ocampo)	☐ Tabasco
☐ Chihuahua	☐ Morelos	☐ Tamaulipas
☐ Coahuila (de Zaragoza)	☐ Nayarit	☐ Tlaxcala
☐ Colima	☐ Nuevo Léon	☐ Veracruz (-Llave)
☐ Distrito Federal	☐ Oaxaca	☐ Yucatán
☐ Durango	☐ Puebla	☐ Zacatecas
☐ Guanajuato	☐ Querétaro (de Arteaga)	☐ Other (specify):_____

Ecuador

☐ Azuay	☐ Los Ríos
☐ Bolívar	☐ Manabí
☐ Cañar	☐ Morona-Santiago
☐ Carchi	☐ Napo
☐ Chimborazo	☐ Orellana
☐ Cotopaxi	☐ Pastaza
☐ El Oro	☐ Pichincha
☐ Esmeraldas	☐ Sucumbíos
☐ Galápagos	☐ Tungurahua
☐ Guayas	☐ Zamora-Chinchipe
☐ Imbabura	☐ Other (specify):_____
☐ Loja	

Pakistan

☐ Bahawalpur	☐ Lahore	☐ Sahiwal
☐ Faisalabad	☐ Larkana	☐ Sargodha
☐ Gujranwala	☐ Mardan	☐ Shekhupura
☐ Gujrat	☐ Multan	☐ Sialkot
☐ Hyderabad	☐ Okara	☐ Sukkur
☐ Islamabad	☐ Peshawar	☐ Sahiwal
☐ Jhang Maghiana	☐ Quetta	☐ Sargodha
☐ Karachi	☐ Rahimyar Khan	☐ Shekhupura
☐ Kasur	☐ Rawalpindi	☐ Sialkot
		☐ Sukkur
		☐ Other (specify): _____

Bangladesh

☐ Bandarban	☐ Narsingdi	☐ Lalmonir Hat
☐ Barguna	☐ Jamalpur	☐ Satkhira
☐ Barisal	☐ Gopalganj	☐ Narail
☐ Bhola	☐ Kishorganj	☐ Rajshahi
☐ Brahmanbaria	☐ Madaripur	☐ Bogra
☐ Chandpur	☐ Netrakona	☐ Naogaon
☐ Chittagong	☐ Rajbari	☐ Nator
☐ Comilla	☐ Narayanganj	☐ Kurigram
☐ Cox's Bazar	☐ Shariatpur	☐ Nawabganj
☐ Dhaka	☐ Sherpur	☐ Nilphamari
☐ Dhaka	☐ Tangail	☐ Pabna
☐ Faridpur	☐ Khulna	☐ Sylhet
☐ Feni	☐ Kushtia	☐ Habiganj
☐ Gazipur	☐ Magura	☐ Maulvi Bazar
☐ Jhalakhati	☐ Khulna	☐ Panchagarh
☐ Khagrachari	☐ Meherpur	☐ Sunamganj
☐ Lakshmipur	☐ Manikganj	☐ Dinajpur
☐ Noakhali	☐ Bagerhat	☐ Rajshahi
☐ Patuakhali	☐ Chuadanga	☐ Rangpur
☐ Pirojpur	☐ Jessore	☐ Sirajganj
☐ Rangamati	☐ Munshiganj	☐ Gaibanda
	☐ Mymensingh	☐ Jaipur Hat
	☐ Jhenida	☐ Thakurgaon
		☐ Sylhet
		☐Other (specify):_____

India

☐ Assam	☐ Mahārāshtra
☐ Bihār	☐ Manipur
☐ Chandīgarh	☐ Meghālaya
☐ Chhatisgarh	☐ Mizorām
☐ Dādra & Nagar Haveli	☐ Nāgāland
☐ Damān & Diu	☐ Orissa
☐ Delhi	☐ Pondicherry
☐ Goa	☐ Punjab
☐ Gujarāt	☐ Rājasthān
☐ Haryāna	☐ Sikkim
☐ Himāchal Pradesh	☐ Tamil Nādu
☐ Jammu & Kashmīr	☐ Tripura
☐ Jharkhand	☐ Uttaranchal
☐ Karnātaka	☐ Uttar Pradesh
☐ Kerala	☐ West Bengal (Bangla)
☐ Lakshadweep	☐ Other (specify):_____
☐ Madhya Pradesh	

Appendix IX
Assessment Interview Form
Minnesota Department of Health

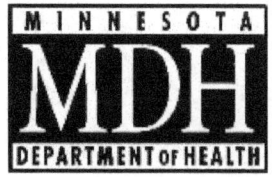

RISK ASSESSMENT INTERVIEW FORM

Date:_____ Case #: _____

Child's Name:_____ Date of Birth:_____

Parent's Name(s):_____ Person interviewed:_____

Address: _____

Phone # (include area code):_____

1. Are there any other children under the age of six? Yes_____ No_____

    Names: _____   _____

    _____   _____

    Have they been tested for lead? Yes_____ No_____

2. How long have you lived at this address?_____ Own_____ Rent_____

    Year built:_____

    If rented, landlord's name, address and phone number:_____

    _____

    If less than 12 months, list previous address for past 12 months:_____

    _____

3. Has any renovation of the residence taken place within the past year? Any furniture renovation? Please specify:

    _____

    _____

4. Does child spend several hours each week in another location such as a day care facility, grandparent's home, babysitter's home, playgrounds, neighbor's home, other neighborhood areas? If so, what are those addresses?:

    1. _____ Average time each week:_____hrs.
    2._____ Average time each week:_____hrs.

5. Occupations of adults in household:_____

6. Are there pets living at the residence that are allowed outdoors? Yes_____ No _____

7. Are there areas of bare soil near the residence? Yes _____ No _____

   Is there a sand box or play area near a street or alley, or next to the house or garage? Yes _____ No _____

8. Is car repair done at the residence? Where? _____

9. Note the condition of the surrounding neighborhood. Are there areas of potential lead exposure?

   _____

   _____

10. Where does the child play inside and outside the residence? _____

    _____

Where does the child like to hide? _____

11. Has the child been given folk medicines such as:

   Greta (Hispanic) _____   Azarcon (Hispanic) _____   Surman (Asian) _____   Pay-loo-ah(Hmong) _____

12. Does the child have contact with or access to:

   car batteries[1] _____   pesticides[4] _____   bullets, gunshot or reloads[8] _____
   solder[2] _____   painted, antique or foreign toys[5] _____   pewter items[9] _____
   lead sinkers or other fishing   pool cue chalk[6] _____   ceramic dishes or food
   supplies _____   colored newsprint[7] _____   containers[11] _____
   stained glass[3] _____   paint, varnish or supplies[10] _____

13. Does the child:

   suck the thumb _____   eat soil/mud pies _____   chew/suck on miniblinds _____
   put fingers in mouth _____   eat crayons _____   spend time at windows _____
   eat paint chips _____   chew/suck on matches _____   chew/suck on windowsills or
   pick at paint _____   chew/suck on furniture _____   sashes _____

14. Where do parents think lead exposure is occurring? _____

    _____

Foot Note:
1. Car batteries are made of lead.
2. Solder used for electrical or plumbing work may contain lead.
3. Leaded solder is typically used to hold the stained glass together at the seams.
4. Some older pesticides may contain lead arsenate, usually in powder form.
5. Antique toys or those produced in another country may have lead paint.
6. Some brands of green pool cue chalk may contain lead.
7. Colored newsprint, more likely glossy print, may be printed with ink containing lead.
8. Bullets and shot used for reloading are made of lead and the dust from reloading may also be a hazard.
9. Pewter contains lead.
10. Old paint and varnish may contain lead.
11. Paint and glaze used on ceramics and pottery may contain lead.

Appendix X
Lead Based Paint Risk Assessment Form
Minnesota Department of Health

Lead-Based Paint Risk Assessment Report

for the Property located at

[ADDRESS]
[CITY, Minnesota, ZIP]

Conducted by

[RA signature on line (*delete this*)]

_____

[RISK ASSESSOR'S NAME], [LICENSE NUMBER (LR####)]

Minnesota Department of Health
[ADDRESS]
[CITY, Minnesota, ZIP]
[PHONE]

[REPORT DATE]

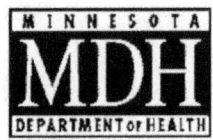 **LEAD RISK ASSESSMENT REPORT**

[ADDRESS]
[CITY, MINNESOTA, ZIP]

Case: [CASE NUMBER]

I. AUTHORITY

Minnesota Statutes 144.9504, subdivision 2, sub-subdivision (a) requires the Minnesota Department of Health (MDH) to conduct a lead risk assessment on a property according to the venous blood lead level of a child or pregnant female residing at the property.

II. BACKGROUND

(Pick one of the following paragraphs, delete the rest)

MDH conducted a lead risk assessment at the property located at [ADDRESS] in [CITY], Minnesota, on [DATE OF RISK ASSESSMENT]. The property was constructed in [YEAR] and is owned by [PROPERTY OWNER NAME, PROPERTY OWNER ADDRESS, PROPERTY OWNER CITY, STATE, ZIP, PHONE NUMBER].

(If unable to determine the year of construction)
MDH conducted a lead risk assessment at the property located at [ADDRESS] in [CITY], Minnesota, on [DATE OF RISK ASSESSMENT]. MDH was unable to determine the year of construction. The property is owned by [PROPERTY OWNER NAME, PROPERTY OWNER ADDRESS, PROPERTY OWNER CITY, STATE, ZIP, PHONE NUMBER].

(If unable to determine the year of construction or the phone number of the property owner)
MDH conducted a lead risk assessment at the property located at [ADDRESS] in [CITY], Minnesota, on [DATE OF RISK ASSESSMENT]. MDH was unable to determine the year of construction. The property is owned by [PROPERTY OWNER NAME, PROPERTY OWNER ADDRESS, PROPERTY OWNER CITY, STATE, ZIP. MDH was unable to determine the phone number of the property owner.]

III. FINDINGS

MDH observed deteriorated lead-based paint in these areas: [LIST OUT ROOMS OR AREAS].

- Kitchen
- Child's bedroom
- Parent's bedroom
- Bare soil on west side of house

(Use one of the following sentences: MDH did not observe any dust or debris in the property. *OR* MDH observed dust and debris in the following areas [THEN LIST OUT ROOMS OR AREAS]:

- Child's bedroom
- Parent's bedroom

IV. METHODS

The lead risk assessment was conducted with an x-ray fluorescence (XRF) analyzer, dust wipe sampling [and soil sampling]. MDH used a [BRAND AND MODEL] XRF (Serial #####) to analyze painted surfaces. The specific testing locations are located in Appendix A. Analytical results from the XRF testing are located in Appendix B. Dust wipe samples [and soil samples] were collected and sent to [LAB NAME, LAB ADDRESS, LAB CITY, LAB STATE, LAB PHONE NUMBER, (EPA ID#)] for analysis. The analytical results of the dust wipe samples [and soil samples] are located in Appendix C. *(If snow cover prevents soil sampling, delete soil sampling from the paragraph and add this sentence:* Due to snow cover, soil sampling was unable to be completed at this time, but will be done as soon as conditions allow. An amended report will be issued with the soil sampling results.)

V. DISCLOSURE REQUIREMENT

Code of Federal Regulations, title 24, section 35.88, and title 40, section 745.107, requires that a copy or a summary of the lead risk assessment report be provided to current lessees and future tenants if renting the property; or to the purchaser of the property at the time of sale of this property.

VI. RECOMMENDATIONS

The following table identifies the location, type and severity of lead hazards observed at the property. They are prioritized with the items at the top of the table having the most immediate health impact while those near the bottom of the table will impact health to a lesser extent.

Lead Hazards			
Location	**Component**	**Color**	**Severity**
Child's Bedroom	All Windows	Blue	Poor
Parent's Bedroom	Closet Door	Brown	Poor
Living Room	All Windows	White	Poor
Kitchen	Door Casing	Green	Poor
Front Porch	Floor	Red	Poor
Front Porch	Railing	Red	Poor
Rear Porch	Railing	Red	Poor
Back Yard	Bare Soil	N/A	Poor
Parent's Bedroom	All Windows	White	Intact

Kitchen	Window Sash by Sink	White	Intact
Rear Porch	Car Batteries	N/A	Intact

(Expand or contract the table as necessary. Keep the severity at intact or poor.)

Areas where lead hazards are identified should be washed with a household detergent and rinsed with clean rinse water.

Paint identified in poor condition is a lead hazard. Options to reduce lead hazards on sound or non-rotting components include, but are not limited to:

- Wet scraping and repainting
- On- or off-site paint stripping
- On- or off-site component planing
- Covering with an impermeable material, such as vinyl or aluminum coil stock
- Component replacement

Options to reduce lead hazards on unsound or rotting components include, but are not limited to:

- Component repair
- Component replacement

(If bare soil is a lead hazard, use the following sentence. If no bare soil was observed, delete it)
Bare soil may be covered with sod, wood chips, sand or other non-living material after all visible paint chips are removed from the bare soil area.

[LIST OUT ANY OTHER UNUSUAL COMPONENTS AND RECOMMENDATIONS FOR THEM i.e. The car batteries on the rear porch should be removed to an area where they are inaccessible to the child.]

Appendix A

Testing Locations

Appendix B

XRF Testing Results

Paint Standard

≥ 1.0 milligram per square centimeter (≥ 1.0 mg/cm^2)

If a paint sample equals or exceeds the standard, it is considered a lead hazard.

Explanation of Column Headings

(The following items will have to be edited depending on what the XRF print-out looks like)

XRF# - Machine generated sequence number

Insp/XRF – Initials of the inspector and the serial number of the machine

Floor – Floor level

Wall – Wall side of the room starting with A on the street side and going clockwise

Room – Room being tested

Structure (and Feature) – What is being tested

Substrate – The composition of the tested component

Condition – Condition of the paint

Color – Color of the paint

DI – Depth Index – the larger the number the deeper the lead-based paint layer

Result – The result of the test

PbC – The total combined lead in the layers of paint

PbC Error – The error of the total combined lead level

Appendix C

Dust Wipe and Soil Sample Results

Dust Wipe Standards
Floor Wipe – 40 micrograms per square foot ($\mu g/ft^2$)
Window Sill – 250 $\mu g/ft^2$
Window Well – 400 $\mu g/ft^2$

If a dust wipe sample equals or exceeds the standard, it is considered a lead hazard.

See the attached City of Minneapolis Public Health Laboratory Chain of Custody Form for sampling results.

(If soil samples were not collected, delete this)
Soil Standard
100 parts per million (ppm)

If a soil sample equals or exceeds the standard, it is considered a lead hazard.

See the attached City of Minneapolis Public Health Lab Chain of Custody Form for sampling results.

Appendix XI
Primary Prevention Information Form
New York Department of Health and Mental Hygiene

NEW YORK CITY DEPARTMENT OF HEALTH AND MENTAL HYGIENE
LEAD POISONING PREVENTION PROGRAM

Primary Prevention Information Form (PPI)

Instructions: Fill out the information on the first page using the Referral Form. The information on this page will be double-checked beginning on Page 2.

Child Name: _____ _____ _____
                          Last   *Middle*   *First*

BLL (if known) at assignment (µg/dL): _____ **Test Date:** ____/____/____

Mother's BLL (if known) at delivery: _____ **Test Date:** ____/____/____

Child DOB: ____/____/____   **Child Age:** _____
                                                      (Days/wks/mos/yrs)

Instructions: Prior to conducting the inspection, the primary language for the visit should be determined. If necessary, an interpreter from the family, the LPPP office, or the Language Line can be used to assist in gathering information.

Language scheduled: *(Instructions: Check the scheduled interview language.)*

☐ English ☐ Spanish ☐ Russian ☐ Bengali ☐ Hindi

☐ Haitian-Creole ☐ Urdu ☐ Other: _____

Interpreter Scheduled: ☐ No ☐ Yes>>

If yes >> **Type of interpreter scheduled:**

   ☐ Family member (specify): _____ ☐ Friend

   ☐ Language line ☐ LPPP staff ☐ Other: _____

NAME OF INSPECTOR: _____

INTERVIEW DATE: _____ **TIME STARTED:** _____

A. CONTACT AND DEMOGRAPHIC INFORMATION

1. **Is this the address where [child's name] currently lives?**

☐ Yes >> *Continue*   ☐ No >> *Stop* >> *Determine current address*

I would like to find out your name and make sure the information we have in our records is correct.

2. **What is the exact spelling of <u>your</u> name?**

LAST NAME	FIRST NAME

2a. What is your relationship to [child's name]?
   ☐ Mother ☐ Father ☐ Grandparent ☐ Legal Guardian ☐ Foster Parent>> ☐ Other: _____

3. **What is the exact spelling of the child's full name?** *Instructions: Ask for exact spelling of name.*

LAST NAME	FIRST NAME	MIDDLE NAME	☐ NA

3a. *Instructions: Enter child's sex if known. If sex unknown, ask>>*

Is [child's name] a boy or a girl?   ☐ Male   ☐ Female

3b. How old is [child's name]?   Age: _____ (days/wks/mos/yrs)

3c. When is [child's name]'s date of birth? _____/_____/_____

Month   Day   Year

4. **Please confirm this address.** *Instructions: Ask for spelling of street and specific apartment #.*

STREET		APT. #

BOROUGH	STATE	ZIP

4a. How long has he/she lived at this address?

_____ mo(s) and _____ day(s)   ☐ Since birth

5. **Please tell me the telephone number of this address:**

Telephone number: (_____) _____ – _____

5a. If you have a cell phone, please tell me your cell   (_____) _____ – _____   ☐ Not Provided

phone number:

5b. If you work, please tell me your work phone number: (_____) _____ – _____   ☐ Not Provided

5c. Which phone number is the best to reach you?   ☐ Home   ☐ Cell   ☐ Work

5d. Which days of the week are the easiest to reach you?

☐ Mon   ☐ Tues   ☐ Wed   ☐ Thurs   ☐ Fri   ☐ Sat   ☐ Sun   ☐ Any day

5e. When is the best time of day to reach you? _____   ☐ AM   ☐ PM   ☐ Any time

6. **Which of the following best describes your child's race or ethnicity? I'm going to first read out all the categories. You can tell me more than one category.**

Instructions: Read out all categories first. Check as many as reported. Do not read Refused response out loud.

☐ African American or Black   ☐ Hispanic or Latino

☐ American Indian or Alaska Native   ☐ Native Hawaiian or Other Pacific Islander

☐ Asian   ☐ White or Caucasian

☐ Other group not listed, *Instructions: Ask to describe and write in response*

_____

☐ Refused

7. **In what country was [child's name]'s birth <u>mother</u> born?** _____

☐ Don't know   ☐ Refused

7a. **In what country was [child's name]'s birth <u>father</u> born?** _____

☐ Don't know   ☐ Refused

B.   ALTERNATE CONTACT INFORMATION

I would like to ask for a contact person in case we cannot reach you by telephone.

8. **Is there another adult <u>living at this address</u> whom we can contact, in case we cannot reach you?**

☐ No   ☐ Yes>>

8a.	*If yes >>* **Please tell me his/her name.** *Instructions: Ask person to spell name.*		
ALTERNATE CONTACT LAST NAME		ALTERNATE CONTACT FIRST NAME	☐ REFUSED

8b. **What is this person's relationship ot the child?**

☐ Mother/Father   ☐ Sibling   ☐ Aunt/Uncle   ☐ None

☐ Legal Guardian   ☐ Foster Parent   ☐ Grandparent   ☐ Other: _____

8c. **Is there <u>another person, like a family member or friend, who lives at a different address</u>, whom we could contact?**

☐ No   ☐ Yes>>

8d. *If yes >>* **Please tell me his/her name and telephone number.**

ALTERNATE CONTACT LAST NAME		ALTERNATE CONTACT FIRST NAME
HOME NUMBER ( )	WORK NUMBER ( )	CELL NUMBER ( )

8e. **What is this person's relationship ot the child?**

☐ Mother/Father   ☐ Sibling   ☐ Aunt/Uncle

☐ Grandparent   ☐ Other: _____

Instructions: Inform interviewee that she/he should notify alternate contacts that we may contact them if we cannot get in touch with the interviewee.

9. **Please give me the name and contact information for the landlord or owner?**

Instructions: Ask interviewee to spell landlord's name and address.

MANAGEMENT COMPANY			
LAST NAME		FIRST NAME	
STREET			APT #
BOROUGH	STATE	ZIP	TELEPHONE NUMBER ( )

C. PAINT INSPECTION AND DUST SAMPLING

10. **In which rooms in the house does [child's name] <u>sleep, play or spend time</u>?**

Instructions: Check off all that apply.

☐ Child's bedroom   ☐ Parent's bedroom   ☐ Other bedroom(s) (specify) _____

☐ Living room   ☐ Kitchen   ☐ Other room(s) (specify) _____

Instructions: Make a visual inspection of the unit. Perform inspection as per protocol. Show person area(s) that need remediation.

D. INTERVIEW LANGUAGE

Interview Language:

☐ English   ☐ Russian   ☐ Hindi   ☐ Urdu

☐ Spanish   ☐ Bengali   ☐ Haitian-Creole   ☐ Other: _____

Interpreter <u>used</u>:   ☐ No   ☐ Yes>>

If yes >> **Type of interpreter <u>used</u>:**

☐ Family member (specify): _____

☐ Friend   ☐ Language line   ☐ LPPP staff   ☐ Other: _____

G. COUNSELING AND EDUCATION

Follow up with your child's doctor

☐ Blood lead tests are necessary to monitor your child's exposure to lead. How often these tests need to be done depends on your child's lead level, length of exposure and risk for further exposure.

☐ Generally, the higher the blood lead level and the longer the exposure, the more time it will take for the lead to leave your child's body, and the longer your child will need to be monitored by your doctor.

Reduce your child's exposure to lead

☐ Keep your child away from the lead paint hazards noted in your home. Consider having your child stay somewhere else while hazards are being corrected.

☐ Wash floors and windowsills often using a damp mop or damp cloth.

☐ Wash your child's hands, toys, pacifiers and bottles often to remove lead dust, especially before your child eats or sleeps.

☐ If someone in your home has a job or hobby that involves contact with lead, have them remove their shoes before entering your home. Wash their work clothes separately from family laundry.

☐ Avoid using medicines, spices, foods, cosmetics, jewelry, and painted toys from other countries. They are more likely to contain lead than products made in the U.S.A.

☐ Avoid using clay pots and dishes from other countries to cook, store or serve food. Do not use pottery that is chipped or cracked.

☐ Do not let your child eat or mouth non-food items that may contain lead or lead dust.

☐ Use cold tap water only for making baby formula or baby cereal, and for drinking or cooking. Let water run for a few minutes before you use it. Lead can get into water through old plumbing.

Help your child to eat healthy

☐ It is important for your child to eat a healthy diet with enough calcium, iron and vitamin C.

☐ Talk to your doctor to make sure your child is eating foods with enough calcium, iron, and vitamin C in them.

Get other household members tested for lead

☐ This is especially important for children younger than 6 years of age, children with developmental problems and pregnant women.

☐ Older children and adults should be tested if they may have had contact with lead.

For more information about lead poisoning

☐ Speak with your doctor
Contact your case coordinator at 212-676-6379

☐ Call 311 and ask for the BAN-LEAD information line

☐ Go to www.nyc.gov/lead

Provide information packet. Ask if there are any questions.

TIME ENDED: _____ DATE: _____

SUPERVISOR NAME: _____

Appendix XII
Child Risk Assessment Form
New York City Department of Health and Mental Hygiene

P

NEW YORK CITY DEPARTMENT OF HEALTH AND MENTAL HYGIENE
LEAD POISONING PREVENTION PROGRAM
Child Risk Assessment Form (CRA)

PRIMARY ADDRESS

P

Child Name: _____ _____ _____
                                    Last   *Middle*   *First*

BLL at case assignment (µg/dL): _____   **Drawn Date:** ____/____/____

Child DOB: ____/____/____

Information will be confirmed at the inspection.

Instructions: __In the office__, the primary language for the visit should be determined. If necessary, an interpreter from the family, the LPPP office, or telephone interpreting services can be used to assist in gathering information.

Interview language __scheduled__: *(Instructions: Check off the primary language for the visit.)*

☐ English   ☐ Spanish   ☐ Russian   ☐ Bengali   ☐ Hindi

☐ Haitian-Creole   ☐ Urdu   ☐ Other: _____

Interpreter __scheduled__: ☐ No   ☐ Yes >>

If yes >> **Type of interpreter __scheduled__:**

☐ Family member (specify): _____   ☐ Friend

☐ Telephone interpreting services   ☐ LPPP staff   ☐ Other: _____

Name of PHS: _____   **Time Started:** _____

A. ENVIRONMENTAL ADDRESS

Is this the address where [child's name] currently lives?

☐ Yes >> *Continue*   ☐ No >> *Go to supplement form*

B. CONTACT INFORMATION

I would like to find out the child's name and make sure the information we have in our records is correct.

1. **What is the exact spelling of the __child's full name__?** *Instructions: Ask for middle name.*

LAST NAME	FIRST NAME	MIDDLE NAME	☐ NA

1a. *Instructions: Enter child's gender if known. If gender unknown, ask >>*

Is [child's name] a boy or a girl?   ☐ Male   ☐ Female

1b. What is [child's name]'s date of birth? ____/____/____
                                            Month Day Year

2. **Please confirm the __child's address__.** *Instructions: Ask for spelling of street and specific apartment #.*

STREET		APT. #

CITY/BOROUGH		STATE	ZIP

Inspection Date: ____/____/____

3. What is the exact spelling of **your** name?

LAST NAME	FIRST NAME

3a. What is **your** relationship to [child's name]?

☐ Mother   ☐ Father   ☐ Aunt   ☐ Uncle   ☐ Grandmother   ☐ Grandfather   ☐ Foster Parent>>

☐ Other: _____

3b. *Instructions: If foster parent, ask for the following information:*
Please tell me the name and telephone number of the foster agency:

FOSTER AGENCY	PHONE NUMBER	☐ NOT PROVIDED

4. Please tell me the telephone number of this address:

Environmental address telephone number: (____) _____ – _____   ☐ Not Provided

4a. If you have a cell phone, please tell me your cell number: (____) _____ – _____   ☐ Not Provided

4b. If you work, please tell me your work number: (____) _____ – _____   ☐ Not Provided

4c. Which phone number is the best to reach you?   ☐ Home   ☐ Cell   ☐ Work

4d. Which days of the week are the easiest to reach you?
☐ Mon   ☐ Tues   ☐ Wed   ☐ Thurs   ☐ Fri   ☐ Sat   ☐ Sun   ☐ Any day

4e. When is the best time to reach you? _____   ☐ A.M.   ☐ P.M.   ☐ Any time

4f. Do **you** reside at this address   ☐ No   ☐ Yes

4g. How long has [child's name] lived at this address? _____ yr(s) _____ mo(s) _____ day(s) ☐ Since birth >> *go to Q. 5*

If more than 3 months at current address >> go to Q. 5
If less than 3 months at current address >> go to Q. 4h

4h. In the past 3 months, where else has the child lived?

STREET		APT. #

CITY/BOROUGH	STATE	ZIP	PHONE NUMBER	☐ NOT PROVIDED

If prior address is in NYC >> Plan to inspect previous address as supplement.

C. CHILD'S MEDICAL INFORMATION

I need to write down contact information for [child's name]'s doctor and for his/her current health insurance. If you have a card, letter or bill from the doctor or health insurance, I can copy down the information.

Instructions: Ask to see card and write down information. If no information shown, ask for spelling of name and address.

5. What is the contact information for your child's doctor?

CLINIC NAME

DOCTOR'S LAST NAME	FIRST NAME

STREET	CITY/BOROUGH	STATE	ZIP

TELEPHONE NUMBER	☐ DOCUMENTS SHOWN ☐ NO DOCUMENTS SHOWN

LP 125 (6/07) Child Risk Assessment

Inspection Date: _____/_____/_____

6. Does [child's name] currently have <u>any type</u> of health insurance such as Medicaid or Child Health Plus (CHP)?

☐ No >> *go to Q. 7*   ☐ Yes >>   ☐ Don't know >> *go to Q. 7*

If yes >> Instructions: Ask to see insurance card and write down information. If no card provided, ask for any information available.

MEDICAID # __ - __ - __ - __ - __ - __ - __ - __	OTHER PLAN NAME	ID #	☐ CARD SHOWN ☐ CARD NOT SHOWN

7. In the past, were you ever told that your child had a high blood lead level or had your child been diagnosed with lead poisoning?

☐ No >> *go to Q. 8*   ☐ Yes >>   ☐ Don't know >> *go to Q. 8*

If yes >>

7a. What was the blood lead level? _____ µg/dL   ☐ Don't know

7b. In what city and state was the blood test performed?   City: _____   State: _____

8. Has a doctor or other health care provider ever told you that [child's name] has a learning or behavior problem?

☐ No   ☐ Yes >> **Please describe:** _____

☐ Don't know

Early Intervention

If child < 36 months of age, offer Early Intervention Program Referral and Information.   ☐ Accepted   ☐ Rejected

CHILD 12 MONTHS OR YOUNGER [*If child is older than 12 months, go to Section D.*]

9. Is [child's name] regularly fed infant formula mixed with tap water?   ☐ No   ☐ Yes

10. Are you [child's name]'s birth mother?   ☐ No >> *go to Section D*   ☐ Yes >>

10a. *If yes >>* Did you have a blood test for lead   ☐ No >> *go to Section D*
when you were pregnant with [child's name]?   ☐ Yes >> ☐ Don't know >> *go to Section D*

10b. *If yes >>* What was the blood lead level?   _____ µg/dL   ☐ Told it was high   ☐ Don't know

D. COUNTRY OF BIRTH/FOREIGN TRAVEL

Now I have a few questions about where [child's name] was born, lived and any trips s/he may have taken outside of the U.S. This information can help us identify possible ways your child may have been exposed to lead. I am not interested in [child's name] or your family's immigration status.

11. In what country was [child's name] born? _____

☐ Don't know >> *go to Q. 12*   ☐ Decline to answer >> *go to Q. 12*

*Instructions: If child was born in **Bangladesh, Dominican Republic, Haiti, Mexico,** or **Pakistan** show list at the end of the form (Appendix A).*

11a. Where in [*Bangladesh, Dominican Republic, Haiti, Mexico, or Pakistan*] was [child's name] born?

Bangladesh: _____   Dominican Republic: _____

Haiti: _____   Mexico: _____

Pakistan: _____

☐ Don't know >> *go to Q. 11b*

Instructions: For ALL children born <u>outside of the U.S.</u>

11b. How long did s/he live in that country? _____ (in years)

11c. When (what month and year) did [child's name] come to the U.S.?   Month: _____   Year: _____

Instructions: For ALL children, including US-born children.

12. <u>In the last 12 months</u>, has [child's name] spent any time outside of the U.S.? This includes any traveling, visiting family or friends or living in another country.

☐ No >> *go to Q. 13*   ☐ Yes >>

If yes >> Instructions: Write down all information about time spent outside the U.S. Ask for all visits. If more than 3 times, write below.

	#1	#2	#3
Country			
When did s/he stay there? (start with most recent)	____ / ____ Month Year	____ / ____ Month Year	____ / ____ Month Year
How long did s/he stay?	____ Week(s) ____ Month(s)	____ Week(s) ____ Month(s)	____ Week(s) ____ Month(s)
Comments: (e.g. How often does s/he travel there?)			

13. Which of the following groups best describes <u>your child's</u> race or ethnicity? First, I'm going to read out all the categories. You can tell me more than one category.
Instructions: Read out all categories first. Check as many as reported.

☐ African American or Black   ☐ American Indian or Alaska Native
☐ Asian   ☐ Hispanic or Latino
☐ Native Hawaiian or Other Pacific Islander   ☐ White or Caucasian

Instructions: Do not read aloud.
☐ Other group not listed – If mentioned, write in response: _____
☐ Declined to answer

14. In what country was [child's name]'s birth <u>mother</u> born? _____
☐ Don't know   ☐ Declined to answer

14a. In what country was [child's name]'s birth <u>father</u> born? _____
☐ Don't know   ☐ Declined to answer

E.   PAINT HAZARDS

15. In which rooms in the house does [child's name] <u>sleep, play or spend time</u>?

Instructions: Check off all that apply.

☐ Child's bedroom   ☐ Parent's bedroom   ☐ Other bedroom(s) (specify) _____
☐ Living room   ☐ Kitchen   ☐ Other room(s) (specify) _____
☐ Bathroom   ☐ All rooms

16. Does [child's name] play or spend time in the building basement, hallways, foyers, stairways, or other areas in the building?   ☐ No >> *go to Q. 17*   ☐ Yes >>

16a. *If yes >>* Please tell me the area(s) inside the building where your child spends time.

_____

Instructions: Find out floor and specific area(s) inside the building.

17. Does [child's name] play outside in locations where there is bare soil, such as the front or backyard, a neighborhood playground, or park?

☐ No >> *go to Q. 18*   ☐ Yes >>

17a. *If yes >>* **Please describe.**		
	#1	#2
Description		
Address/Location		
Plays in bare soil?	☐ Yes ☐ No	☐ Yes ☐ No
Sample Taken	☐ Yes ☐ No	☐ Yes ☐ No

Instructions: See sampling guidelines. Complete Non-Dust Chain of Custody Form.

18. In the past 12 months, has there been water damage, deteriorated plaster or paint <u>in this home</u>? neighborhood playground, or park?

☐ No >> *go to Q. 19*   ☐ Yes >>   ☐ Don't know >> *go to Q. 19*

18a. *If yes >>* **Can you please show me and describe the damage?**

Location/Room	Describe damage	When did this occur? (month/year)	Current status
		_____/_____ Month Year	

19. In the past 12 months, has there been any renovation or repair work <u>in this home</u>?

☐ No >> *go to Q. 20*   ☐ Yes >>   ☐ Don't know >> *go to Q. 20*

19a. *If yes >>* **Please tell me what type of work and when the work was done.**

	#1	#2
Location/Room		
Work Description		
When was the work done? (month/year)	_____ Month _____ Year	_____ Month _____ Year
Current status		

20. In the past 12 months, has there been any renovation or repair work in <u>other areas of the building or in the neighborhood</u> where [child's name] spends time?

☐ No >> *go to Q. 21*   ☐ Yes >>   ☐ Don't know >> *go to Q. 21*

20a. *If yes >>* **Please tell me what type of work and when the work was done.**

	#1	#2
Location		
Work Description		
Address		
When was the work done? (month/year)	_____ Month _____ Year	_____ Month _____ Year
Current status		

21. Does [child's name] currently spend more than five hours a week anywhere other than this home? For example, spending time at a day care center, school, babysitter, or another home.

☐ No >> *go to Q. 22*   ☐ Yes >>   ☐ Don't know >> *go to Q. 22*

Inspection Date: _____/_____/_____

21a. *If yes >>* **Please tell me the locations.**

	#1	#2	#3
Location/Description			
Children less than 6 yrs reside in location?	☐ No (SNC) ☐ Yes (SC) ☐ Don't know	☐ No (SNC) ☐ Yes (SC) ☐ Don't know	☐ No (SNC) ☐ Yes (SC) ☐ Don't know
# hrs/week			
Address			
Contact Name *(Ask for spelling)*			
Phone Number			
Work Number			
Cell Number			

F. IMPORTED PRODUCTS

Now I am going to ask you about some product(s) [child's name] may have used or come in contact with, such as medications and health remedies, foods or spices. Some of these products may be made in other countries and may contain lead. They could be products:

- sent by friends and family
- bought in local stores
- brought back from trips you may have taken
- or given to you by friends or family

I want to find out if [child's name] used or was given any of these products during the past 12 months.

Instructions: Ask parent/guardian to show you products in the kitchen and medicine cabinets, Take note of any product(s) that may contain lead. If yes to Questions 22-25, ask to see product(s). See sampling guidelines. Complete Non-Dust Chain of Custody Form.

22. [Imported Medicines] Has your child been given imported...

Product	No	Yes >>	Sample Taken	Comments/Observations
Medicines? (e.g. Remedies for teething, colic, fever, stomachaches or diarhea)			☐ Yes ☐ No	
Ayurvedics? (e.g. Remedies based on traditional Indian medical system)			☐ Yes ☐ No	
Vitamins?			☐ Yes ☐ No	
Powder or pills?			☐ Yes ☐ No	
Herbs?			☐ Yes ☐ No	
Tea?			☐ Yes ☐ No	
Any other imported remedies?_____			☐ Yes ☐ No	

23. [Imported Cosmetics] Has your child used any imported...

Product		Sample Taken	Comments/Observations
Cosmetics? (e.g. Eye makeup)	☐ Yes ☐ No	☐ Yes ☐ No	
Deodorant? (e,g, Litargirio)	☐ Yes ☐ No	☐ Yes ☐ No	
Any other imported cosmetics?_____	☐ Yes ☐ No	☐ Yes ☐ No	

Inspection Date: _____/_____/_____

24. [Imported Food] Has your child eaten any imported...			
Product		Sample Taken	Comments/Observations
Spices? (e.g. orange or red spices)	☐ Yes ☐ No	☐ Yes ☐ No	
Foods?	☐ Yes ☐ No	☐ Yes ☐ No	
Snacks or candies? (e.g. candy spiced with chili or sold in clay pots)	☐ Yes ☐ No	☐ Yes ☐ No	
Any other imported foods?_____	☐ Yes ☐ No	☐ Yes ☐ No	

25. [Imported Pottery] Has your child been served food in or eaten from imported, antique or painted...			
Product		Sample Taken	Comments/Observations
Clay pots?	☐ Yes ☐ No	☐ Yes ☐ No	
Ceramic dishes, bowls, pitchers, or cups?	☐ Yes ☐ No	☐ Yes ☐ No	
Any other imported containers? _____	☐ Yes ☐ No	☐ Yes ☐ No	

G. NON-FOOD ITEMS

Some products that children play with or wear, such as toys, crayons, jewelry, or candy wrappers, may contain lead. If the child puts these items in his/her mouth, she/he can get lead into his/her body.

Instructions: Be specific when entering responses to 'How often?' (e.g. # times per day, week, or month)

26. **Does [child's name] eat, chew on, or put items in his/her mouth, such as toys, mini-blinds, crayons, candy wrappers, jewelry charms or other jewelry?**

☐ No >> *go to Q. 27*   ☐ Yes >>   ☐ Don't know >> *go to Q. 27*

26a. *If yes >>* **Please show me.**

	Item Name/Description	Country of Manufacturer	How Often? (Be specific)	Sample Taken	Comments/Observations
#1			_____times per _____	☐ Yes ☐ No	
#2			_____times per _____	☐ Yes ☐ No	
#3			_____times per _____	☐ Yes ☐ No	
#4			_____times per _____	☐ Yes ☐ No	
Instructions: See sampling guidelines. Complete Non-Dust Chain of Custody Form.					

LP 125 (6/07) Child Risk Assessment

Inspection Date: _____/_____/_____

27. Does your child mouth or chew on any surfaces or furniture? For example, windowsills, walls, chairs, or cribs.

☐ No >> *go to Q. 28*   ☐ Yes >>   ☐ Don't know >> *go to Q. 28*

27a. *If yes >>* **Please show me.**

	Item Name/Description	How Often? (Be specific)	Sample Taken	Comments/Observations
#1		_____times per _____	☐ Yes ☐ No	
#2		_____times per _____	☐ Yes ☐ No	
#3		_____times per _____	☐ Yes ☐ No	
#4		_____times per _____	☐ Yes ☐ No	

Instructions: See sampling guidelines. Complete Non-Dust Chain of Custody Form.

28. Does [child's name] eat, chew on, or put paint chips, plaster, soil, or clay in his/her mouth?

☐ No >> *go to Section H*   ☐ Yes >>   ☐ Don't know >> *go to Section H*

28a. *If yes >>* **Please show me.**

	Item Name/Description	Location/Room	How Often? (Be specific)	Sample Taken	Comments/Observations
#1			_____times per _____	☐ Yes ☐ No	
#2			_____times per _____	☐ Yes ☐ No	
#3			_____times per _____	☐ Yes ☐ No	
#4			_____times per _____	☐ Yes ☐ No	

Instructions: See sampling guidelines. Complete Non-Dust Chain of Custody Form.

H. OCCUPATIONS AND HOBBIES

Now I'd like to ask you about the jobs, hobbies or activities of people in the houusehold.

29. In the past 12 months, has anyone in this household done any of the following jobs, hobbies or activities?

Job/Hobby/Activity	Person's Relationship to Child	Time/Period/ How Long? (wks/months)	Comments Section/ Current Status
Bridge painting or repair work ☐ Yes ☐ No		_____ weeks _____ months	
Commercial building renovation or demolition ☐ Yes ☐ No		_____ weeks _____ months	

Inspection Date: _____/_____/_____

Home renovation, repair or repainting in buildings built before 1960	☐ Yes ☐ No		_____ weeks _____ months	
Torch cutting or burning steel, welding	☐ Yes ☐ No		_____ weeks _____ months	
Cable splicing, soldering, electronics repair	☐ Yes ☐ No		_____ weeks _____ months	
Metal or car battery recycling; working in a scrap yard; radiator repair	☐ Yes ☐ No		_____ weeks _____ months	
Working in a firing range; target shooting	☐ Yes ☐ No		_____ weeks _____ months	
Jobs/Crafts like furniture refinishing, jewelry making, stained glass, pottery, ceramics, glass blowing; making fishing weights, bullets, or lead figures	☐ Yes ☐ No		_____ weeks _____ months	
Other: _____	☐ Yes ☐ No		_____ weeks _____ months	

I.   HOUSEHOLD INFORMATION

I'd like to find out about other children in your household because they may also be exposed to lead.

30.   Other than [child's name], how many children under age 18 live here? _____
Instructions: If no other children, go to Section J.

Please give me the name(s) and age(s) of the other child(ren). Let's start with the youngest child.
Instructions: Write in information. If more than 5 children, write below.

	Full Name (ask for spelling)		Date of Birth	Relationship to child?	Date & BLL if available
#1	LAST:	FIRST:	___/___/___ Mo Day Year	☐ Brother ☐ Sister ☐ Cousin ☐ Twins ☐ Other: _____	_____ µg/dL ___/___/___ Mo Day Year
#2	LAST:	FIRST:	___/___/___ Mo Day Year	☐ Brother ☐ Sister ☐ Cousin ☐ Twins ☐ Other: _____	_____ µg/dL ___/___/___ Mo Day Year
#3	LAST:	FIRST:	___/___/___ Mo Day Year	☐ Brother ☐ Sister ☐ Cousin ☐ Twins ☐ Other: _____	_____ µg/dL ___/___/___ Mo Day Year
#4	LAST:	FIRST:	___/___/___ Mo Day Year	☐ Brother ☐ Sister ☐ Cousin ☐ Twins ☐ Other: _____	_____ µg/dL ___/___/___ Mo Day Year
#5	LAST:	FIRST:	___/___/___ Mo Day Year	☐ Brother ☐ Sister ☐ Cousin ☐ Twins ☐ Other: _____	_____ µg/dL ___/___/___ Mo Day Year

Instructions: Tell parent/guardian that all children should have blood lead tests.

J.   ALTERNATE CONTACT INFORMATION

Finally, I would like to ask for a contact person in case we cannot reach you by telephone.

31.   Is there another adult living at this address whom we can contact, in case we cannot reach you?

☐ No >> *go to Q. 32*   ☐ Yes >>

31a. *If yes >>* **Please tell me his/her name and telephone number.**
Instructions: Ask person to spell name.

ALTERNATE CONTACT LAST NAME	ALTERNATE CONTACT FIRST NAME	☐ NOT PROVIDED
WORK NUMBER ☐ NOT PROVIDED	CELL NUMBER	☐ NOT PROVIDED

31b. What is this person's relationship ot the child?
☐ Mother ☐ Father ☐ Grandmother ☐ Grandfather ☐ Brother ☐ Sister ☐ Aunt
☐ Uncle ☐ Family Friend ☐ Foster Parent ☐ Other: _____

32. Is there <u>another person, like a family member or friend, who lives at a different address</u>, whom we could contact?

☐ No >> *go to Q. 33*   ☐ Yes >>

32a. *If yes >>* **Please tell me his/her name and telephone number.**

ALTERNATE CONTACT LAST NAME	ALTERNATE CONTACT FIRST NAME	☐ NOT PROVIDED
HOME NUMBER ☐ NOT PROVIDED	WORK NUMBER ☐ NOT PROVIDED	CELL NUMBER ☐ NOT PROVIDED

32b. What is this person's relationship ot the child?
☐ Mother ☐ Father ☐ Grandmother ☐ Grandfather ☐ Brother ☐ Sister ☐ Aunt
☐ Uncle ☐ Family Friend ☐ Foster Parent ☐ Other: _____

Instructions: Inform person that s/he should notify alternate contacts that we may contact them only if we cannot get in touch with him/her.

K. LANDLORD INFORMATION

33. Can you please give me the name and contact information for the landlord or owner?
Instructions: Ask to see rent bill or lease. Ask person to spell landlord's name and address.

MANAGEMENT COMPANY		☐ NOT PROVIDED
LAST NAME	FIRST NAME	
STREET		APT #
CITY/BOROUGH	STATE	ZIP
TELEPHONE NUMBER ☐ NOT PROVIDED	CELL NUMBER	☐ NOT PROVIDED
Record where landlord information was obtained from:		

TIME ENDED: _____

L. PAINT INSPECTION AND DUST SAMPLING

INSTRUCTIONS: First conduct a visual inspection of the apartment. After visual inspection, perform an XRF inspection, if required, as per protocol. Show the person the area(s) with lead paint violations.

If lead paint violations are identified, consider obtaining temporary address information AND consider obtaining "Request for Safe House Placement" information.

LP 125 (6/07) Child Risk Assessment

Inspection Date: ____/____/____

250

Provide the following information:

34. **Lead paint hazards were found in your home. We recommend that [child's name] not stay at this address during repair work. Staying at a temporary address, such as with a friend or with relatives, is advised. Please call us to request a visual inspection for lead paint hazards <u>before</u> your child moves to a temporary address.**

If [child's name] does not have another place to stay and you would like information about staying at a Lead Safe House, please call us. The phone number is in the packet with the other materials that I will review with you.

(The phone number is 212-676-6379).

Release Supplement/Temporary Address Information

LAST NAME		FIRST NAME	
STREET			APT #
CITY/BOROUGH		STATE	ZIP

TEMPORARY ADDRESS PHONE NUMBER	☐ NOT PROVIDED

CONTACT WORK NUMBER	☐ NOT PROVIDED	CONTACT CELL NUMBER	☐ NOT PROVIDED

☐ Safe House Offered   ☐ Safe House Accepted   ☐ Safe House Rejected

35. **Is there anything else you would like to tell me about how your child may have been exposed to lead?**
Instructions: Ask if there are any questions.

_____

_____

_____

M. INTERVIEW LANGUAGE

Interview Language: *(Instructions: Check off the primary language for the visit.)*

☐ English   ☐ Russian   ☐ Hindi   ☐ Urdu
☐ Spanish   ☐ Bengali   ☐ Haitian-Creole   ☐ Other: _____

Interpreter <u>used</u>:   ☐ No   ☐ Yes>>

If yes >> **Type of interpreter <u>used</u>:**

☐ Family member (specify): _____   ☐ Friend
☐ Telephone interpreting services   ☐ LPPP staff   ☐ Other: _____

N. COUNSELING AND EDUCATION

Follow up with your child's doctor

☐ Blood lead tests are necessary to monitor your child's exposure to lead. How often these tests need to be done depends on your child's lead level, length of exposure and risk for further exposure.

☐ Generally, the higher the blood lead level and the longer the exposure, the more time it will take for the lead to leave your child's body, and the longer your child will need to be monitored by your doctor.

Reduce your child's exposure to lead

☐ Keep your child away from the lead paint hazards noted in your home. Consider having your child stay somewhere else while hazards are being corrected.

☐ Wash floors and windowsills often using a damp mop or damp cloth.

☐ Wash your child's hands, toys, pacifiers and bottles often to remove lead dust, especially before your child eats or sleeps.

☐ If someone in your home has a job or hobby that involves contact with lead, have them remove their shoes before entering your home. Wash their work clothes separately from family laundry.

☐ Avoid using medicines, spices, foods, cosmetics, jewelry, and painted toys from other countries. They are more likely to contain lead than products made in the U.S.A.

☐ Avoid using clay pots and dishes from other countries to cook, store or serve food. Do not use pottery that is chipped or cracked.

☐ Do not let your child eat or mouth non-food items that may contain lead or lead dust.

☐ Use cold tap water only for making baby formula or baby cereal, and for drinking or cooking. Let water run for a few minutes before you use it. Lead can get into water through old plumbing.

Help your child to eat healthy

☐ It is important for your child to eat a healthy diet with enough calcium, iron and vitamin C.

☐ Talk to your doctor to make sure your child is eating foods with enough calcium, iron, and vitamin C in them.

Get your household members tested for lead

☐ This is especially important for children younger than 6 years of age, children with developmental problems and pregnant women.

☐ Older children and adults should be tested if they may have had contact with lead.

For more information about lead poisoning

☐ Speak with your doctor

☐ Call 311 and ask for the BAN-LEAD information line

☐ Contact your case manager at 212-676-6379

☐ Go to www.nyc.gov/lead

Ask if there are any questions.

Inspection Date: _____/_____/_____

APPENDIX A: Questions 11a. Instructions: Please show this list to parent/guardian and ask him/her to tell you/point to the area where the child was born. If the area is not on the list, please write in the area and ask for the spelling.

Mexico

- ☐ Aguascalientes
- ☐ Baja California
- ☐ Baja California Sur
- ☐ Campeche
- ☐ Chiapas
- ☐ Chihuahua
- ☐ Coahuila (de Zaragoza)
- ☐ Colima
- ☐ Distrito Federal
- ☐ Durango
- ☐ Guanajuato
- ☐ Guerrero
- ☐ Hidalgo
- ☐ Jalisco
- ☐ México
- ☐ Michoacán (de Ocampo)
- ☐ Morelos
- ☐ Nayarit
- ☐ Nuevo Léon
- ☐ Oaxaca
- ☐ Puebla
- ☐ Querétaro (de Arteaga)
- ☐ Quintana Roo
- ☐ San Luis Potosí
- ☐ Sinaloa
- ☐ Sonora
- ☐ Tabasco
- ☐ Tamaulipas
- ☐ Tlaxcala
- ☐ Verazruz (-Llave)
- ☐ Yucatán
- ☐ Zacateca
- ☐ Other (specify): _____

Haiti

- ☐ Aribonite (Gonaïves)
- ☐ Centre (Hinche)
- ☐ Grand'Anse (Jérémie)
- ☐ Nord (Cap-Haïtien)
- ☐ Nord-Est (Fort Liberté)
- ☐ Nort-Quest (Port-de-Paix)
- ☐ Quest (Port-au-Prince)
- ☐ Sud (Les Cayes)
- ☐ Sud-Est (Jacmel)
- ☐ Other (specify) _____

Pakistan

- ☐ Bahawalpur
- ☐ Faisalabad
- ☐ Gujranwala
- ☐ Gujrat
- ☐ Hyderabad
- ☐ Islamabad
- ☐ Jhang Maghiana
- ☐ Karachi
- ☐ Kasur
- ☐ Lahore
- ☐ Larkana
- ☐ Mardan
- ☐ Multan
- ☐ Okara
- ☐ Peshawar
- ☐ Quetta
- ☐ Rahimyar Khan
- ☐ Rawalpindi
- ☐ Sahiwal
- ☐ Sargodha
- ☐ Shekhupura
- ☐ Sialkot
- ☐ Sukkur
- ☐ Other (specify) _____

Dominican Republic

- ☐ Azua
- ☐ ABahoruco
- ☐ Barahona
- ☐ Dajobón
- ☐ Distrito Nacional (incl. Santo Domingo)
- ☐ Duarte
- ☐ El Seibo
- ☐ Elias Piña
- ☐ Espaillat
- ☐ Hato Mayor
- ☐ Independencia
- ☐ La Altagracia
- ☐ La Romana
- ☐ La Vega
- ☐ María Trinidad Sánchez
- ☐ Monseñor Nouel
- ☐ Monte Cristi
- ☐ Monte Plata
- ☐ Pedernales
- ☐ Peravia (incl. San José de Ocoa)
- ☐ Puerto Plata
- ☐ Salcedo
- ☐ Samaná
- ☐ San Cristóbal
- ☐ San Jose
- ☐ San Pedro de Macorís
- ☐ Sánchez Ramírez
- ☐ Santiago
- ☐ Santiago Rodriguez
- ☐ Valverde
- ☐ Other (specify): _____

Bangladesh

- ☐ Bandarban
- ☐ Barguna
- ☐ Barisal
- ☐ Begerhat
- ☐ Bhola
- ☐ Bogra
- ☐ Brahmanbaria
- ☐ Chandpur
- ☐ Chuadanga
- ☐ Chittagong
- ☐ Comilla
- ☐ Cox's Bazar
- ☐ Dinajpur
- ☐ Dhaka
- ☐ Faridpur
- ☐ Feni
- ☐ Gaibanda
- ☐ Gazipur
- ☐ Gopalganj
- ☐ Habiganj
- ☐ Jamalpur
- ☐ Jaipur Hat
- ☐ Jessore
- ☐ Jhalakhati
- ☐ Jhenida
- ☐ Kishorganj
- ☐ Khagrachari
- ☐ Khulna
- ☐ Kurigram
- ☐ Kushtia
- ☐ Lalmonir Hat
- ☐ Lakshmipur
- ☐ Maulvi Bazar
- ☐ Madaripur
- ☐ Magura
- ☐ Meherpur
- ☐ Manikganj
- ☐ Munshiganj
- ☐ Mymensingh
- ☐ Narayanganj
- ☐ Naogaon
- ☐ Nator
- ☐ Narsingdi
- ☐ Narail
- ☐ Nawabganj
- ☐ Nilphamari
- ☐ Noakhali
- ☐ Netrakona
- ☐ Pabna
- ☐ Patuakhali
- ☐ Panchagarh
- ☐ Pirojpur
- ☐ Rangamati
- ☐ Rajshahi
- ☐ Rajbari
- ☐ Rajshahi
- ☐ Rangpur
- ☐ Shariatpur
- ☐ Sherpur
- ☐ Satkhira
- ☐ Sylhet
- ☐ Sanamganj
- ☐ Sirajganj
- ☐ Tangail
- ☐ Thakurgaon
- ☐ Other (specify) _____

NOTES

Question #	Comments/Observations
_____	_____
_____	_____
_____	_____
_____	_____
_____	_____
_____	_____
_____	_____
_____	_____
_____	_____
_____	_____

LP 125 (6/07) Child Risk Assessment   Inspection Date: ____/____/____

Appendix XIII
Nutritional Reference Information

Nutrition Reference Information

RECOMMENDED INTAKE AND COMMON FOOD SOURCES

The Dietary Reference Intakes are nutrient reference values established by the Food and Nutrition Board of the National Academy of Sciences' Institute of Medicine (IOM 1997, 2000, 2001). Reference values are population specific and vary by sex and life cycle group and during pregnancy or lactation. The type of reference values established differ based on the quantity and quality of the research used to establish recommendations. The Recommended Dietary Allowance (RDA) is the nutrient intake level that is used as a goal for an individual and represents an intake level which is sufficient to meet the nutrient requirements of nearly all healthy individuals in the population (IOM 1997, 2000, 2001). If insufficient clinical data is available to establish an RDA, an Adequate Intake (AI) is established. The AI is a level that is felt to meet the needs of all individuals in the group (IOM 1997, 2000, 2001). Pregnant and lactating women should aim to meet established RDA or AI levels for through dietary intake. Vitamin or mineral supplementation is recommended for those women who are unable to meet nutrient requirements through dietary sources.

Calcium

The Adequate Intake level of calcium is 1,300 mg/day for pregnant and lactating women 18 years and younger and 1,000 mg/day for pregnant and lactating women 19 years and older (IOM 1997). The richest and most absorbable sources of calcium are dairy products including: milk, cheese, and yogurt. However, many ethnic groups avoid dairy products because of lactose intolerance which has been estimated to have a high prevalence in Asians (100%), African Americans (75%), Native Americans (100%), and Hispanics (53%)(Jackson and Savaiano, 2001). Calcium-set tofu and calcium-fortified fluids such as orange juice, soymilk, almond milk, and rice milk, are also rich sources of calcium. Calcium is also found in some vegetables such as broccoli, bok choy, and kale; however, the calcium found in plant foods is less bioavailable than the calcium in dairy products and fortified foods.

Iron

The Recommended Dietary Allowance of iron is 27 mg/day for all pregnant women, 10 mg/day for lactating women 18 years and younger, and 9 mg/day for lactating women 19 years and older (IOM 2001). The amount of iron from food that is absorbed by the body is dependent on the source of the iron. Heme iron is readily absorbed by the body and is found in meat, poultry, and fish. Nonheme iron is found in iron-fortified foods such as bread, cereal, and grain products, beans/legumes, vegetables, and iron supplements. The absorption of nonheme iron is enhanced when eaten at the same time as vitamin C rich foods or with an animal product such as meat or poultry.

Selenium

The Recommended Dietary Allowance of Selenium is 60 µg/day for all pregnant women and 70 µg/day for all lactating women (IOM 2000). Selenium is found in: meats, especially organ meats, seafood, and Brazil nuts. The selenium content of fruits, vegetables, nuts, and grains is dependent on soil selenium content and therefore varies substantially based on the plant's origin.

Zinc

The Recommended Dietary Allowance of zinc is 12 mg/day for pregnant and 13 mg/day for lactating women 18 years and younger and 11 mg/day for pregnant and 12 mg/day lactating women 19 years and older (IOM 2001). Red meat and shellfish are rich sources of bioavailable zinc. Zinc is also found in: nuts, legumes, fortified cereals, and whole grains.

Vitamin C

The Recommended Dietary Allowance of vitamin C is 80 mg/day for pregnant and 115 mg/day for lactating women 18 years and younger and 85 mg/day for pregnant and 120 mg/day lactating women 19 years and older (IOM 2000). Vitamin C is found in: plant products such as citrus fruits, fruit juice, tomatoes, tomato juice, potatoes, cauliflower, broccoli, strawberries, cabbage and spinach.

Vitamin D

The Recommended Dietary Allowance of vitamin D is 200 IU/day for all pregnant and lactating women (IOM 1997). Recommendations for higher dietary intakes of pre-formed vitamin D have also been made (Prentice 2003; Hollis 2005). In nonpregnant adults, daily supplementation with 400 IU vitamin D increases 25(OH)D by 7.0 nmol/L (2.8 ng/ml) (Heaney). Supplementation of a pregnant woman with 400 IU vitamin D, as in prenatal vitamins, has little effect on her 25(OH)D concentration (Wagner 2008). The AAP recommends that pregnant women maintain a 25(OH)D level of ≥80 nmol/L (32 ng/ml) (Wagner 2008). Dark-skinned individuals require exposures about 5-10 times as long as light-skinned individuals to achieve similar levels of cutaneous vitamin D production. (Holick 2004). At latitudes above 35°N and below 35°S ultraviolet B photons do not penetrate of the earth's surface in winter months, making cutaneous vitamin D production negligible in those months; additionally sun exposures outside the peak sun hours of 10 AM to 3 PM in the spring, summer and fall has limited impact on cutaneous vitamin D synthesis (Holick 2003). Clinicians should note that obesity is a risk factor for low 25(OH)D and that sunscreen blocks cutaneous production of vitamin D (Holick 2007). The AAP recommends that exclusively and partially breastfed infants receive supplements of 400 IU/day of vitamin D shortly after birth and continue to receive these supplements until they are weaned and consume ≥1,000 mL/day of vitamin D-fortified formula or vitamin D-fortified milk (Wagner).

Food sources of vitamin D (25-hydroxy vitamin D) include: fortified milk, fortified orange juice, fortified cereal, some fatty fish (such as salmon and sardines), fish liver oils, and some eggs. UV radiation exposure stimulates vitamin D synthesis (through activation of the pro-vitamin D precursor 7-dehydrocholesterol present in skin), so vitamin D needs can also be met through sun exposure though dark-skinned women require more time exposed to sunlight for the same benefits and, thus, more vitamin D to be obtained from the diet (Holick, 2004).

In the United States 98% of fluid milk is estimated to be fortified with vitamin D (Anderson and Toverud, 1994), however, one study found that only 47.7% of milk samples were appropriately fortified with most of the out-of-compliance milk samples being under-fortified (Murphy et al., 2001). In 2003, the Food and Drug Administration approved food fortification with vitamin D of calcium-fortified juices and juice drinks (FDA, 2003). This may provide enhanced sources of dietary vitamin D to ethnic groups who avoid dairy products because of lactose intolerance. Strategies to increase vitamin D intake, especially for non-Caucasians, emphasize dietary supplements and these vitamin-D enriched non-dairy products.

Vitamin E

The Recommended Dietary Allowance of vitamin E is 15 mg (22.5 IU)/day for all pregnant women and 19 mg (28.5)/day for all lactating women (IOM 2000). Foods rich in vitamin E include: vegetable oils (olive, sunflower, and safflower oils), nuts, whole grains, green leafy vegetables, and meats.

ASSESSMENT OF NUTRIENT STATUS AND INTAKE

Biochemical Indicators

Blood hemoglobin levels are routinely measured to screen for iron deficiency anemia (IOM 2001) and serum concentration of 25(OH)D is the best indicator of vitamin D status (IOM 1997). Biochemical assessment of nutrient status is not routinely performed for all vitamins and minerals, however, because reliable and valid laboratory tests of nutritional status are not available for many nutrients such as zinc and calcium (reference needed).

In the absence of biochemical assessment options, dietary assessment methods are utilized to estimate usual dietary intake and to screen for possible dietary inadequacies. The most commonly used dietary assessment methods include: 24-hour recalls, food (diary) records, and food frequency questionnaires.

24-Hour Recall

During a 24-hour recall, an individual is asked to report food and fluid intake information for the previous day (Hu 2008). The individual is probed for additional information about the food or beverage consumed, including preparation the portion size eaten. A brief qualitative assessment of the recall is usually conducted by the clinician performing the assessment. Common qualitative assessments conducted include: estimation of the number of servings of fruits/vegetables eaten or for the inclusion so of iron-rich or calcium-rich foods. The 24-hour recall is the dietary assessment method most commonly utilized in clinical settings because they can be conducted in a short amount of time and they do not require advanced preparation or complicated scoring. Limitations of the 24-hour recall include: reliance on memory, difficulty in estimation of portion sizes, underreporting of food intake, and intentional omission of nutrient-poor foods. In addition, food consumed in the previous day may also not be representative of usual dietary intake.

Food Record

The food record (diary) method requires that an individual record in detail all the foods and beverages consumed over one or more days (typically between 3 and 7 days) (Hu 2008). The individual completing the food record is typically taught about recording procedures such as portion size estimation prior to completing the records. Quantitative analysis of completed food records are typically completed by a Registered Dietitian so dietary inadequacies and excesses can be identified. Although food records are typically considered the "gold standard" of dietary assessment, there are a number of limitations to this approach. Food records are time and labor intensive to both the individual completing the record and the individual conducting the dietary analysis. Individuals may also alter their food intake while completing the food record.

Food Frequency Questionnaire

Food Frequency Questionnaires (FFQs) were developed to assess long-term dietary intake and are often used in epidemiologic studies (Hu 2008). Numerous food frequency questionnaires have been developed and validated for use in specific populations. A food frequency questionnaire consists of a list of food items and beverages. Individuals are asked to report their usual consumption over a specified period of time from a list of frequency categories. The average intake over the designated time period of an assortment of nutrients is calculated based on the individual's responses. FFQs have a number of advantages in epidemiologic studies such as minimal respondent burden and low costs. However, since FFQs lack the detail of dietary records or 24-hour recalls, they provide less accurate estimates of absolute intake.

TABLE XII-1 **Recommended Dietary Intake and Common Food Sources of Selected Nutrients**

Recommended Intake and Common Food Sources of Selected Nutrients				
Nutrient	Recommended Intakes		Food Sources	Nutrient Content
	(RDA/AI) Pregnancy	**(RDA**/AI) Lactation		
Calcium (mg)	**1,300** (≤18 years) **1,000** (>19 years)	**1,300** (≤18 years) **1,000** (>19 years)	Fortified ready-to-eat cereals (various), 1 oz	236-1043
			Plain yogurt, low-fat (12 g protein/8 oz), 8-oz container	415
			Soy beverage, calcium fortified, 1 cup	368
			Fruit yogurt, low-fat (10 g protein/8 oz), 8-oz container	345
			Swiss cheese, 1.5 oz	336
			Ricotta cheese, part skim, ½ cup	335
			Mozzarella cheese, part-skim, 1.5 oz	311
			Cheddar cheese, 1.5 oz	307
			Fat-free (skim) milk, 1 cup	306
			Sardines, Atlantic, in oil, drained, 3 oz	325
			1% low-fat milk, 1 cup	290
			Low-fat chocolate milk (1%), 1 cup	288
			Whole milk, 1 cup	276
			Tofu, firm, prepared with nigari , ½ cup	253
			Spinach, cooked from frozen, ½ cup	146
Iron (mg)	**27** (All ages)	**10** (All ages)	Clams, canned, drained, 3 oz	23.8
			Fortified ready-to-eat cereals (various), ~ 1 oz	1.8 -21.1
			Oysters, eastern, wild, cooked, moist heat, 3 oz	10.2
			Fortified instant cooked cereals (various), 1 packet	4.9-8.1
			Soybeans, mature, cooked, ½ cup	4.4
			White beans, canned, ½ cup	3.9
			Blackstrap molasses, 1 Tbsp	
			Lentils, cooked, ½ cup	3.5
			Spinach, cooked from fresh, ½ cup	

Nutrient			Food	Amount
			Beef, chuck, blade roast, lean, cooked, 3 oz	3.3
			Prune juice, ¾ cup	3.2
			Shrimp, canned, 3 oz	3.1
			Ground beef, 15% fat, cooked, 3 oz	2.3
				2.3
				2.2
Selenium (µg)	60 (All ages)	70 (All ages)	Brazil nuts, dried, unblanched, 1 ounce	544
			Tuna, light, canned in oil, drained, 3 ounces	63
			Beef, cooked, 3½ ounces	35
			Cod, cooked, 3 ounces	32
			Turkey, light meat, roasted, 3½ ounces	32
			Chicken Breast, meat only, roasted, 3½ ounces	20
			Noodles, enriched, boiled, 1/2 cup	17
			Egg, whole, 1 medium	14
			Cottage cheese, low fat 2%, 1/2 cup	12
			Oatmeal, instant, fortified, cooked, 1 cup	12
			Rice, white, enriched, long grain, cooked, 1/2 cup	12
			Rice, brown, long-grained, cooked, 1/2 cup	10
			Bread, enriched, whole wheat, commercially prepared, 1 slice	10
Zinc (mg)	12 (≤18 years) 11 (>19 years)	13 (≤18 years) 12 (>19 years)	Beef shank, lean only, cooked 3 oz	8.9
			Beef tenderloin, lean only, cooked, 3 oz	4.8
			Breakfast cereal, complete wheat bran flakes, 3/4 c serving	3.7
			Chicken leg, meat only, roasted, 1 leg	2.7
			Pork tenderloin, lean only, cooked, 3 oz	2.5
			Yogurt, plain, low fat, 1 c	2.2
			Baked beans, canned, with pork, 1/2 c	1.8
			Cashews, dry roasted w/out salt, 1 oz	1.6
			Pecans, dry roasted w/out salt, 1 oz	1.4
				1.3
				1.3
				1.1
				1.1

			Raisin bran, 3/4 c	
			Chickpeas, mature seeds, canned, 1/2 c	
			Mixed nuts, dry roasted w/peanuts, w/out salt, 1 oz	
			Cheese, Swiss, 1 oz	
Vitamin C (mg)	**80** (≤18 years) **85** (>19 years)	**115** (≤18 years) **120** (>19 years)	Red sweet pepper, raw, ½cup	142
			Kiwi fruit, 1 medium	70
			Orange, raw, 1 medium	70
			Orange juice, ¾ cup	
			Green pepper, sweet, raw, ½ cup	61-93
			Grapefruit juice, ¾ cup	60
			Vegetable juice cocktail, ¾ cup	
			Strawberries, raw, ½ cup	50-70
			Brussels sprouts, cooked, ½ cup	50
			Cantaloupe, ¼ medium	49
			Broccoli, raw, ½ cup	48
				47
				39
Vitamin D (IU)	**200**	**200**	Cod liver oil, 1 tablespoon	1,360 360
			Salmon, cooked, 3.5 ounces	345 200
			Mackerel, cooked, 3.5 ounces	250
			Tuna fish, canned in oil, 3 ounces	98 60
			Sardines, canned in oil, drained, 1.75 ounces	40 20
			Milk, nonfat, reduced fat, and whole, vitamin D-fortified, 1 cup	15 12
			Margarine, fortified, 1 tablespoon	
			Ready-to-eat cereal, fortified with 10% of the DV for vitamin D, 0.75-1 cup	
			Egg, 1 whole (vitamin D is found in yolk)	
			Liver, beef, cooked, 3.5 ounces	
			Cheese, Swiss, 1 ounce	
Vitamin E (mg)	**15 mg**	**19 mg**	Fortified ready-to-eat cereals, ~1 oz	1.6-12.8
			Sunflower seeds, dry roasted, 1 oz	7.4
			Almonds, 1 oz	

			Sunflower oil, 1 Tbsp	7.3
			Cottonseed oil, 1 Tbsp	5.6
			Safflower oil, 1 Tbsp	
			Hazelnuts (filberts), 1 oz	4.8
			Mixed nuts, dry roasted, 1 oz	4.6
			Turnip greens, frozen, cooked, ½ cup	
			Peanut butter, 2 Tbsp	4.3
			Tomato puree, ½ cup	3.1
			Canola oil, 1 Tbsp	
			Wheat germ, toasted, plain, 2 Tbsp	2.9
			Peanuts, 1 oz	2.5
			Avocado, raw, ½ avocado	2.5
				2.4
				2.3
				2.2
				2.1

Appendix XIV
Template for Letter to Construction Employer re: Occupational Exposure

Template for Letter to Construction Employer re: Occupational Exposure

TEMPLATE FOR HEALTH CARE PROVIDER LETTER TO EMPLOYER
Prior to issuing such a letter, the healthcare provider should discuss the contents with the affected employee and obtain her authorization.

Physician Provider Letterhead

Month XX, 20XX

Employer
Company Name
Company Address
City, State XXXXX

Re: Medical Opinion Regarding Occupational Lead Exposure of [NAME OF PATIENT]

Dear Employer:

On [DATE], I conducted a medical evaluation of Ms. [NAME OF PATIENT], who reports being an employee of your company. Based on the information provided by Ms. [NAME OF PATIENT], she performs work at your company that may expose her to lead. A laboratory test performed on [DATE] reported a blood lead concentration of [ENTER RESULT] micrograms per deciliter (μg/dL).

My evaluation of Ms. [NAME OF PATIENT] indicates that she is pregnant or planning to conceive. Lead exposure has been associated with adverse reproductive outcomes, including an increased risk of miscarriage, hypertension during pregnancy, decreased fetal growth, and developmental problems in children born to lead-exposed mothers. The U.S. Centers for Disease Control and Prevention recommends that women who are or may become pregnant limit their exposure to lead.

In accordance with the OSHA Lead Standards [1910.1025(j)-(k), and 1910.1025 App C – Section I. Medical Surveillance and Monitoring Requirements for Workers Exposed to Inorganic Lead, or 1926.62(j)-(k)], this letter represents my medical opinion that Ms. [NAME OF PATIENT] should be removed from lead exposure at your company. This removal should remain in effect until such time that she is no longer pregnant or no longer trying to conceive a child. In the interim, Ms. [NAME OF PATIENT] is capable of continuing to work at a job task or location associated with her employment that would not be expected to result in a blood lead concentration of ≥ 5 μg/dL. I am available to discuss the acceptability of any alternative work assignments for the patient with you or one of your representatives.

I have also attached a brochure that discusses the health effects of lead exposure and outlines steps that may be taken to reduce workplace exposure.

Sincerely,

[PHYSICIAN NAME]

Appendix XV
Workplace Hazard Alert for Lead
Occupational Lead Poisoning Prevention Program
California Department of Health

New Health Dangers from Lead

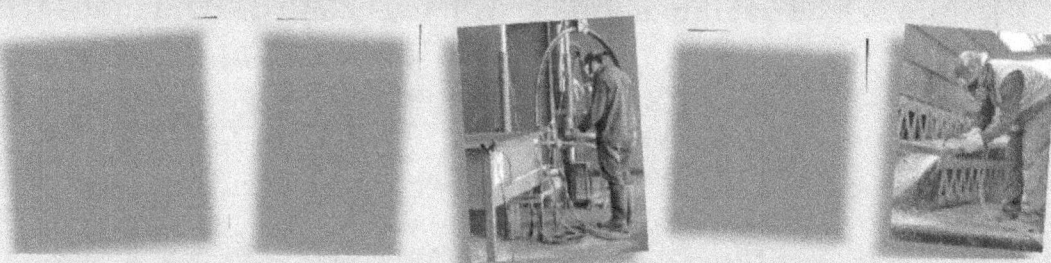

Levels of lead once thought harmless now shown to be toxic

If you work with lead you need to:

➡ Find out how much lead is in your blood.

➡ Talk to your doctor about lead and your health.

➡ Take steps to protect yourself at work.

What health damage can low levels of lead cause?

Studies in recent years show that low levels of lead in adults can:

➡ **increase blood pressure**— may increase your chances of having a heart attack or stroke.

➡ **decrease brain function**— making it more difficult to think, learn, and remember.

➡ **decrease kidney function**— making it more difficult to get rid of toxic waste products through your urine.

➡ **harm the physical and mental development of your baby** before it's born.

➡ **increase chances of having a miscarriage.**

Health damage from lead:

✳ **Can be permanent.**

✳ **Can be occurring even if you have no symptoms.**

✳ **May not show up until many years later.**

You may work with lead if you:

● Make or repair radiators

● Make or recycle batteries

● Recycle scrap metal or electronics

● Melt, cast, or grind lead, brass, or bronze

● Make or glaze ceramics

● Work at a shooting range

● Remove paint or coatings

● Remodel homes and buildings

● Tear down buildings, bridges, or tanks

This is not a complete list. If you are unsure if you work with lead, ask your employer.

California Department of
Publi Health

OLPPP
Occupational Lead Poisoning Prevention Program

How does lead get into my body?

Lead gets into the body through the air you breathe. You can also swallow lead without knowing it if lead dust gets onto your hands or face or on food you eat.

How do I know how much lead is in my body?

Get a blood lead level test. This test measures the amount of lead in a person's blood. Blood lead test results are reported as micrograms of lead per deciliter of blood (μg/dL or mcg/dL). The typical blood lead level for adults in the U.S. is less than 2 μg/dL. Even if you feel fine, you should get tested.

> ✳ **Know your number.**

What level of lead is harmful?

Some of the harmful effects of lead have been seen at very low levels. Scientists and doctors now recommend that blood lead levels be kept below 10 μg/dL. Pregnant women or women considering pregnancy should not have a blood lead level above 5 μg/dL.

> ✳ **Blood lead levels should be kept below 10.**

Will my health be damaged?

No one can predict for sure whether your health will be damaged at a low blood lead level. Your risk (chance) of suffering from health damage increases with the amount of lead in your blood and the length of time you have been exposed. It will also depend on whether you have any health conditions that place you at higher risk of damage from lead.

If your blood lead level has been above 10 μg/dL for more than a year, the most important thing you can do is take steps to lower your exposure in the future. Information on how you can protect yourself is on pages 4 and 5.

You should also talk to your personal doctor about whether you have any medical conditions that may make you more sensitive to the harmful effects of lead.

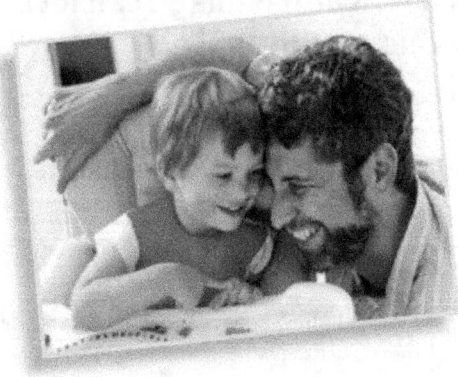

> ✳ **Can lead at work harm my family?**
>
> **YES.** You take lead dust from your job to your family when you wear your work clothes and shoes home. Lead dust can get in your car. It can get on furniture, floors, and carpets. Your child can swallow this lead dust and be poisoned. The steps you take to protect yourself will also keep you from bringing lead home to your family. See pages 4 and 5 for more information on what you can do.

2

What should I tell my doctor?

Your doctor needs to know if you work with lead. Your doctor can order a blood lead level test if you need one. Also, you may have a medical condition that makes you more sensitive to the harmful effects of lead.

Tell the doctor:

➡ What you do at work.

➡ How long you have been at your job.

➡ Any lead jobs you've had in the past.

➡ If you've ever had a blood lead level test.

➡ If you've had to be moved to a different job or be off work because your lead level was high.

➡ If you think working with lead is making you sick.

Women should also tell their doctor if they are pregnant or considering becoming pregnant.

Ask the doctor if you:

➡ Have any medical conditions that may make you more sensitive to the effects of lead.

☐ High blood pressure
☐ Kidney disease
☐ Brain or nerve disease
☐ Other

➡ Need any follow-up medical tests to see if lead is affecting your health.

☐ Recheck blood pressure
☐ Kidney function tests
☐ Cognitive evaluation
☐ Other

See the attached clip-off form to fill out and take to your doctor.

My blood lead level has been high for years. Should I find other work?

Whether you continue to work with lead is a personal decision. It is often a tough decision to make. When making this decision, consider:

➡ Are there steps you can take to lower your exposure to lead? See pages 4 and 5 for steps you can take to protect yourself.

➡ Do you have any health conditions that may make you more sensitive to the harmful effects of lead?

➡ If you have a medical condition that places you at higher risk, can you transfer to another job without lead at the same company?

➡ If you change jobs will you receive the same salary and benefits? If not, can you and your family afford a lower paying job?

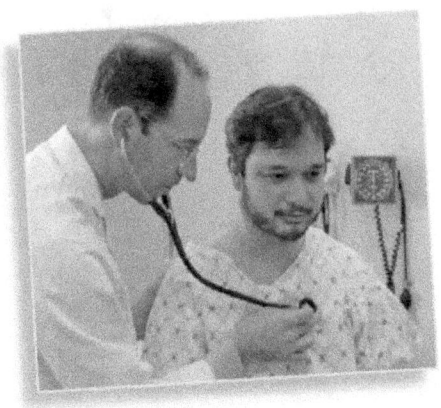

For industrial workers

What can I do to protect myself?

Make sure you don't accidentally swallow lead.

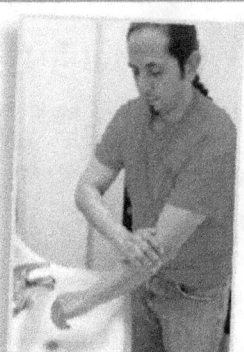

➡ **Wash your hands and face** with soap and water before eating or drinking and before leaving work.

➡ **Do not eat, drink, or smoke** in the work area.

➡ **Take a shower and wash your hair** as soon as you get home. (It's better to shower at work if you can.)

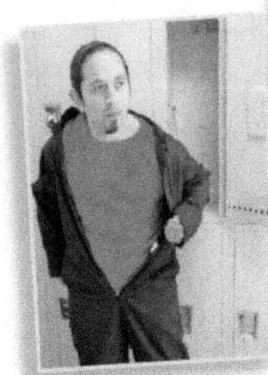

➡ **Change into clean clothes and shoes at work** before you go home. Keep dirty work clothes and shoes separate from clean street clothes. If you don't have a storage locker, keep your dirty clothes and shoes in a plastic bag.

➡ **Use wet cleaning methods.** Wet wipe surfaces and mop or HEPA vacuum the shop floor daily.

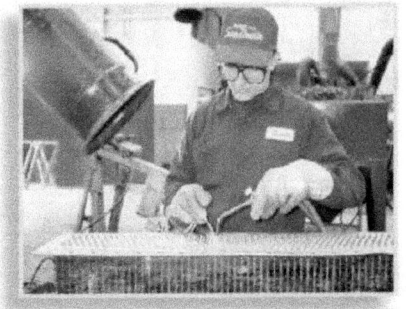

Do what you can to lower the amount of lead you breathe in.

➡ **If you have local exhaust ventilation,** turn it on and position it correctly while you work with lead.

➡ **Ask your employer for a respirator** to wear while you work with lead. If you already wear a respirator, ask whether there is another type of respirator that will protect you better. If you use a respirator, your employer has to pay for a doctor to evaluate whether you can wear one safely. Your employer must also provide you with a fit-test to make sure that the respirator fits you well.

Get a blood lead level test at least every 6 months.

➡ **Ask your employer for a blood lead level test.** If you have significant lead exposure at work, your employer must provide you with a test and pay for it.

➡ **Ask your personal doctor for a test** if your employer doesn't provide one.

✳ **Get tested at least every 6 months.**

4

For construction workers

What can I do to protect myself?

Make sure you don't accidentally swallow lead.

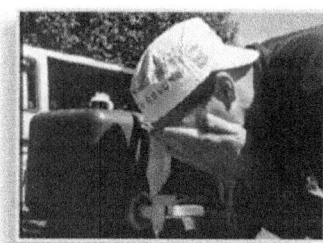

➡ **Wash your hands and face** with soap and water before eating or drinking and before leaving work. Use a portable plastic container with a spigot if running water is not available.

➡ **Do not eat, drink, or smoke in the work area.** Move to a clean area for lunch or breaks.

➡ **Take a shower and wash your hair** as soon as you get home. (It's better to shower at the job site if there are portable showers.)

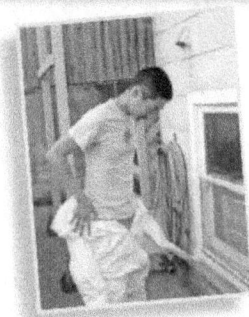

➡ **Change into clean clothes and shoes at the job site** before you go home. Keep dirty work clothes and shoes separate from clean street clothes. Dirty clothes and shoes can be stored in a plastic bag.

➡ **Use wet cleaning methods.** Wet wipe surfaces and wet clean or HEPA vacuum the work area daily.

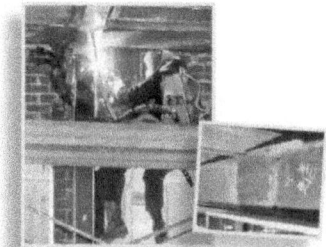

Strip back paint before cutting or welding.

Do what you can to lower the amount of lead you breathe in.

➡ Use work methods that keep dust and fume levels down.

➡ **Ask your employer for a respirator** to wear while you work with lead. If you already wear a respirator, ask whether there is another type of respirator that will protect you better. If you use a respirator, your employer has to pay for a doctor to evaluate whether you can wear one safely. Your employer must also provide you with a fit-test to make sure that the respirator fits you well.

Get a blood lead level test at least every 6 months.

➡ **Ask your employer for a blood lead level test.** If you have significant lead exposure at work, your employer must provide you with a test and pay for it.

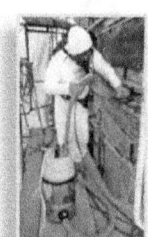

Attach power tools to a HEPA vacuum.

➡ **Ask your personal doctor for a test** if your employer doesn't provide one.

> ✳ **Get tested at least every 6 months.**

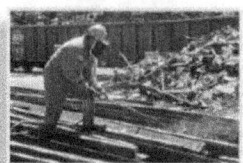

Use a long-handled torch and stand upwind.

5

Are there any laws that protect me if I work with lead?

Yes. Your employer must follow special laws to protect you from lead hazards on the job. These laws are called the Cal/OSHA Lead Standards.

The Lead Standards contain many important requirements to protect you from lead. However, because they were written many years ago they are not based on the most recent scientific information. You can have a blood lead level above 10 µg/dL even if your employer follows the standards. That's why it's important for workers and employers to do everything they can to lower the amount of lead in the workplace.

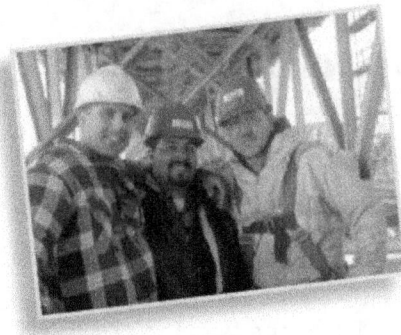

To find out more about the Cal/OSHA Lead Standards, call the Lead in the Workplace Helpline (866/ 627-1587) or visit www.cdph.ca.gov/programs/olppp .

Talk to your employer if you think there is a lead problem at your job. If your employer does not fix the problem, you can call Cal/OSHA and ask for an inspection. Cal/OSHA will not tell your employer who made the call. Call the Cal/OSHA office in your area or call Cal/OSHA headquarters at (510) 285-7000.

6

RESOURCES

Toll-free to California callers.

- **For information about lead safety:** (866) 627-1587

- **For information about other workplace hazards:** (866) 282-5516

- **California Relay Service:** (800) 735-2929 or 711

- **www.cdph.ca.gov/programs/ohb**

To obtain a copy of this document in an alternate format, please contact: (510) 620-5757. Please allow at least ten (10) working days to coordinate alternate format services.

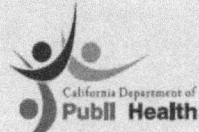
California Department of **Publi Health**

OLPPP
Occupational Lead Poisoning Prevention Program

California Department of Public Health
Occupational Health Branch
850 Marina Bay Parkway, Building P, Third Floor
Richmond, CA 94804

Arnold Schwarzenegger, Governor
State of California

Kimberly Belshé, Secretary
Health and Human Services Agency

Mark B. Horton, MD, MSPH, Director
California Department of Public Health

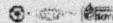

Worksite Evaluation Form

What your employer should do to protect you

The best thing that your employer can do is to get rid of lead and lead-containing materials. If it's not possible to get rid of the lead, your employer should take steps to keep the amount of lead in the workplace as low as possible. Your employer should:

☐ **Train you to work safely with lead.**

☐ **Provide wash-up and shower facilities.**

➡ If you work in construction these may be portable wash stations and portable showers.
➡ Your employer should provide you sufficient time to wash up before breaks, lunch, and going home.

☐ **Provide clean areas for eating and changing.**

☐ **Provide work clothes and work shoes** that stay at the job site.

☐ **Provide a HEPA vacuum or tools for wet cleaning** the work area.

☐ **Install local exhaust ventilation** whenever possible.

➡ If there is already local exhaust ventilation your employer should check it regularly to make sure it works well.

☐ **Provide you with the right tools to keep lead dust and fume levels down** such as power tools attached to a HEPA vacuum and long-handled torches.

☐ **Separate lead work areas from non-lead work areas.**

➡ In construction, plastic sheeting can be used to isolate dusty work from the surrounding area.

☐ **Provide you with a respirator** to give you even more protection.

➡ If you use a respirator, your employer has to pay for a doctor to evaluate whether you can wear one safely. Your employer must also provide you with a fit-test to make sure that the respirator fits you well.

☐ **Provide you with a blood lead level test** at least every six months.

OLPPP
Occupational Lead Poisoning Prevention Program
California Department of Public Health, Occupational Health Branch
850 Marina Bay Parkway, Building P, Third Floor, Richmond, CA 94804

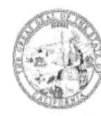
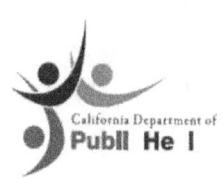
California Department of
Publl He l

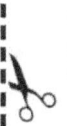

Lead Health Evaluation Form

To the worker:

Fill out the upper part of this form as completely as you can and share the form with your doctor. The lower part of the form has information for your doctor on body systems and health conditions that may be affected by lead. Talk to your doctor about any concerns you have.

Your name _____ Date of birth _____

Your employer's name _____

What job do you do now? _____ How long have you been at this job? _____

Have you worked with lead at other jobs in the past? _____

Have you had a blood lead level test done in the past? *(List the date(s) and the test results if you know them.)* _____

_____

Have you ever had to be moved to a different job or be off work because your blood lead level was high? _____

Do you think working with lead is making you sick? If yes, explain. _____

_____

To the healthcare provider:

Recent studies show that persistent low-level lead exposures are associated with an increased risk of hypertension, subtle effects on renal function, subclinical cognitive dysfunction, and adverse female reproductive outcome. Please review the following with your patient:

☐ Any blood pressure concerns   ☐ Any kidney function concerns

☐ Any brain function concerns   ☐ Pregnancy concerns (for female patients of reproductive age)

Follow-up recommendations:

☐ Recheck blood pressure?   ☐ Test kidney function with BUN/Cr?

☐ Cognitive evaluation?   ☐ Other?

For health care providers with questions about medical management of lead-exposed California workers, please call Dr. Ray Meister of the Occupational Lead Poisoning Prevention Program at (510) 620-5731.

OLPPP
Occupational Lead Poisoning Prevention Program

California Department of Public Health, Occupational Health Branch
850 Marina Bay Parkway, Building P, Third Floor, Richmond, CA 94804

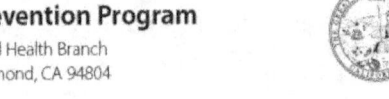

California Department of
Publl He l

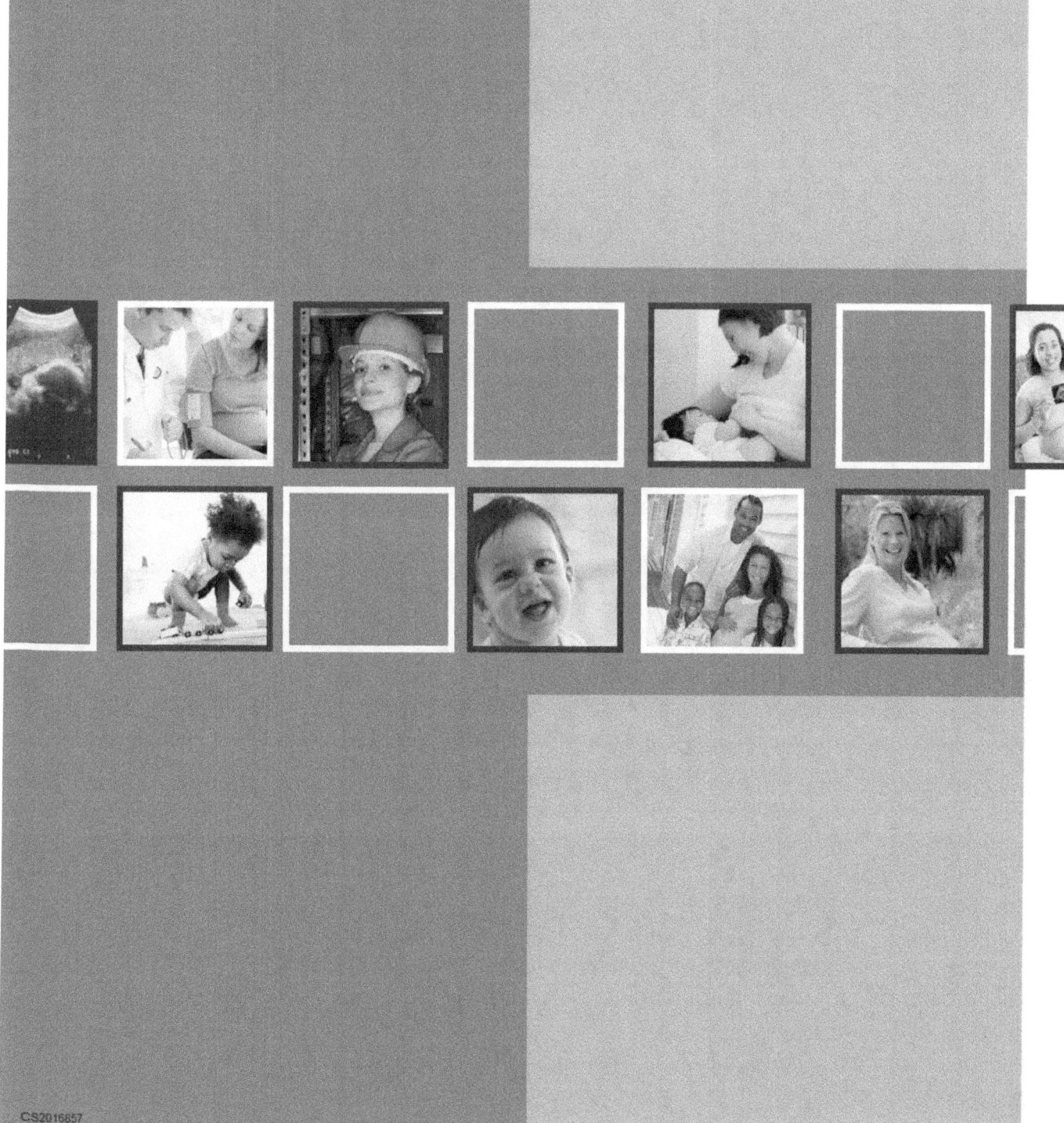